Medical Humanities Series

Theodore R. LeBlang, *Editor*

Glen W. Davidson, *Senior Consulting Editor*

The Medical Humanities Series is sponsored by the Department of Medical Humanities at Southern Illinois University School of Medicine in Springfield. The series is devoted to publication of original materials that contribute insights from the humanities on medicine, including medical education, clinical practice, and health care delivery.

The Editor encourages submission of manuscripts in the areas of anthropology, ethics, health policy, history, law, literature, philosophy, psychosocial care, religious studies, and the visual arts.

Inquiries should be directed to the Editor, Department of Medical Humanities, Southern Illinois University School of Medicine, Box 19230, Springfield, IL 62794-9230.

DR. GEORGE

An Account of the Life of a Country Doctor

George T. Mitchell, M.D.

Southern Illinois University Press
Carbondale and Edwardsville

97 96 95 94   4 3 2 1

Library of Congress Cataloging-in-Publication Data

Mitchell, George T.
    Dr. George: an account of the life of a country doctor / George T.
Mitchell.
        p. cm.
    Includes index.
    1. Mitchell, George T. 2. Physicians (General Practice)—Illinois—
Biography. 3. Medicine, Rural—Illinois. 4. Mitchell, George T. I. Title.
II. Title: Doctor George.
    [DNLM: 1. Physicians—personal narratives. 2. Delivery of Health
Care—history—Illinois. WZ 100 M6814 1994]
    R154.M648A3 1994
    610'.92—dc20
    [B]   93-16589
    ISBN 0-8093-1915-2   CIP
    ISBN 0-8093-1916-0 pbk.

Excerpts from "Rural MDs, 1970-Style," *American Medical News,* October 19,
1970. Reprinted with permission of American Medical News. Copyright
1970 American Medical Association.

Excerpts from "Cooperation Insures Quality Medical Care in Rural Illinois
Area," by George T. Mitchell, *Family Practice News,* August 15, 1973.
Reprinted with permission of Family Practice News.

Dedicated to Millie,
my loving wife,
and our daughters
Linda and Mary Kay

Contents

Plates

Foreword

READERS OF *Dr. George* are in for a treat! The author, Dr. George Mitchell of Marshall, Illinois, shares reflections that span several generations of life in the Midwest, from the days of horse and buggy to the space age.

Educated and degreed in both medicine and mechanical engineering, Dr. Mitchell provides the reader with more than the reflections of a casual observer. First and foremost, he is a clinician trained to look beyond what others only see. Dr. Mitchell also retains an engineer's fascination with how things—and people—are organized. More, as a pragmatist in the American mold idealized by Ralph Waldo Emerson, he has been responsible for leading his community in the establishment of some of the stalwart institutions that embody so much of what people value in mid-America.

Readers of *Dr. George* will experience a little nostalgia for the good of the old days but also encounter some sobering reminders of the bad that make us grateful for the new days. A physician for more than fifty years, and the son of a physician and a nurse, Dr. Mitchell helps readers place many problems of the present into historical context. His stories are not just of the transition from horse-and-buggy medicine to high-tech healing but also of how the values that lead some people to choose a rural or small-town life-style—even if doing so means forgoing access to high technology—are formed and identified.

Residents of Marshall and southeastern Illinois know the author as an activist. When he becomes concerned about something, particularly the welfare of his patients, Dr. Mitchell takes action. For example, when elderly people living in the more sparsely settled areas of Clark County chose to remain in their own homes, even if doing so meant living alone, Dr. Mitchell contacted the president of the General Telephone Company to help change the level of service in the county. A representative from the company headquarters met with a group of citizens Dr. Mitchell had assembled to hear complaints. Soon thereafter, a large force of workers completely refurbished the county's telecommunications system, eliminating, among other things, multiparty lines and, therefore, the isolation of significant parts of the area.

Another example of his activism occurred when Interstate 70 had been completed across Indiana to the Illinois state line, and across

Illinois except for the fifty miles near Marshall. Officials of the State Department of Highways announced that it would be five years before that stretch of the interstate would be completed. The two-lane remainder of Route 40 became one of the most dangerous stretches of highway in the country. No "No Passing" zones had been designated along the route, and incidents of tragedy skyrocketed. Dr. Mitchell used his political connections to contact the governor and demand action. With data in hand, Dr. Mitchell organized a large petition drive with a local newspaper editor. The governor was moved to announce a "crash program" to finish the interstate immediately, despite what the citizenry had been told earlier. Dr. Mitchell received the distinguished service award from the United States Jaycees for his efforts.

Whether organizing physical examinations and immunization programs for school children, or establishing an ambulance service staffed by emergency medical technicians, or recruiting health care personnel to the area, Dr. Mitchell has been able to motivate people to address community needs.

Dr. Mitchell's most lasting contribution, other than being a model for community service, will probably be the development of a modern health care delivery system that respects the values of the community. The system, revolutionary at the time, called upon physicians to work together in a clinic designed for the county and consisted of the building of two medical centers, one in Marshall and the other in Casey on the west side of the county, with donated funds—no government or invested monies. It was a new concept in rural medicine that received national attention and as recently as 1992 was used as the most successful model for primary care in rural mid-America. His expertise led to his appointment as cochair of the Access to Health Care Committee of the Illinois State Medical Society in 1990, the mission of which is to work toward improving access to health care throughout the unserviced areas of the state.

In 1972, Dr. Mitchell was recognized by the American Academy of Family Physicians for his contributions to primary care and by the University of Illinois for "commitment and unselfish effort in founding the School of Basic Medical Sciences." In 1978, Illinois Blue Cross and Blue Shield awarded him special recognition for his contributions to the "improvement of health care services." Many honors have followed: from the Illinois State Medical Society in 1981 and again in 1986; from the Illinois Department of Public Health in 1987; and from the Illinois General Assembly in both 1989 and 1992.

Perhaps the most touching recognition Dr. and Mrs. Mitchell have received was that held on October 17, 1981, by the people of Marshall and the surrounding areas—"Dr. George and Millie Mitchell Day"—marked by a barbecue and dedication program.

Despite the responsibilities of the daily care of Millie and his other patients, Dr. Mitchell has not confined his community service to health care. He served twelve years on the local board of education and fourteen years as a member of the Board of Trustees of Lake Land Community College. He has been a member of the Marshall Rotary Club for more than forty-seven years and was elected a Paul Harris Fellow; he is active in the First United Methodist Church, the Marshall Chamber of Commerce, the American Legion, the Masons and Shrine, the Clark County and Illinois Farm Bureaus, the Clark County Historical Society (of which he was founding president), as well as many other community organizations.

The 1990s have brought new accolades to Dr. Mitchell from his colleagues around the state. In 1993 he was named Rural Health Practitioner of the Year by the Illinois Rural Health Association as well as Physician of the Year by the Illinois Academy of Family Physicians.

As a "country doctor," Dr. Mitchell has traveled through ice, snow, and other storms, sometimes requiring the use of farm tractors and rowboats. He has performed home deliveries, sometimes by lamplight. At the time he ceased obstetrical deliveries, he had assisted more than fifteen hundred citizens into the world. Through it all, he collected many of the stories and reflections that await the reader of *Dr. George*.

The Southern Illinois University Press Medical Humanities Series was created, among other reasons, to bring readers original works that investigate the interfaces between cultural values and the health sciences. *Dr. George* is a worthy addition to the series. My sole regret in its publication is that the book is only half the length of the author's original manuscript. The economics of publishing, however, should not dissuade scholars and other readers from access to the entire manuscript. A complete copy is archived in Special Collections, Southern Illinois University School of Medicine Library, in Springfield.

Glen W. Davidson
Senior Consulting Editor, Medical Humanities Series

Preface

As our daughters Linda and Mary Kay were growing up, they were my audience—listening to stories I had to tell concerning my life as a boy growing up in the small town of Marshall, to stories about family members who came before, and to stories about my experiences as a country doctor.

After they reached adulthood, our girls strongly urged me to record all of these stories. So I began. I have been fortunate in having a vivid memory of events that have occurred throughout my life and can picture them clearly in my mind. Over a period of nearly fourteen years, I wrote from time to time until I completed what is now presented to you.

I want to express my gratitude to all those who listened as I related stories about my life as a country doctor and asked, "Why don't you write a book?" To the many who over the years transcribed my words from scribbled longhand. To Barbara Reedy, secretary of the First United Methodist Church, who labored long and hard at the word processor. To Vivian McClelland, my high school classmate, herself a published author, who after reading my manuscript insisted that I seek a publisher. To Dr. James Turner, Dr. Steven Macke, and all of the loyal staff of the Cork Medical Center, especially my conscientious friend Doris Curran. To Dick Ott of the Illinois State Medical Society, who put me in touch with Dr. Glen W. Davidson of the Southern Illinois University School of Medicine. To Dr. Davidson, who took over the editing of my manuscript and guided me through the maze to publication. To Mary Ellen McElligott, who so skillfully edited the final draft. To Susan Wilson and Natalia Nadraga of Southern Illinois University Press, and to freelance copyeditor Ruth Kissell. To Dr. Don Tingley, professor emeritus of history at Eastern Illinois University, and Dr. Thomas Bonner, Distinguished Professor of History at Wayne State University, for reading the manuscript and recommending publication. And last, but not least, to Drew Casteel, my old friend in Marshall, who graciously provided pictures from his vast collection.

G.T.M.

1

My Dad, the Doctor

DAD DECIDED IN 1891, at the age of twelve, that he wanted to be a doctor. His decision was reached in an unusual way. He learned that a man who lived not far away was to have a leg amputated, and, as was the custom in those days, the surgery was performed in the home. On the given day (in the heat of summer), he went to the house, a small log cabin, where the surgery was to be performed.

When Dad arrived, there was already a large crowd assembled. A number of buggies and wagons were parked in a nearby grove of trees, and the people were crowded around the house peering through the windows and open door. He worked his way through the crowd until he was able to see through a window. The patient was lying on the kitchen table. The doctor was ready to get about the business of amputating the leg. A volunteer was administering the chloroform anesthetic. As the doctor made the incision, blood began to spurt. The people looking on began to faint. Suddenly the volunteer anesthetist also fainted. Dad, the little boy of twelve years, ran around to the door and took over the job of anesthetist. At this point he made his decision. Roscoe Addison Mitchell wanted to be a doctor.

In the ensuing years, he continued farming with his father. For a time he was a mule skinner. He had a fine span of mules, and he began hauling logs to Shawneetown, on the Ohio River. These trips took two days. He also became interested in playing the fiddle. At age sixteen, he purchased a fiddle (which I still have, framed and hanging in my den). He spent many enjoyable hours playing at square dances in his area. In time he saved his money and finally bought a good horse and buggy.

If Dad were to realize his dream of becoming a doctor, he knew he must accumulate more than he could on the farm. He had a relative who ran a general store in Kentucky. He contacted this man, who agreed to hire him as a clerk in his store. Dad took his horse and buggy, his fiddle, and other meager possessions and made the trip to

Kentucky. He enjoyed his new job. He was a handsome young man with coal black hair. When the young ladies found out there was an eligible, handsome young man clerking in the store, business soon increased. Dad told me that although all he had was a few clothes, he was always well groomed, his clothes neat and clean. Like the other clerks, he wore a pair of scissors suspended on a ribbon around his neck to cut yard goods for the customers. It was not long before he was receiving numerous invitations to fiddle dances.

Sometime later he heard about a man named Wasson of Harrisburg, Illinois, who had a patent medicine business and was a member of the Wasson family engaged in the coal mining business. Dad contacted Mr. Wasson and was offered a job traveling and selling patent medicine and notions house to house. The products offered for sale were numerous, ranging from "King of Pain" liniment to vanilla extract.

Dad gave up his clerk's position and returned to Harrisburg, where he began the new position with Mr. Wasson. His territory was western Indiana and eastern Illinois. He would leave Harrisburg with his buggy loaded down with Wasson products, cross into Indiana, and work his way north. He stopped at every farmhouse and attempted to sell his products to the homemaker. This was before the days of good roads, good transportation, and supermarkets. Country folk did not get to town often for supplies, so the itinerant peddler and his wares were a welcome sight. In order to keep expenses down, he devised a plan to receive meals and lodging in return for the products he had for sale. The first time into a new territory, he selected the most promising house to put up in for the night. He was always on the lookout for one with a good cook and a good housekeeper. Keep for his horse was included in the deal. Over the years he became good friends with these people, and they were always happy to see him. An overnight guest afforded the people an opportunity to catch up on news from other localities. A traveler was the radio, television, and newspaper of that day. Of course, Dad always had his fiddle and in the evening he entertained his hosts with good fiddlin' music.

He eventually extended his travels north to Indiana. He recounted one experience at Vincennes, the largest town he had ever seen. When he and Old Joe, his horse, drove into town, they encountered something they had never seen before—a streetcar. This horrible contraption was coming right at them. Dad was terrified—a house on wheels was loose. Old Joe stopped, laid back his ears, and took off at top speed across a vacant lot. After that, they avoided any town that had streetcars. Dad would stop outside of town, leave Old Joe in a barn, and proceed on foot.

After passing through Vincennes and Terre Haute, Dad worked his way west across the Wabash River into Illinois. He came to the town of Marshall, the county seat of Clark County. He liked this little town and its people the best of any he had seen. He did a good business in Marshall and the surrounding countryside. One old man, since deceased, told me that Dad stayed many times in his home. The old gentleman was a boy then and told me how he looked forward to those overnight visits. He said the first thing Dad did in the morning was to go to the barn and check on his horse. He would ask Old Joe, "Did you sleep well last night? What, you have a toothache! A little 'King of Pain' will fix that."

Dad has often told me that he thought good grooming, neatness, cleanliness, and politeness were the most important factors in dealing with the public. He tipped his hat so much that he wore a hole in the hat brim. He also told me he had so much confidence in his ability to sell that he was sure he could make a good living selling nothing but toothpicks. He became the top salesman and was making so much in commissions that the owner placed him on a good salary.

After he had saved a considerable amount of money, the time had come to get on with his dream. He came back to southern Illinois and had a talk with his family. Grandpa told him he could offer no financial support except for a hundred dollars. Dad felt that with his earnings and working his way through school he could make it.

He still didn't know where to go to medical school. He had heard there was one in Indianapolis. He decided to travel there to find out if he would be accepted. The trip involved taking a new mode of transportation—a train. He had never been on a train, and he was a little apprehensive about riding something that traveled so fast. His mother packed him a little suitcase and a basket lunch, and he set off to the depot. The station agent told him he could ride either a passenger train or the caboose of a freight train. He settled on the freight because it traveled much slower, and he thought it would be safer. He rode north several miles, then transferred to another line that ran east to Indianapolis. The train that he boarded traveled through two towns about sixteen miles apart with similar names. Dad mistakenly got off at the wrong station. Instead of waiting for the next train, however, he proceeded to walk the sixteen miles.

Finally, he arrived in the big city of Indianapolis and received directions to the Central College of Medicine. This country boy, carrying his little valise and lunch basket, walked to the school. He located the dean's office and was given an audience. The dean listened sympathetically, but upon learning this young man did not have a high school diploma (a prerequisite for admission), told him he did not qualify for admission. Dad's dream had been shattered. Yet, his earnestness and enthusiasm so impressed the dean that he finally told Dad that if he passed an exam covering all subjects of the four-year high school curriculum, he would be permitted to enter. Dad asked for a list of the subjects to be covered and inquired about where he could get the necessary textbooks. He purchased used books and returned to southern Illinois to study. He studied hard for three months and returned to Indianapolis to take the examinations. You can be sure he was nervous, but at the same time he had confidence in himself. He took the examinations, and when his grades were tallied, he had a general average of 96.5 percent. He was presented a small certificate listing all the subjects covered with the average grade obtained and bearing the signatures of the examining committee, composed of members of the medical school faculty. I believe that Dad was prouder of that certificate than any other recognition he ever received. It was framed and hung on the wall of his office as long as he lived.

Dad was so eager to get started that he was one of the first students to arrive on campus. He was standing on the steps of the school when a large young man approached, carrying a straw suitcase. It was fairly apparent he was not a city boy. He had a round face and rosy cheeks and took in the whole scene with wide-eyed wonderment. It was evident that his clothes had received much wear. The sleeves were a little short, the pants were a little short, and it was apparent he had added considerable weight since he had first worn the suit. Dad stuck out his hand and introduced himself. "I assume you are contemplating entering medical school," he said. ("Contemplating" was a new word he had learned but had not had occasion to use until now.) "Yes," the young man said, "my name is Roy Egbert, and I'm from the state of Kansas." A lifelong friendship was born on the spot.

The next four years were difficult. In order to finance his education, Dad not only continued to travel the territory for Wasson but also worked while going to school. He fired furnaces in a number of homes and waited tables in a boardinghouse. In order to get all of his work done, he rose each morning at three o'clock.

Some of his more affluent classmates always seemed to run short of money before their monthly check arrived from home. They soon discovered that Dad always had a little extra cash, so it was natural that he became their banker.

Because of his responsibilities at school in the winter and the necessity to be on the road selling during the summer, Dad did not get home to visit very often. He made up for this by writing frequently and, in turn, received long, interesting letters from his mother. One summer day he went to the post office in Terre Haute to get his mail. He had just written a long letter to his mother in response to one from her a week before. He picked up the mail, and there was a letter from his dad. The letter stated that his mother had awakened a week before with severe breathing difficulty. She went to the front porch and fell over dead. The funeral already had taken place. Dad collapsed.

During his first year in school Dad became quite impressed with a member of the faculty whose brother was a dentist. This started him thinking, "Wouldn't it be nice if I had a brother who was a dentist and we could practice together?" Which brother would it be? Clarence was the one. He was a few years younger, but that would work out fine. Furthermore, if he could get started, then they could graduate together. (Dental school was a three-year program.) He wrote Clarence and told him to get things together because he was going to be a dentist. Dad arranged for him to go to work for Wasson. They agreed to meet in Vincennes.

Clarence and Dad had not seen each other for a year. When the train arrived, a gangly youth, dressed in a suit with pant cuffs halfway to his knees and coat cuffs halfway to his elbows, stepped off carrying a straw suitcase. His hair was unkempt. Suddenly Dad realized this country bumpkin was brother Clarence. He took him in hand down the street to the barbershop. After a haircut, followed by a bath in the back room of the barbershop, he was taken to a clothing store for a new suit of clothes. Clarence was accepted by the School of Dentistry, and the two brothers completed their training at the same time.

During his senior year, Dad served as an intern at City Hospital. He spent considerable time riding the horse-drawn ambulance. One night a call for an ambulance came from the interurban station in downtown Indianapolis. Through the city streets, horses running at top speed, gong clanging, went the ambulance rocking from side to side with Dad holding on for dear life. The patient was a young girl who had taken an overdose of morphine. In those days morphine was an over-the-counter product. The patient was loaded into the ambulance, and they raced to the hospital at top speed.

There were no drug antidotes in those days. The treatment consisted of continual external stimulation to keep the patient awake. As soon as they reached the hospital, the patient was unloaded, placed in a room, disrobed, and walked around in a circle. The doctors applied external stimulation in the form of towels soaked in ice water. They walked the patient all night, flipping her constantly with icy towels. She made an uneventful recovery.

Responding to another ambulance call, Dad found a woman ready to give birth. Her husband, a big bruiser, made it plain she was not going to have the baby at home. The patient was quickly loaded, and a mad dash was made for the hospital. Dad was in back with the patient and her husband. The "big bruiser" kept reminding Dad that if his wife had the baby before she reached the hospital, he would kill him. Dad spent the whole trip praying and pressing a rolled-up towel against the baby's head with all the strength he had. They made it.

One day while attending a clinic at Central State Hospital (a mental institution), his eyes fell on a pretty brown-haired, blue-eyed student nurse who was also there to attend a clinic. It was love at first sight. From then on they were together frequently. Alma Trice was her name.

In June 1907, Dad saw the culmination of his dream. He received his M.D. degree from Indiana University (Central School of Medicine had become the School of Medicine of Indiana University). Commencement exercises were held at the main campus in Bloomington. Alma, of course, was present for this important ceremony. After receiving his diploma, Dad was so happy that he ran down the hill and attempted to jump across the Jordan River, a small creek winding through the campus. He failed. Instead, he severely sprained his ankle and spent the next several days walking on crutches.

Dad had decided long ago that the little town of Marshall, Illinois, was the place he wanted to live and practice his profession. He rented rooms on the second floor of a building on North Hamilton (now North Sixth) Street. Access to these rooms was by an outside stairway. He was soon joined by his brother Clarence, who opened his dental office in the same building.

Starting a medical practice was not easy. There were several other well-established doctors in Marshall. Most were cooperative and did their best to help their young colleague get a good start. Dr. Prewitt, the epitome of the old family doctor, frequently referred patients to Dad. Dr. Prewitt was most dignified in manner, and his very presence instilled confidence. According to one story, he made daily calls on a patient who lived out in the country. Each day as he returned, a man who lived along the road hailed him with questions concerning the patient. Dr. Prewitt knew the man was stone deaf. He answered the questions by moving his lips, never uttering a sound. The man would say, "Is that so?" or "My goodness! Well, I hope he continues to improve."

Another colleague, Dr. Edward Pearce, had a favorite expression, "So it is, so it is" or "So he did, so he did." One day, while driving down the road to make a house call, Dr. Pearce met a funeral procession. Drawing his buggy to the side of the road, he stopped and doffed his hat, showing proper respect for the deceased in the passing hearse. When he was told who it was, he said, "So it is, so it is. I was just going down to see him." With that, he turned his buggy around and headed back to town.

Dad worked hard all the summer of 1907 getting his practice established and preparing for a bride. He selected a small house in the southwest part of Marshall. He began making payments to the Building and Loan Association for their little cottage, as he called it. He furnished it, and all was in readiness.

On December 6, 1907, he and Alma Trice were married in Indianapolis. The wedding party, which included his old friend and classmate Roy Egbert, had a wedding supper at the Claypool Hotel, the leading hostelry at that time. Later they boarded a train at Union Station, arriving in Marshall at about midnight. It was a mild winter. There had not been a deep freeze, and so the ground was soft. From the train they boarded a jitney—a miniature horse-drawn streetcar with a step and a door at the rear. A seat ran along each side, and an oil lamp hung in a bracket at the front. The jitney was pulled by a team of horses, and the driver sat on a seat high up front on the outside. The streets were knee-deep in mud, and when the bride saw the muck, she could think only of her home back in Indiana where they had good, firm gravel roads. The thought went through her mind that she had come to the "Jumping-Off Place," as she told me later, and she considered getting right back on the train.

The bride and groom arrived at their new home only to have a jolting surprise. Unbeknownst to Dad, brother Earl (the youngest member of the family), Grandpa Stephen Mitchell, and sister Lou and her children had moved in, bag and baggage. Lou had separated from her husband! If it had not been for the deep and abiding love my mother had for my dad, this would have been a very short marriage.

My mother was one of seven children, six girls and one boy. Her father, David Trice, came to Indiana from Maryland, having lived on the eastern shore of Chesapeake Bay. Grandpa Trice had been orphaned and was "contracted out" to a family in Henry County, Indiana. Grandma Trice was a native of Henry County, Indiana. Her maiden name was Sara E. Ball. Grandpa was a hardworking farmer. They were members of a Quaker meeting, and Mom attended the Quaker Academy in Spiceland, Indiana. Grandma always prepared all the food for Sunday a day early, as was the Quaker custom.

At a Quaker meeting, the families sat quietly for an hour. The silence was broken only when someone was moved by the Spirit to speak or sing. Sitting quietly for an hour without talking or squirming was surely an ordeal for a child. Grandma discovered that Mother would be very still if she could munch on a baked sweet potato so each Saturday she baked a small sweet potato, which was wrapped carefully in a clean white handkerchief and carried to church the next day. When the first bit of squirming started, the potato would appear and Mom stayed very quiet throughout the rest of the meeting, happily munching her sweet potato.

Mother's maternal ancestors came west from North Carolina. She had an iron pot that had been brought to Indiana around 1817 in an ox cart. She often spoke of her great-aunt, who made the trip as a child walking most of the distance. Mother grew up not far from the Old National Road (the Cumberland Trail), the first federal highway to be built westward from the East Coast. Its eastern terminus was Cumberland, Maryland, and the road ended in the west at Vandalia, Illinois. She remembered the covered wagons carrying families westward. The road was almost impassable in both the rainy season and the winter months. In order to stabilize the surface and afford better traction, logs were laid crossways. Such "corduroy roads" provided a much better driving surface but also a very rough ride over the logs. There were tollgates at intervals along the way, and a long pole, hinged to a post, was kept lowered across the highway. When a traveler came along, it was necessary for him to pay his toll to the tollkeeper, who would then raise the pole, allowing the traveler to proceed.

Mom developed seasonal hay fever and asthma, and by the time she became a teenager, her condition worsened and she could hardly breathe during the months of August and September until the first frost had killed the goldenrod and ragweed. In those days there was no specific treatment for allergies, so the only relief to be obtained was by changing climates. When she was about sixteen years old, her parents arranged for her to travel each year to northern Michigan, where the air was cooler and free of the pollens that caused her problem. She boarded a train at Richmond, Indiana, and traveled north to Mackinaw City, Michigan.

On one of those trips, the train she was riding was involved in a head-on collision with another passenger train—two trains made up of wooden coaches, each traveling at a speed of sixty miles an hour through the night and meeting head-on in a cornfield. Mom was sitting by a window near the middle of the car but had just gotten up to go to the toilet when the crash occurred. She was catapulted through the air to the front of the car. She was unconscious for a period of time but recovered. Many others were not so fortunate. Both trains were completely destroyed, and onlookers saw only a massive pile of shattered wood and crushed steel. They hauled the dead and injured away on hayracks. In those days there were few rules governing train safety. There were no automatic block signals. The movement of trains was regulated by written orders given to the train crew and semaphore signals operated by a man in a tower or wayside station.

This was before the eight-hour workday. Railroad men worked as long as twenty to twenty-four hours without relief. On that particular night, a towerman had fallen asleep after being on duty nearly all day. The telegraph buzzer was going full blast. Finally, he awakened as the northbound train roared by. The message he received was to stop the train, but it was too late. There was no other point at which the train could be stopped. The towerman disappeared and was never seen again.

My mother wanted more than anything to become a nurse. Her family was not well-to-do, but they encouraged her and helped all they could. She was accepted as a student at the Stearn's Sanitarium in Indianapolis. After three years of study and hard work, she became a registered nurse.

After the traumatic experience of arriving at their house on their wedding night to find a house full of relatives, Mom and Dad began to adjust to their marriage. Dad was busy with his practice, and Mom was working hard to make their little cottage a home. On one occasion, while eating supper, Dad proudly displayed a ten-dollar gold piece he had received in payment for a delivery. Aunt Lou reached over and said she would take it. "No, you won't," said Dad, "this goes as payment on the house." It was not long until Dad asked Aunt Lou and family to leave. However, Grandpa Mitchell and Earl continued to live with them. Earl was entering high school. During his high school years, Mom became his second mother, cooking meals, washing clothes, and offering advice.

Earl went on to college and later graduated from the Indiana University School of Medicine. His two brothers, Dad and Clarence, financed his education.

Dad worked long hours, making house calls in all kinds of weather and at all hours day and night. His good bedside manner and knowledge of medicine did not go unnoticed. He gained the respect and confidence of the people, which he retained throughout his life. This was long before the days of good roads and modern transportation. The mode of transportation was the horse and buggy, but when the roads became impassable, the doctor resorted to riding horseback, and when the horse could not travel through the mud, it became necessary to walk. In time, Dad added another horse to form a team. He also acquired a bicycle, which he used in good weather.

One Saturday night, during his early days in practice, he received a call from a family living north of Marshall who were unable to reach their regular physician. Dad set out in his horse and buggy. The people living in the area were of Irish descent. After ministering to the patient, Dad started home. Along the way he came upon a large square dance in progress in the front yard of a farmhouse. Dad couldn't pass it up. He tied the horse to a fence and proceeded to join the crowd. He was not acquainted with any of the people, but he slowly worked his way through the crowd, smiling and introducing himself as he went.

At intermission he struck up a conversation with the fiddler, who invited him to join in on the next set. Nothing could have made Dad happier. When the next set started, a new fiddler, Dr. R. A. Mitchell, was stroking the bow. He stayed until the dance was over and arrived home early in the morning to a worried wife. When he told her what he had been doing, she was not too happy. Those people who had seen and heard the young doctor playing the fiddle took him to their hearts. From then on, as long as he lived, they were his loyal patients.

Living across the street from my parents was a large family named Grieson. Mr. Grieson was a hardworking man who ruled the family with an iron hand. In fact, it appeared his wife and children lived in fear of him. One day, Mrs. Grieson asked my mother if she could borrow some horse liniment. Mom got the liniment from the barn and asked why she wanted it. Mrs. Grieson stated that her young son Richard, while playing barefoot, had stepped on a stubble. Mom asked to have a look. What she saw was a massively swollen, reddened foot. The boy was feverish, and it was evident he was quite ill. The accident had occurred several days before, and he had not been seen by a doctor. With her knowledge as a nurse, Mom knew the child needed immediate medical attention. Mrs. Grieson stated she had begged her husband to call the doctor, but he had refused. It was not long before the boy developed the dreaded tetanus. At this point the father finally consented to have the doctor see the boy, but it was too late. His fever went higher and convulsions set in. His muscles became rigid, finally contracting until the boy stiffened into an arc, with his legs and head drawn backwards. His pain was terrible, the convulsions continued, and eventually he died. Mom stayed with the child until life finally ceased. She never forgot this incident and in later years told me about the boy's horrible death.

Being progressive in his thinking, Dad was ready to try a motorcycle when that mode of transportation became available. He purchased a Harley-Davidson and eventually learned to ride, although he was not particularly skilled in handling such a machine. One night he received a call from south of town, where a couple had been involved in a horse-and-buggy runaway. Dad took off on his trusty Harley-Davidson. This was his first attempt at night riding. The means of illumination was an acetylene gas headlight. Dad was going down the dirt road at a good rate of speed when suddenly the light went out. Just at that time he struck a large rock. He flew through the air and came down with a terrific crash. Fortunately, he received only

bumps, bruises, and scrapes, but the motorcycle was dem<
When he finally arrived on foot to minister to the victims
runaway, he found they were in better shape than he was. T]
the end of the motorcycle experiment.

By 1910 Dad's practice had grown so that the quarters on North
Hamilton Street had become too small. Clarence also needed more
room for his dental practice. They decided to build a new office on a
lot purchased on the west side of the Courthouse Square on Fifth
Street. Dr. Bradley already was practicing medicine in a building he
owned to the south, and Dr. L. J. Weir's offices were to the north across
the alley.

Dad and Clarence built a handsome, two-story, brick building. The
lower floor had a common waiting room to the front with a large plate
glass window. To the rear there were two rooms on the north and two
rooms on the south. Dad occupied the two south rooms. The room
opening from the waiting room was his treatment and consultation
room. The room to the rear was the drug room, which contained a
large, solid, black walnut drug cabinet with a counter for mixing and
dispensing prescriptions. Above the counter were shelves that held
bottles of pills and liquids. Beneath the counter were drawers for
supplies. The cabinet was constructed from native black walnut taken
from the large stand of timber near Walnut Prairie south of Marshall.
(This cabinet now has been refinished and is a beautiful bookcase in
my family room.)

The two rooms on the north side of the building were used by
Clarence for his dental office and laboratory. The building had central
heating and inside plumbing. The upper floor was made into an
apartment. Of course, there was need for a building to house Dad's
horse and buggy during office hours, so a small barn was constructed
on the rear of the lot. The two brothers were finally located in their
own fine, modern office building, practicing their profession together
just as they had dreamed in Indianapolis years before.

Dad became quite interested in the automobile. His first car was a
Hupmobile Roadster, which resembled the small sports car of today.
It could carry only two people and was started by twisting a crank. He
was very proud of this little car and the speed with which he could get
about—in dry weather. He called it his "Hoopie."

One summer Sunday, Dad was returning from a call north of town,
and as he mounted the bridge over the Vandalia tracks, he saw a huge,
black cloud of smoke over downtown Marshall. He knew something
terrible had happened. He entered town at top speed, and on Main
Street he saw a horrible sight.

A garage occupied the middle of the block on the south side of the
street directly across from City Hall. (This building is now Tom's

Cafe.) The garage was closed on Sunday, but three men, Mr. Eaton, Mr. Jones, and Mr. Huston, had gone there to look at an auto parts catalog. One of the men lighted a cigar, and there was a terrible explosion caused by a gas leak. The entire front of the building was blown out, and the three men were blown across the street. Their horribly burned and mangled bodies were lying on the street when Dad arrived. The men were still alive. He attended to them at the scene and then had them transported to their homes. (Hospitals were not readily available then to people outside the cities.) He did all he could in caring for them the next few days, but the doctors' armamentarium in those days was very limited. In spite of all his efforts, all three died, each leaving a family.

2

1914–1920

I WAS BORN on a wintery day in January 1914. Mother had been in labor for hours and hours. She was very, very tired, and the long labor took its toll. The attending physician, Dr. Stephen Bradley, was becoming quite concerned. He had sat with his patient throughout the long night. A decision had to be made soon as to whether to permit labor to continue or to intervene. It was evident that I was quite large, and my mother was small. There was no possibility she could be moved to a hospital. The distance was too great, and there was no transportation. Without X-ray equipment, the doctor was unable to get an accurate measurement of the pelvis. He was completely on his own. Finally, he made his decision. Forceps would have to be applied. This was not the routine procedure it is today, but instead constituted a final desperate means of delivering the baby. Frequently the baby would be stillborn, or the forceps would cause injury to the mother by lacerating the cervix or the soft tissue around the outlet. Lacerations could result in severe hemorrhage and death of the mother. It was also necessary to administer chloroform, which could be dangerous to both the mother and the baby.

Finally, the forceps were carefully put in place. Traction on the forceps was applied and slowly, slowly, ever so slowly, the head began to move down. At last the crown appeared and then the complete head. The forceps were removed, and slowly the shoulders and arms were delivered, followed by the rest of the body. A sharp spank on the rear and then a loud cry. I weighed ten pounds. Mother was completely exhausted, but when she awoke and saw me, her strength returned. She had been amply rewarded. Dad's emotional euphoria lasted for several days. He had a son.

Earl was then away at college and working in the summer, so he was not living with Mom and Dad. Grandpa found a lady friend, a widow named Emma Murphy. She was the classical grandmother type—of medium height with ample girth and a round, friendly face that readily broke into a smile. They were married and moved to a house on South Eighth Street. Dad and Mom, with their new son, were the only occupants of the cottage. After about six months, they decided that they needed a larger house.

They found just what they needed: a spacious two-and-a-half story Victorian house at the corner of South Sixth and Cherry streets. For the first time they had inside plumbing but no central heating. Heat was supplied by coal stoves, augmented by fireplaces in the living room, parlor, and bedrooms. The new house had a small garage for the "Hoopie," but there was no barn for the horses, which still provided the major means of transportation. Consequently, a lot was purchased across Cherry Street and a new barn constructed. The barn had horse stalls, a hayloft, and room for a milk cow, chickens, and the buggy.

new home after George born

Mother fed the livestock and milked the cow. As soon as I could toddle, I went with her to do chores. One day, while she was in the barn, I wandered into the barnyard with the chickens. I was wearing a red sweater to which a large rooster immediately took offense.

Suddenly there was a loud scream. Mom rushed out and found me sprawled in the dirt, the rooster busily using his beak and spurs on me. She quickly rescued me. Close inspection revealed no physical damage, but I never forgot the experience. From then on I was terrified by anything that looked like a chicken. Mom put my fear to good use. Anything she didn't want me to touch, she simply laid a feather on—I refused to pass through a doorway or climb a step if a feather was there. For some reason or other, a hot water bottle partially filled with water also stopped me. My folks had feathers and hot water bottles scattered throughout the house!

When I was nearly two years old, I was entered in a Better Babies Contest sponsored by the *Ladies' Home Journal.* The contest was open to all babies in the county. Each baby was given a thorough physical examination by a panel of doctors. (Dad was not among them.) The contest narrowed to a tie between two finalists. The panel reexamined the two finalists, and I was the winner. It seems the other finalist, Howard Johnson (now Dr. Howard Johnson of Casey), was a bit overweight—he had failed to have a bowel movement that day.

One spring day, when I was two years old, I was outside with Mom while she worked in the garden. The sun had been shining brightly, but large clouds began rolling in from the west. The sky became darker and darker until it seemed that night had fallen. The air was warm and still. In the house it was so cool a fire had been started in the fireplace. The thunder rolled and the lightning flashed. We were in the house with the doors and windows tightly shut. The wind began to blow so hard it seemed as though the roof was going to go. The trees appeared to bend to the ground. Then the hail came, and it seemed a miracle the windows weren't shattered.

Dad was gone most of the night. When he came home, he was exhausted from taking care of people injured in a tornado that came in from the northwest part of town. It completely demolished the village of Livingston. A baby in Livingston had been blown from a house and was found dead hanging in the top of a tree.

Typhoid vaccine had not been developed yet, and that dreadful disease occurred in epidemic proportion far too often. One such epidemic occurred when I was quite young. Mother had made some spare rooms upstairs into an apartment, which was occupied by Mr. and Mrs. Howard Rubel and their daughter Peggy. One day Mrs. Rubel became very sick. Dad made a diagnosis of typhoid fever. She became delirious, and died after several days. She left a grief-stricken husband and daughter. Mom stepped in and gave Peggy the same love and care she gave to me. Peggy and I played together and shared our toys. I was overjoyed because I now had a sister. Once when Mom came into the kitchen, Peggy was sitting patiently and quietly on the floor while I spooned flour from the bin in the kitchen cabinet onto her head. Eventually, Mr. Rubel rented a house and hired a housekeeper. I lost my sister.

As a youngster I liked to play outside in our yard, but there was no fence to keep me from getting out into the street. Dad solved the problem by enclosing the yard with a four-foot woven-wire farm fence. Some of the children taught me to scale the fence, however, so Dad added another three feet of chicken wire. The seven-foot fence confined me. Our postman Arthur Deaner kidded me about being kept in a horse lot. I responded that if he kept teasing me I'd tell Dad: "He's the Board of Health and you'll be sorry." Despite the fence, I spent many happy hours building sand castles and digging tunnels.

My mother administered justice. Depending on the seriousness of the misdemeanor, the punishment might be a scolding, being put to bed in the daytime, sitting in a chair, or a good switching. Mom's favorite switch came from a peach tree standing to the south of the house. I resolved to cut that tree down when I got big enough. When I was about seven years old, I was given a hatchet! The hated tree had become diseased, so when I began hacking away with my new hatchet, Mom and Dad didn't object. I doggedly stayed at it until finally I had the tree down.

Ours was a big, old-fashioned kitchen with a kitchen cabinet where the flour and spices were kept. There were shelves for the pots and pans. Across the room was the table where we ate most of our meals. In the corner was the icebox. Ice was delivered by the iceman. Each household was provided with a card with large numbers printed in each corner—25 lbs., 50 lbs., 75 lbs., and 100 lbs. The card would be hung in the window with the number showing for the amount of ice needed. The iceman, seeing the card, would stop and deliver the proper size cake of ice. Under the icebox was a large pan to catch the dripping water. Occasionally, the pan was allowed to overflow, and then the floor would be covered with water. The centerpiece of the kitchen, the center of operations, was the big, old-fashioned coal cookstove, which occupied one side of the room. (Coal was hauled from the coal pile on one end of the back porch.) Below the black cooking surface was the oven, and above was the warming oven. On one end was the reservoir, which was filled with rainwater from the cistern. The water was kept hot by the stove and was always available for shampooing and other activities requiring soft water.

One day I was in the kitchen while Mom was getting dinner. A big pot of beans—my favorite food—was simmering on the stove. I had been smelling the aroma and could hardly wait. I asked Mom repeatedly when the beans would be done. Suddenly the phone in the hall rang out, and Mom hurried to answer. I was unable to wait any longer: I pushed a chair up to the stove and planted one foot on the stove in order to take a look in the kettle of beans. A loud scream brought Mom running. The little foot encased in a sandal was terribly burned. The bottom of the foot was one large blister, and the footprint was charred into the shoe sole. Mom kept the shoe among her mementos as long as she lived.

Until about 1916 the unpaved dirt streets of Marshall turned into knee-deep mud in the winter and spring and into dust in the summer and fall. It was decided to pave Main Street between the east and west city limits, and also Sixth Street between the north and south city limits. The south and west sides of the Courthouse Square also were paved. The new surface was to be of large paving bricks, set by hand in concrete. A large steam-powered concrete mixer did the work. That horrible monster, breathing fire and smoke, worked in front of our house while I hid behind the garage terrified, occasionally taking a quick peek to see if it had gone away.

IN 1916 war clouds were gathering over the United States. The war in Europe had been declared, and German U-boats were making it hazardous for our ships to traverse the ocean. The die was cast when the *Lusitania* was sunk, with great loss of American lives. As a result, the United States declared war on Germany.

It was not long before Dad entered the service and became an officer in the Army Medical Corps. He was assigned for training to Fort Harrison in Indianapolis. Mom and I also went to Indianapolis, where we lived in one room. Dad had to live on base and rarely could come into town, but Mom and I visited him at camp often. We rode out and back on a streetcar. Dad was eventually transferred to Camp Greene at Charlotte, North Carolina, and we followed him there. He had the rank of captain and was assigned chief of a medical ward.

He was not required to live in camp, so the three of us lived in one room in a rooming house. Housing was practically nonexistent, and we were lucky to have that much space. We had to go a block or two down the street to a boardinghouse to get our meals. Apparently, boardinghouse food did not agree with me because I became ill, developing colitis. Dad was home only at night, so a kindly neighbor stayed with me while Mom went out to eat at noon. I could tolerate nothing but soft food and liquids, but even my tolerance to that diet was limited. I was confined to bed. There were no cooking facilities so Mom prepared my food over a small alcohol burner. Even with my parents' expert care, I grew weaker and weaker. Dad consulted with the doctors at the hospital, but they were as puzzled as he was. Just when it looked as if I were going to die, a new doctor, a pediatrician from Boston, was assigned to the hospital. He prescribed a new treatment, and I began to improve slowly. After months in bed, I learned to walk all over again. Finally, Dad was able to get another place to live. This time it was a bigger room in a large old frame house down by the railroad, but we did have cooking privileges. After we moved in, we found the place was infested with rats. We could hear them chewing on Dad's boots at night. Occasionally, we found a rat sitting on the rim of the bathtub or on the toilet seat. I came down with the measles shortly after moving in, so we were stuck there until I recovered, nearly six weeks later. Again I was very sick and had a long convalescence.

As soon as I was able, my parents and I moved into a duplex. The new quarters were indeed a luxury. We had a kitchen, living room, bedroom, dining room, and bath. The duplexes were arranged in a U-shape around a mall. I remember Mom ordering groceries from the commissary, the deliveries being made by soldiers in an army truck.

During the time we were in Charlotte, Dad was advised to have a tonsillectomy. He was hospitalized at the base, and Mom and I visited him daily. The experience was strange for me, seeing Dad lying in a hospital bed, wearing an ice collar around his neck.

At the hospital I ran into a little boy who was peddling papers to patients. I struck up a conversation with him. "How would you like to help me?" he asked. "Sure," I replied. "Here, take these papers and go through the ward and see how many you can sell and be sure and get the money—a nickel for each paper." I felt very important as I made my way through the ward full of ailing soldiers. As a small boy, I was unfamiliar with homesickness, but every one of these men was afflicted. One soldier with tears in his eyes grabbed me and gave me a big hug. Somewhere he had a little boy like me. "Nurse, get me my billfold," he said. The nurse came back, and the man took out a dollar; he asked the nurse for a safety pin and pinned it to my undershirt, gave me a final hug, lay back in bed, and closed his eyes. Mom had been looking everywhere for me. After turning the extra papers and money over to the paperboy, she led me back to Dad's room. I unbuttoned my blouse and proudly showed them the dollar bill pinned to my undershirt.

Dad had a uniform and army coat made for me. It was decorated with a captain's insignia and officer's braid at the sleeves. Frequently, we walked downtown at night. The streets were filled with soldiers; as they met us, they would salute. I returned the salute the same as Dad.

Flu was rampant, and pneumonia was the usual complication. There was no specific treatment for pneumonia, just aspirin, cough medicine, pneumonia jackets, and prayer. The mortality rate from 1917 through 1918 was high. On our walks downtown, we passed the railroad station. I'll never forget seeing the long rows of caskets encased in wooden shipping boxes stacked four high, stretching for a city block along the railroad platform—just one day's shipment.

The tide had turned, and the Americans and their allies were winning. Rumors were rampant. Early in November 1918, rumor spread that the armistice had been declared; but the rumor was false, and our high hopes were dashed. On November 11, however, the armistice was signed and the war was over.

I'll always remember that night. It was bitterly cold, but no one noticed the weather. Everyone was downtown. The streets were filled with people—men, women, children, and soldiers. It was so crowded you could hardly walk. Horns and whistles were blowing; bells were ringing. People were shouting and crying tears of joy. They were dragging effigies of the German Kaiser up and down the streets. It was utter chaos. I can still remember the three of us standing on a street corner, our backs against a building away from the streaming humanity, loving every minute of it.

In a few weeks Dad received his honorable discharge, and we started our trip home. He thought we should have a vacation before returning to Marshall. Before the war he and three others—his brother Clarence, his cousin Lucian Blackman, and his friend Olen Clements—had purchased about two hundred acres of land near Lakeland, Florida, and started an orange and grapefruit grove. Consequently, we went to Lakeland for our vacation. Each day we traveled the ten or twelve miles by train out to Haskell. The tenant met us in the spring wagon pulled by a mule, and we rode through the pine woods to the farm. Still wearing his uniform, Dad hitched a mule to a walking plow and plowed all day; I walked along beside him.

AFTER OUR Florida vacation, we returned to Marshall. The flu epidemic was still raging, and Dad was welcomed home with open arms. Only the very old doctors had remained home during the war, and they were physically exhausted. Very few people were well, and Dad was constantly on the go. He spent little time in the office because most people were too sick to get there.

Transportation was by horse and buggy because the roads were knee-deep in mud. Dad hired a driver who also took care of the rig. Being relieved of driving permitted Dad to catch a few winks while traveling from one farm to the next. Mom acted as dispatcher and, as the calls came in, relayed messages, sending him from one house to another.

Telephones were still primitive. There were two separate systems—one for farmers, and one for the rest of the populace. Calls could not be transferred from one system to the other, so it was necessary to have two phones at the house and office. The farmers' system covered the rural area, and the citizens' system included the area within the town of Marshall. The farmers were all on a party line, and each phone had a code system of long and short rings. The phones were crank operated, and each person on the line could communicate by turning the crank, which then sent out the required long and short rings for the individual on the receiving end. The telephone operators were paid the large sum of ten cents per hour. In our house, there were two phones in the hallway near the foot of the stairs. On one of the rare nights when Dad was at home, the phone rang and he started downstairs. He did not turn on a light, and suddenly there was a loud crash. Mom ran out of the bedroom and down the stairs. Dad was piled up on the floor by the phone. "What in the world happened?" she asked. "Well, I wanted to be able to go right back to sleep," Dad answered, "so I kept my eyes closed and I missed that damned top step." The next day the bed was moved to a room on the main floor just off the lower hall near the phones. They never slept upstairs again.

There were days on end during which Dad never got home to sleep. It was a constant, grueling pace that he kept, going from house to house, day and night. When it was cold, he bundled up in a fur coat, fur hat, and gloves. In the buggy, a large, woven, heavy lap robe covered him up to his chin. The robe was handsomely decorated with the image of a bear, complete with glass eyes. On wintery days he also used a foot warmer, fueled by charcoal bricks.

Despite all the influenza, babies were still coming into the world, and the obstetrical cases took an extra amount of time. There was no such thing as prenatal care, and often the first the doctor knew about such a case was when he received a call: "Hurry, Doc, my wife is painin'." The doctor usually had help from a grandmother and a neighbor woman. Having a baby meant boiling a lot of water, supplying lots of clean sheets and towels, and sitting and waiting. Complications were the rule rather than the exception—eclampsia, with its convulsions (usually fatal), hemorrhage (usually fatal), and stillbirths. Infant and maternal mortality rates were high, not through any fault of the doctor, but because of the lack of facilities, equipment, and medications.

It was the rule that if a doctor were having trouble, he always called another in consultation. Although the procedure did not necessarily benefit the patient, the old adage of two heads being better than one seemed to be appropriate. Besides, it made the doctor feel better to have a colleague share his misery.

I became a victim of the flu and once again was confined to bed. Dad was torn between caring for his patients and trying to take care of me. I was fortunate in having a nurse for a mother. She spent many sleepless nights sitting by my bed, checking on my breathing, giving me medicine for my racking cough and aspirin for my high fever, sponging my face, and praying for my recovery. After nearly three months in bed, I was able to be up again, but the flu had taken its toll. I was unable to shake my cough and was so weak that I could hardly walk.

I GRADUALLY REGAINED my strength, and in the fall of 1919 at age five I was enrolled at the South Side School. Although my sixth birthday was not until the following January, Dad prevailed on the school board to let me enter in September. I was not happy about going to school: I liked it the way it was, being at home with Mom and playing all day.

When I went to school that first morning, I felt like I was walking the last mile. This was the end. I was unused to being with all those strangers. I was scared. At noon the teacher, Miss Washburn, told me she had been informed I was too young and I was not to come back that afternoon. I had to wait another year. My mood changed immediately. As I left school, I told my new acquaintances I would not return. I didn't have to go to school. When I got home, Dad was there, and I told him my good news. "We'll see about that. I'll call the president of the school board." While he was talking on the phone, I was under the bed in the adjoining bedroom screaming and beating my fists and feet on the floor. He came in and dragged me from under the bed and said, "Young man, you will go back to school this afternoon!" This ended my stay of execution. A very downcast little boy dragged himself back to school that afternoon to face his classmates, who, only an hour before, had been told, "I don't have to go to school."

I wanted my mother. I couldn't seem to let go of the apron strings. The teacher spent a good part of her time holding me on her lap. Finally, I began to make friends and show interest in the daily activities. It seemed as if we spent a lot of time sitting at our desks outlining letters, which had been drawn by the teacher on a sheet of paper by sticking holes with a pin through the paper along the lines of the letter.

Spankings were frequent. The ritual consisted of the culprit lying across a desk at the front of the room as the teacher administered punishment with a board paddle. My best friend, Gene Spotts, was the victim on one occasion. The first room and second room across the hall shared one paddle, and it had been used last in the second room. With Gene in position on the front desk, the teacher discovered she had no paddle. "George," she said, "go get the paddle across the hall." This was like asking me to furnish the gun to shoot my best friend. Afterwards, the teacher told Mom that my face turned "white as a sheet." I slowly walked to the cloakroom and then started to walk to the hallway door, but stopped. I stood and listened as she lectured Gene until finally I could tell she was running out of steam. After I thought it was safe, I went on to the second room and got the paddle. When I returned, she had changed her mind. Gene did not get paddled.

I still suffered the effects of the flu. It seemed as if I coughed constantly, ran a fever, and always had to carry a bottle of cough medicine and pills. I was able to be in school only about three months that first year. Nevertheless, I managed to stay with my class, and the next year I was in the second grade with Miss Green. I was not the timid, scared little boy I had been. Instead, I was into everything. I occasionally fought with another boy, and it seemed as if the teacher had me staying in at recess most of the time. She would threaten to spank me, and I'd talk her out of it.

DANNY GARWOOD was Dad's driver. Dad always said that if Danny couldn't get him through, no one could. Danny was a short, sturdy fellow who drove fast and furiously and loved every minute of it. Regardless of the weather, he was always on the job and always had a grin. He was my hero. Danny always wore a short-billed cap and a vest. I wanted to dress like him, but of course had no vest. Mom took one of Dad's old vests and altered it so that it fit me. She took a picture of Danny and me standing on the front steps, with me wearing a short-billed cap and my coat thrown open so the vest was in plain view—my thumbs in my vest pockets, my feet spread apart, and a grin on my face just like Danny's.

One day in early spring, I was standing in the living room looking out the north window. Danny had gone to the barn across the street and hitched the horse to the buggy. The horse, a little on the wild side, had been restricted to the barn for some time. The long confinement had failed to ameliorate his disposition. Horse and buggy came roaring out of the barn onto the street and, just as the buggy was opposite the house, the horse raised up on its hind legs until it was standing straight up, pawing the air. I thought it was going to fall backwards onto the buggy, crushing poor Danny; but just at that moment, it fell forward on all fours and took off at full speed straight across Sixth Street. Through it all, Danny sat straight in the seat roaring with laughter.

When the roads improved somewhat, the horse was given a rest, and the Model T Ford was brought out. Danny was just as handy with the car as he was with the horse and buggy. He kept the car serviced and repaired the flat tires, which occurred far too often. A flat tire meant crawling under the vehicle to place the hand jack under the axle. Danny never hesitated—dust, rain, or snow, under he would go. After the car was lifted, the tire had to be pried loose from the rim of the wheel with tire tools. Then the inner tube was removed and the can of tire patches and glue was brought out. If the puncture hole was not readily apparent, the tube was pumped up with a hand pump and placed in a tub of water. Air bubbles coming up through the water pinpointed the puncture. The tire repair kit included a small round piece of metal with holes punched through, making for a rough surface on one side like a rasp. The tool was used to scrape the surface at the puncture site, a procedure that roughened the rubber surface. Then, glue was applied and the rubber patch was placed on. A small clamp was then placed over the patch and tightened. Once the patch was secure and the clamp removed, the tube was stuffed into the tire, and the tire forced back on the rim. These were called clincher rims. After the tire was finally in place, the hand pump was attached to the valve and the tire reinflated. The jack was lowered with the hope that the job was done. The average elapsed time to perform the entire procedure was between forty-five minutes and one hour.

Even in so-called good weather, heavy rains turned the dirt roads into a sea of mud. Danny hit these mud holes at full speed, with Dad hanging on for dear life. The old Model T was open to the weather, but if the weather became too bad, side curtains were dragged out and put in place. Of course, if a sudden downpour occurred on the road, Danny and Dad both became soaked before the curtains could be put up. Since there was no heater, the charcoal foot warmer was moved from the buggy to the Ford. On occasion, the lap robe was also necessary.

The Ford had no gearshift; instead, there were three pedals on the floorboard. The left pedal put the car in low gear, the middle pedal was reverse, and the pedal to the right was the brake. On the left side of the driver was a hand lever. When pulled clear back, it became the parking brake; when pushed forward, it put the car in high gear. There was no footfeed. There were two hand levers mounted on the steering column just under the steering wheel. Each lever was mounted on a quadrant. The one on the left was the spark, and the one on the right was the accelerator (better known as the gas). Two choke wires, one located on the front of the car next to the crank and the other sticking out of the left side of the dash, were used to prime the engine.

There was no instrument panel—no speedometer, gas gauge, or oil gauge—and no self-starter. The ritual for starting the Ford was to push the spark lever up, pull the gas lever down a little, make sure the brake lever was back, go to the front of the car, pull the choke wire out, grasp the crank and spin it. If you were lucky, the car started. You then ran back and adjusted the spark lever until the motor was running smoothly. If you were unlucky, which too often was the case, the thing "kicked"—the crank spinning backwards and possibly striking the wrist and fracturing it.

Once in the driver's seat, the throttle was pulled down, the lever at the left was advanced slightly to release the parking brake, while the left foot pushed the left pedal to the floor. After the car was moving at a fair pace, the lever on the left side was pushed full forward and the foot removed from the pedal. The car now was in high gear. Driving at top speed, the occupants had "both ears down." This colloquialism meant that both the spark lever and the throttle lever were all the way down. Top speed was about thirty-five miles an hour. To stop, the lever on the left was pulled part way back, the spark and throttle lever were pushed up, and the foot was applied to the right floor pedal. To reverse, the parking brake was released, the foot was applied to the middle pedal, and the throttle lever was pulled down. To stop the engine, the throttle and spark levers were pushed up, and the choke wire was pulled. The procedure flooded the engine and stopped it. There was no battery. Instead, magneto coils were mounted in a box under the dash. By twisting the crank, a revolution of the crankshaft activated the magneto coils causing electricity to be generated that ran to the spark plugs.

The first really major improvement in cars was a change in the ignition system. The wet-cell battery became the source of electrical power, and an electric generator was attached to the engine to keep the battery charged. Along with these two improvements came the self-starter. There was a dramatic decrease in the number of fractured wrists with the advent of the self-starter. The starter button was mounted on the floorboard just in front of the driver's seat. It was still necessary to use the choke, but the driver could start the car without leaving the seat. A major improvement was a special low gear for added power. The low gear was mounted in the center of the floorboard with a gearshift lever to the right of the driver. When the mud was quite deep and, in spite of full pressure on the foot pedal, the car was unable to move, the low gearshift lever was pulled and the lower gear ratio went into play. With the extra power the car moved forward.

A common joke was that a Ford came in any color desired—as long as it was black. No other color was available. Of course, when the rain fell, the color was changed from black to muddy brown. The wheels had wooden spokes, but, after traveling through the mud, they became solid disc wheels.

I could hardly wait until I was big enough to try my hand at driving. When I was about eight years old, Dad finally let me get behind the wheel. I had watched him drive and knew every movement that was required. It was not long before I could circle the block without any trouble at all. The adventure became a daily ritual. When Dad came home for lunch, he parked on the street in front of the house. I hurriedly ate my lunch, then ran out and climbed into the car, stepped on the starter, and away I'd go around the block. I was especially happy when the mud was extra deep and I could use the shift lever for extra low gear. After a time, I ventured around two blocks, then three, then four. When I was ten years old, a crisis required me to take my first trip uptown to Courthouse Square. A man working at our house was seriously cut by a piece of tin. He had a Model T Ford touring car but was in no condition to drive himself to Dad's office. Mom had not yet learned to drive, so I jumped in the man's Ford and drove him to the doctor. After the injury had been attended to, I drove him around the Courthouse Square and back home, wondering all the time why some of my friends weren't on the street to see me proudly driving a car.

Improvements continued to be made on the Model T. New models were added. Now you could purchase coupes and sedans. Side curtains were unnecessary since these models were glass enclosed, and the glass windows could be lowered and raised by a handy strap. The upholstery was cloth, a more comfortable improvement over the cold leather upholstery of the open cars. These models also were equipped with heaters, which, although inadequate, did lessen the chill. The heater consisted of a pipe that ran from the top of the manifold into the interior of the car through either an opening in the firewall below the dash or up through the floorboards. The heater opening had a shutter that could be opened and closed to control the heat flow. There were cases reported of passengers being overcome by carbon monoxide from exhaust fumes seeping in from the engine compartment through the heater tube.

The manufacturer added decoration to the sedans by installing a vase in a holder on each side of the interior next to the door. Flowers were placed in these vases.

Dad eventually traded for a coupe, and that purchase made traveling much easier for him. The roads also had been improved somewhat, so he did not require the services of a driver all the time. Danny was kept on standby, though.

One Sunday afternoon in summer Dad had to make a call in Dennison. I asked if I could go along and take my playmate Sylvia, who lived up the block on the next corner. Dad gave his approval so we got in and started for the country. We had to travel about six miles east on the National Road, then north about three miles—a big trip. The road north from the National Road was deep with dust, so we had to keep the windows up. Dad was wearing his Palm Beach pants (held up by suspenders), white shirt, and black bow tie topped by a straw sailor hat perched at a jaunty angle on his bald head. As always, he was smoking his cigar. We went merrily along to Dennison. We waited in the car while Dad attended his patient. Pretty soon we started home. The sun disappeared from view, and the sky became darker and darker until it was almost black. A storm was approaching. Dad drove faster and faster. Just as we started down a hill, the rain came down so hard that we could hardly see. There was no windshield wiper. What had been deep dust only minutes before was now greasy mud. The car slithered down the hill and across the bridge, and ahead was a hill that we had to climb as steep as the one we had just come down. Dad started up with all the speed he could get out of that machine, but as the grade steepened, the car slowed until he pushed on the left peddle (low gear). We went a few feet farther and stopped. The Model T had gone its limit. We started to roll back down the hill, and Dad applied the brake. We stopped rolling, but the car continued to slide. There was an embankment to the left. The car continued its slide, slowly slipping to the left. Finally, the left rear wheel, followed by the left front wheel, slipped over the edge of the embankment. Dad was gripping the steering wheel tightly, but there was nothing he could do. Over and over we rolled, finally coming to rest in a field below. The car was lying on its left side in the mud. Incredibly, there was no flying glass. Only one window was broken and that, fortunately, was on the right side of the car.

Everything was quiet for a few seconds. Then Dad, who was on the bottom, said, "Let's get out of here." I scrambled out of the broken window and pulled my playmate out. Then Dad's head appeared. He still had his cigar clamped between his teeth and his hat in place; only now one side of the brim had a huge chunk out of it, as if someone had taken a big bite. The rain was pouring down, and the water dripped off the end of Dad's soggy cigar and ran off the rim of his partially demolished hat. He grabbed us by the hand and started up the embankment, slipping and sliding. Finally we were on the road. The surface was like grease. After slipping and falling in the mess several times, we reached the crest of the hill. Just a few hundred feet ahead was a house. We three water-soaked, mud-covered victims sloshed up on the porch and knocked on the door. The door opened, and there stood a woman, obviously shocked by what she saw. She got us inside where it was warm, brought out towels, and we proceeded to dry ourselves.

Dad called my playmate's father and told him of our predicament. It wasn't long until he arrived. The woman gave us each a blanket to ward off chill as we rode back to town. A wrecker was sent out later to retrieve the Model T from the bottom of the embankment. Fortunately, little damage was done other than the broken window and some dents and scrapes.

Mom laundered the blankets, and a few days later, Dad had to make another trip out that way. He took the blankets along to return to the kind lady. He stopped in front of the house and carried the blankets to the door. He knocked several times, and finally the door opened just wide enough so that the woman could peek out. "I am returning the blankets you so kindly provided this past Sunday, and I want to thank you again for your help," said Dad. The woman merely grunted, reached out and grabbed the blankets, and slammed the door in Dad's face. Dad walked slowly back to the car and stood scratching his head, trying to figure out the dramatic change in the woman's behavior. As he was getting into the car, he suddenly picked up a peculiar odor. He had his answer. He rapidly drove back to town and called Jim Turner, the sheriff. "I think there is something you should check out," he said. He then gave Jim the directions to the house from which he had just returned.

The sheriff and his deputy, armed with a search warrant, immediately paid the woman a visit. Going to the barn back of the house, they went in—and there stood a still surrounded by barrels of mash and bottles of the finished product. It was a moonshine operation. The woman and her husband were lodged in jail. The still, mash, and whiskey were confiscated. The old adage "One good turn deserves another" got a little twisted. Or did it? Dad might have saved their lives. They might have been killed by an exploding still or by drinking some of their concoction.

3

Machines

I WAS AND STILL AM fascinated by trains. I could stand for hours by a railroad track or at the station watching trains go by, pulled by the big engines spewing smoke from their stacks and hissing steam from their cylinders, whistles blowing, bells ringing. I remember the engineer dressed in overalls, with a bandanna around his neck, wearing a tall cap with a visor and goggles to keep out the cinders, leaning far out the window staring down the track, his left hand on the throttle lever. If he turned to give me a sideways glance and waved his hand, I was in seventh heaven. The drive rods moving back and forth, the wheels whirling until the spokes became but a blur—this was speed, this was action, this was the true poetry of motion. The slow "chug chug" as the train started—becoming louder, sharper, and closer together until it was a continuous roar—was the sound accompaniment to the nostalgic scene.

Going to Terre Haute was a big event. Most everyone rode the train. Traveling by car in the early 1920s was still an adventure, and with frequent flat tires and slow speed, the train was still the best mode of transportation. Mr. Rector was called. The jitney appeared at the door, and we rode to the Vandalia (Pennsylvania Railroad) station on the northern outskirts of town. There were frequent trains, but our favorite was the "Bob," a local. The "Bob" stopped at McKeen, Dennison, Farrington, and West Terre Haute (Mackville) before arriving at Union Station in Terre Haute.

Union Station was a huge building with towers and turrets. It seemed as if there was always a train in the station, so there was plenty for a little boy who was "train crazy" to see. The Pennsylvania ran east and west, and the Chicago and Eastern Illinois ran north and south. The tracks crossed at the northeast edge of the station. There were trains from St. Louis, New York, Washington, Chicago, Florida, Georgia, Alabama, Tennessee, and Kentucky. There were long trains with Pullman cars and diners, with observation cars in the rear. There were shorter trains with day coaches, baggage cars, and mail cars. It was fun to watch the trains, imagining their points of departure and speculating as to their destinations. Amid the passenger train traffic was an occasional freight, which slipped past on an outside track while passengers were being loaded and unloaded at the platform. The smell of the smoke and warm lubricating oil from the engine was like perfume. In the station, waiting to "run the next lap," the locomotive appeared almost alive as it stood there panting (the sound of air pumps), steam gently hissing from open valve ports. It seemed as if it were resting and catching its breath after a fast run. Covering the tracks at the station was the huge barn-like roof constituting the train shed, which protected passengers going to and from the station and the trains.

It was always necessary to drag me away from the track. I was reminded that we had not come to watch trains but rather to do some shopping in the city. Leaving the train, we went into the station with its enormous waiting room and ceiling three stories high and out the opposite door. Here we boarded a streetcar for the ride down to the Terre Haute business district. After finishing our shopping, we boarded a streetcar downtown and rode back to the door of Union Station. After only a short wait, we caught the train back to Marshall. The faithful driver of the jitney was waiting, and before long we were back home.

Occasionally, Mom and I visited the families of her sisters in Henry County, east of Indianapolis. That trip involved a much greater distance but was still accomplished without any inconvenience. We usually took a train in early evening. After boarding and stowing our luggage in the rack above the seat, we always rode awhile before going to the diner. Eating in the diner was a really big event. We were greeted by the steward in his black cutaway coat, white shirt, and bow tie. With great dignity he seated us at a table covered with snowy linen. The napkins were perched in front of each of us like white tents. The table service was heavy silver. The sugar bowl and creamer were heavy silver plate, and at the side of the table was a glass decanter filled with pure spring water. The menu was filled with good things to eat. Mom wrote our selection on the order slip that the steward had provided. A smiling waiter, dressed in starched white jacket and apron, read the order and checked for accuracy, then took it to the galley at the end of the car.

Some of the finest meals I have ever eaten were prepared in dining cars. Those chefs had to be masters of their art to prepare such delicious meals in cramped quarters while traveling at high speed, swaying and bouncing along the tracks. The waiters also were skilled, carrying huge trays of dishes down the narrow, swaying aisle without spilling a drop of food. The waiter cleared the table and brought us each a finger bowl containing warm water. After dangling my fingers in the water and putting some on my lips and around my mouth, I dried my fingers and patted my mouth with the napkin and started back to my seat in the coach. I stopped at the beautiful sideboard at the end of the car, to pick up a few mints from a bowl and a quill toothpick from the toothpick holder. Dinner in the diner was truly fit for a king—the epitome of gracious living.

Arriving at Union Station in Indianapolis, we took a cab a few blocks to the interurban station. This was railroading of a different kind. The huge interurban station had about ten separate tracks spread across its width. Covering the tracks was a high-roofed train shed a block long. Inside was the big waiting room. A big blackboard was attached to a side wall near the door to the train shed. A man in the uniform of a trainman, the train caller, stood on a platform in front of the board. He had a booming voice. When each train was ready for departure, he called out the number and all of the stops to be made to its destination, ending with the track number and the exclamation "All aboard!" His voice echoed off the high ceiling of the waiting room.

Interurbans actually were overgrown streetcars. The motive power came from electric traction motors; current traveled down the trolley pole from an overhead wire above the track. A wheel on the end of the pole, which extended above the car, ran along the underneath side of the wire. These cars were longer and heavier than streetcars and had toilet facilities. The motorman or driver was in a compartment at the front. A broad window extended across the front of the car. In front of the motorman was a console with a handle fastened in a horizontal position on top. At the end of the handle was a round knob. The motorman grasped the knob and turned the handle either clockwise or counterclockwise. He increased or decreased the speed according to the direction he turned the handle. The other control mounted on top of the console was the air brake lever. Behind the motorman was the baggage compartment, and behind that area were the smoking and nonsmoking compartments, respectively. A sliding door separated the passenger compartment from the vestibule in the rear. The entire train crew consisted of the motorman and the conductor.

The interurban wound its way slowly along the city streetcar tracks through downtown Indianapolis and finally on to East Washington Street and away from downtown. As the traffic became less congested, the motorman increased his speed. Once in the country, with the right-of-way parallel to the highway, the motorman turned his controller to near top speed; a speed of sixty miles per hour was not uncommon. A high-pitched whistle (not like the deep chime whistles of the steam engines) warned of the train's advance at the many grade crossings. Approaching a village or town, the train drastically reduced speed and tiptoed sedately down the middle of the main street. Once again, outside of town and back along the side of the highway, the train accelerated quickly. Arriving at Dunreith, we greeted my aunt and uncle, who took us home in the Buick or Model T. In the 1920s the trip from Marshall took a little more than four hours. With modern interstate highways and powerful automobiles, it takes about three hours. Unfortunately, it is impossible to have dinner in the diner or experience the joy of riding a train through the countryside completely relaxed and not burdened with traffic worries—this is progress?

Visiting Grandpa and Grandma Trice meant taking the train to southern Indiana. Usually we left Marshall on the early morning train, arriving in Terre Haute just in time to board the Milwaukee Railroad train that ran from Terre Haute to Seymour. The train consisted of a combination baggage and mail car plus two coaches pulled by a small steam locomotive. The wooden cars were painted a beautiful shade of orange. They were open platform cars, which meant that passage from one coach to the other was accomplished in the open, not a particularly safe venture when the train was in motion. Bouncing and swaying along with smoke and cinders clouding one's vision made slipping and falling between the cars a real possibility.

The designer of the seats must have determined the angle of the back to the seat cushion to be that which would cause maximum discomfort to the passenger because a trip of more than a few miles usually resulted in a backache for the occupant. The standard color of the mohair upholstery was green. The woodwork of the seats and the car interior was mahogany. Illumination at night was furnished by ornate brass kerosene lights hung from the ceiling over the aisle. Heating was provided by a potbellied stove at the end of each car. The windows were raised in summer to provide a bit of fresh air forced in by the movement of the train. There were no screens in the windows, so fine cinders, along with an occasional puff of smoke from the engine, added to passenger discomfort. The train poked along at an average speed of thirty miles an hour, if the engineer was able to maintain his schedule. Unscheduled stops along the way to pick up a passenger at some road crossing resulted in delays that made a timetable worthless.

Those delays meant nothing to a little boy who loved trains. There was so much to see: the loading and unloading of express baggage and mail; the conductor in his dark blue uniform with brass buttons, watch in hand, standing on the station platform and giving the "highball" signal (hand waved high above his head in daytime and a lantern swung in a high arc at night) to the engineer. On the train, the conductor communicated with the engineer by pulling on the signal cord, which was suspended over the center of the aisle and ran the length of each car. Three long pulls, for example, ordered the engineer to stop the train. The cord produced a high-pitched hissing sound like escaping steam or air under pressure. What the engineer heard was a high-pitched whistle.

Bouncing along on the train, listening to the engineer blowing the whistle at crossings, looking out the window at the ever-changing scenes—a meadow with grazing cows barely heeding the passage of the train; a creek bubbling along over the rocks; the cool, dark woods with birds of many colors flitting among the branches—and up ahead the sharp rhythmic sounds of the exhaust from the engine, slow on the upgrades and accelerating on the downgrades, until it became almost a continuous roar. This was the excitement of riding the train.

The high point of the trip was the tunnel. As the train approached, the lamps in the cars were turned on by the conductor and the windows were closed tightly. Then we were plunged into total darkness. The roar of the sounds of the train reverberating from the rock walls of the tunnel was deafening. The air became heavy with the acrid smell of burning coal. It was frightening but exciting. Then suddenly we burst out of the mouth of the tunnel into bright sunlight.

THE TRAIN PAUSED just a moment at the little station at Heltonville, engine panting and puffing. We would be greeted by Grandma and Grandpa Trice, then suddenly the conductor would shout "All aboard!" and the train huffed off again around the curve and over the bridge, finally disappearing. Grandpa and Grandma were waiting with old Dandy hitched to the buggy. Grandma was dressed in her Sunday best with a high frilly collar, her snow-white hair parted in the middle and brought around to a knot at the rear of her head, topped by a proper hat held in place by a long hat pin. Grandpa was in his good suit and wearing his black broad-brimmed hat. Having stuffed our suitcase into the hinged box at the rear, we squeezed into the buggy. The three adults sat on the seat, and I perched on a box on the floor or on Grandma's lap.

Before going out to the farm, we might stop at the general store, and of course Grandpa saw to it that I got a sack of peppermint candies. Leaving town, we forded the creek, stopping in midstream so Dandy could have a drink, then turned up the road toward home. Along the road I remember a thicket of trees, their branches arching above the road, almost forming a tunnel. In the summertime I dreaded that part of the trip because a horde of horseflies was always lying in wait. Grandpa took an extra firm grip on the lines because he knew a horse being bitten by a bunch of horseflies would start to run. A steady pull back on the reins set the bit tight in the horse's mouth and held him in check. Pulling off the road, we went down the lane across a creek and up to the farm.

Grandpa got out and tied the horse to the white picket fence that encircled the house. To me, the Trice house was a mansion, the finest place in the world. Actually, the house was a log cabin that had been covered with weatherboarding. Inside there were three rooms on the lower floor—a kitchen that also served as the dining room, a living room, and a bedroom. An enclosed back porch served as a pantry. A steep stairway provided access to another—a loft with little square windows set under the eaves that served as the guest room. It contained a dresser, a chair, and big old-fashioned bed with the usual feather mattress. Sleeping on this mattress was true luxury. In the wintertime, with snow deep on the ground and the wind whistling under the eaves, I knew no harm could come to me as I snuggled deep into the feathers with several of Grandma's quilts spread in layers over me.

Under a corner of the back side of the house was a cellar. On a hot summer day, I knew I could find bins of potatoes and other vegetables gathered from the garden. Near the back door was the well. Fresh, cool water was pumped from the well to fill the water bucket, which stood on a table inside the kitchen door, the dipper hanging nearby. Water also was carried to fill the reservoir at the end of the big old wood cookstove. The reservoir provided an ample supply of hot water for washing dishes.

Toilet facilities were in the old outhouse—a "two-holer"—behind the woodshed. Next to the woodshed was a smokehouse, which held smoked hams hanging from the rafters. One end of the smokehouse was used for weekly washing. A large tub and washboard were the utensils used.

Down below the house was a creek that bubbled out from under a ledge of rock. The water was ice-cold, and Grandpa constructed a little house over the spring, which was used for refrigeration. Crocks of milk and butter and other perishables were sunk down into the cold water. Before each meal, a trip was made to that natural refrigerator to get the items necessary. The barn and granary were up the hill from the house. Grandpa's horses were the finest, and he was very particular about their care.

Grandpa decided that at the age of five I should learn to milk cows. Timidly, I followed him into the barn. With a great deal of trepidation, I was coaxed into sitting on a three-legged stool at the rear of a big monster of a cow. I was shown how to push my bowed head into Bossy's right flank and how to grasp the teats. Grandpa fastened his hand over mine and, gently grasping my fingers, squeezed and gently pulled down. To my surprise, a stream of milk came shooting out and into the pail set between my feet. It wasn't long until I got the knack, and soon I was delivering regular streams of milk into the bucket. The old cow, munching her cud, would occasionally turn her head with a big inquisitive eye staring straight at me. Finally, she would turn back to get another mouthful of hay as if she were thinking, "What is that little thing doing to me? Ah well, thus is life."

I loved to roam the woods and along the creek, looking for anything of interest. There was always a tree to climb, a squirrel to watch, or a bird's distinctive song to identify—a killdeer or a bobwhite, a crow with its harsh cackle or a whippoorwill calling in the cool of the evening with the sun's last rays viewed over the hill to the west.

Grandma always baked the pies she knew I liked, and at the end of the day in the coziness of the kitchen, we sat down to a bountiful table. The flickering kerosene light produced a contrast of light and shadows about the room. Grandpa, head bowed, said grace in his singsong voice. After the table was cleared and the dishes washed and dried, the table was set for the next meal. A wire frame was put in place on the table and a clean cloth spread over it so that it looked like a white tent. In the summer when flies were abundant, large strips of "tangle foot" flypaper were hung from the ceiling. Grandpa had made "shoo flies" by tacking strips of paper to the end of a stick. One of my favorite chores was removing flies from the house. With a "shoo fly" in each hand, I walked through the house, waving them like magic wands as I herded flies toward the door. Standing at the door, Grandma would open it at the right instant, and I would furiously wave the flies out the door.

After supper, we would sit a spell in the living room. If I had forgotten to do so earlier in the day, I would drop bits of fishfood wafer into the goldfish bowl. Grandpa might take a nap while the women talked, or maybe Grandma would play the old pump organ. Then it was time for bed because, as Grandpa said, morning comes early.

Wheat harvest was always exciting. For this special job, Grandpa was assisted by a threshing ring, men and women who formed a loosely knit cooperative, going from one farm to another at harvest.

The wheat was cut by the binder. Grandpa hitched the big team to the machine and slowly cut a round next to the fence. After the first round, he could go faster. The big reel, rotating round and round, gently pushed the stalks of wheat, heavily laden with grain, back against the cutter bar, the sickle going back and forth at a blinding rate of speed. The cut stalks fell back and lined up in a neat row and were carried by the binder's canvas belt through the part of the machine that bunched and tied them into neat bundles. The bundles were kicked out onto the ground. It was my job to gather the bundles and place them standing up in a circle to form a shock. Two or three bundles were laid on top as a cap.

After a few days, the big steam threshing machine pulled in up near the barn. Fired by wood, the thresher seemed the next best thing to a train. The engineer—or traction man, as he was called—was the most important person in the whole operation as far as I was concerned. The separator was hooked on behind the engine, which had huge wide wheels with steel cleats, providing the traction to pull the heavy machine. After getting the separator set and level, the steam engine was moved on a distance and turned so that it was directly in line with the separator. A huge belt was unrolled and one end hooked over the big pulley on the separator. Then the belt was twisted, and the other end was hooked over the big pulley on the traction engine. The traction engine was backed up slowly until the belt was tight. The engine wheels were blocked and threshing could begin. Bundle wagons were already in the field, and the men could begin picking up bundles from the shocks. These wagons were flatbeds with long posts and cross planks set at each end.

The man riding the wagon and driving the team was the loader. Pitchers walked on either side of the wagons, pitching bundles from the shock to the loader, who—with great dexterity—wielded his fork to lay the bundles neatly row by row on the flatbed, building his load till it reached the top of the end posts. Driving up to the side of the whirring separator, the loader then pitched the bundles into the open mouth of the monster. Mechanical fingers snatched the bundles and stowed them back into the innards, where knives forced them apart into the separator and across a series of screens where the grain was separated from the straw and chaff by shaking. The clean grain was ejected through a chute into the grain wagon on the other side of the separator. The grain wagon was a leakproof boxbed. The straw and chaff were blown out a long stack at the far end. The separator man stood on top of the machine and manipulated the stack back and forth, up and down, by means of a long rope attached to the end of the pipe. Glistening golden straw was the residue. The water boy busily carried ice-cold water from the well to the men in the field and on the wagons. He usually rode a pony, with stone jugs strapped to the horn of his saddle. The water wagon for the engine had a pump mounted on the tank to pump water from the creek or from a pond. A length of hose attached to the tank was thrown into the water, and the man standing on top of the tank worked a long handle back and forth to operate the pump. If the engineer was urgently in need of water, he blew the whistle. Then the tank man would come at a gallop because he knew a dry boiler meant an explosion. The engineer stoked his boiler, watched the water glass closely, and at the same time kept a close eye on the separator. Wet grain or too large a feed could choke the separator, so he had to be ready to open the throttle quickly for more power if necessary.

At noon everything shut down.

The dust and dirt of the morning's work was washed off in the yard under the shade trees. Rows of wash pans, buckets of water, bars of soap, and lots of big towels were set out. While the men were in the fields, the women had been preparing a big lunch—beef, pork, chicken, mashed potatoes and gravy, sweet potatoes, corn, green beans, lima beans, fresh tomatoes, slaw, pickles, onions, cucumbers, radishes, hot homemade rolls, sweet country butter, apple pie, peach pie, chocolate pie, butterscotch pie, lemon pie, mincemeat pie, coconut pie, pumpkin pie, blueberry pie, rhubarb pie, blackberry pie, raspberry pie, angel food and devil's food cake, coffee, iced tea, and cold milk. After eating, the men would rest a few minutes, then go back to work.

OCCASIONALLY, we followed a different route to my grandparents' farm. Taking the evening train from Marshall, we traveled east to Limesdale, just south of Greencastle. This was the junction where the Monon Railroad, from the north, crossed the Pennsylvania. Riding the evening train out of Marshall provided the opportunity for having dinner in the diner. Usually we had a short wait in the station at Limesdale before boarding the southbound train to Bedford. The right-of-way for the Monon Railroad ran down the main street of every town we passed. We were able to ride right by store windows and watch people as they shopped. Arriving in Bedford, we were met by an aunt and uncle waiting to take us out to the farm in their automobile.

The winter trip to Heltonville was quite different. The landscape was transformed from fields of green grass and growing crops to a winter wonderland blanketed in pristine snow. The bubbling creeks of summer were ice covered in winter. The dark green forest gave way to a vast array of naked trees stretching their arms to the sky. The earth was sleeping under the warm blanket of snow, resting and regaining its strength in preparation for the spring and summer ahead, when the new crops would be drawing life from its bosom. Everywhere was peace and quiet.

Mabel Wray lived across the road. I imagined her as a big sister. Behind Mabel's house was a large hill with a very long slope. In winter, with a thick layer of snow covering the slope, conditions were just right for sledding. Mabel had a homemade sled with wooden runners covered by strap iron. These metal straps were shined until they glistened. Pulling the sled to the top of the slope, she sat me to the front, then giving a push, hopped on behind. Down, down the slope we streaked, snow flying out from under the edges of the runners. At last the sled came to a stop, then back up the hill we went, pulling the sled behind us.

In the spring the sap would start to run in the big grove of maple trees up the hill behind the barn. Grandpa had a maple sugar camp. Located near the middle of the grove was the building that housed the big evaporation pans. The long low building had a gently sloping roof, with openings under the eaves to vent the steam from the evaporating sugar water. Inside was the long furnace built of bricks. The evaporation pan was set on top of the brick furnace. Heat was furnished by wood, which was stuffed in from one end of the furnace. The smoke was emitted through the brick chimney at the other end of the building. With me tagging along, Grandpa made the rounds through the grove, tapping each tree. Using an auger, he bored a hole through the bark into the heart of the tree. After removing the auger, he inserted a wooden spigot into the hole. Slowly, drop by drop, the maple sap would start flowing. He then hung a bucket on the spigot and moved on to the next tree. After all the trees were tapped, he made numerous trips back to check the buckets. As the buckets began to fill, he hitched the team to a wooden sled that had a big tank mounted on top. We then moved slowly through the grove, emptying each bucket into the tank and hanging it back on the spigot. Back to the sugar house we went, the sugar water sloshing in the tank. A huge fire was started in the furnace, and the water was transferred from the tank to the evaporating pan. As the fire became hotter, the water began to simmer, finally coming to a vigorous boil. The sweet-smelling steam rising from the boiling sugar water filled the building and finally found its way to the outside through the opening beneath the eaves. As the boiling continued, the light golden liquid in the pan became thicker. Grandpa always tested the consistency by taking a dipperful outside and pouring a little into the last remaining snow on the ground; the cold snow would quickly solidify the liquid, forming a little cake of maple sugar. This was the part I always anticipated. No candy was any tastier than a freshly made cake of maple sugar. When the syrup was just the right consistency, it was dipped into tin pails. At the end of the season, Grandpa had many gallons of the delicious syrup. An ample supply was kept for home consumption, but there was always a large surplus, which he hauled to the village and sold to storekeepers.

Many, many years later, I found myself in the vicinity of the old farm. I made a side trip from the main highway to seek out the old place. Grandpa and Grandma had been gone many years, and Mom was in her eighties. Driving into the village of Heltonville, I thought the place seemed as if nothing had changed. There was the old railroad station. Up the track a ways was the elevator where Grandpa sold his wheat. I could almost see the big wagon, pulled by a handsome team, and guided by a sturdy man with a big moustache and wearing a big straw hat. Sitting high on the seat next to him was a barefoot boy in overalls with a happy grin on his face. The general store was still there, and driving out to the farm still required fording the creek. Coming to the farm, I was gratified to see the house and barn still standing. They looked tired, as if they were worn out by the years of service. Looking down the lane and across the creek, I could envision Grandma in her long dress, her white hair shining in the sunlight, bent over with a feeding bottle in her hand. A barefoot boy stood beside her, helping to hold the bottle. A little lamb, its neck outstretched and head upturned, was vigorously drinking the warm milk through the nipple. Looking up the hill toward the barn, I could see Grandpa in his felt boots, tramping through the snow to the barn for the evening chores. The same little boy, wearing boots and bundled up in heavy pants and coat, mittens and heavy cap with flaps pulled down to protect his ears, was almost running to keep up.

I tried to tell my own children about these happy times, but what I had in my memory just didn't seem to come out right. The house seemed to have gotten smaller. The paint had long since peeled away from the weatherboarding. Some of the boards had fallen away, showing the old logs beneath. No longer was it the shining castle.

MARK JONES and Howard Hoff, husbands of my mother's sisters, were two of my favorite uncles. Both were farmers and lived in Henry County, Indiana, near the place were Mom was born. Mom and I visited them at least twice a year, at Christmas and during the summer. I believe the reason I liked my uncles so much was that they treated me as an equal even though I was just a little boy.

In the 1920s, Uncle Mark had a gasoline-powered baler with which he did custom baling for neighbors. A team of horses pulled the baler from one farm to another. After the baler was placed next to a stack of hay or straw, the horses were unhitched and driven away. A wooden platform, which was hinged, was unfolded and extended out from the side of the baler. The platform was near the middle of the baler next to the opening of the press. A steel rod attached to the gears moved back and forth, pushing the piston and compressing the straw or hay inside the press. A man stood on the platform with a pitchfork and pushed the straw or hay into the opening in the press. He was called the feeder. An arm with a broad plunger on the end moved up and down in rhythm with the piston pushing the stalks down to the bottom of the press. The arm was synchronized with the piston.

After the piston was drawn back by the rod, the arm with the plunger on the end snapped down into the press, and as the piston advanced, the arm rose, drawing the plunger back out of the hole. A slotted gate holding a thick wooden block was located next to the platform. When the bale in the press chamber was of the right size, the man on the platform swung the gate over the press opening, dropping the block into the chamber and thus separating the bale from the next. The feeder had only a split second to drop the block right at the instant when the piston was back and the arm was still up. If his timing was off, the blade struck the block or the piston caught it before it was fully in place. This would demolish the block and jam the machine. Usually two or three men were required to pitch the hay or straw down from the stack to the platform. The dirtiest and hottest job was that of "poking wires." The bales were held together by baling wire. The wire came in big bundles nearly eight or nine feet long. Each wire had a loop on one end. Grooves were cut across each block—one near the top and the other near the bottom of each side. The man who poked the wire crouched beneath the table and, as a block came through, he pushed a wire through the top and bottom grooves. As the bale was pushed along by the piston, he waited until the other block appeared, then he pushed the other end of the wire through the upper and lower grooves in the next block.

A man on the other side of the baler tied the bales by running the straight end of the wire through the loop at the other end and twisting the end around the wire several times. Occasionally, the man who was poking the wires made a mistake and pushed the wire through the groove on the wrong side of the block, tying the block to the bale. After the bale was tied, it was pushed along by the bales behind until it dropped out at the far end of the baler. The finished bales were either stacked up or loaded onto a wagon and hauled to the barn to be stored in the haymow. Baling was a hot, dirty job that required strong muscles.

When I was about eleven years old, I asked Uncle Mark if I could help with the baling. He initiated me with one of the hardest jobs—forking the straw down to the table. I hadn't done any hard work all summer, and my hands were tender. He handed me a huge straw fork with a handle so big I could hardly get my hands around it. I had no gloves, and it wasn't long till my hands were blistered. I kept doggedly at the job even though the heat was almost unbearable and my hands felt as if they were holding two red-hot coals. Finally, noon came and it was time to eat. Every muscle in my body ached and the palm of each hand was a solid blister, but I wouldn't complain. After dinner I climbed back up on the stack and resumed my job. I thought the day would never end. Taking a bath in the tub in the kitchen that night was a luxury. It felt so good to get the grime and sweat washed off and to be relieved of the scratching from pieces of straw and wheat barbs inside my shirt and pants. The blisters had burst and my hands were raw. Uncle Mark decided I had been properly initiated, so he let me rest for several days until my hands had healed.

When I went back to work, Uncle Mark taught me how to poke wires. This was an easier job, but it was much hotter and dirtier working beneath the table. No air could get beneath the table since it was butted up against the stack. I was surrounded on three sides by straw and the baler itself was in front of me. I just had a small opening through the mound of straw to get into my cubicle. To add to my misery, straw and chaff filtered down through the cracks in the table. I had no time to rest because the bales were moving through the baler at a rapid rate and I was continuously poking wires. The only thought that went through my mind was how good it would feel to peel off my clothes and jump into a cool creek. For my day's work I was paid a dollar.

I helped Uncle Howard with the wheat harvest. His elderly father and I followed the binder, picking up the bundles and placing them in shocks. Howard's dad, an old German, believed that a boy should know everything about farming. Occasionally a bundle would come from the binder without a tie. He went to great lengths to teach me how to make a tie by taking a number of stalks of wheat in each hand and with an intricate maneuver looping them together to form a tie. He gathered up the rest of the loose stalks and formed a bundle. Then, with a quick motion of his hands, he whipped the improvised tie around the bundle and tied it. It took me quite a while to master the craft, but he was most patient. After a while, I could tie the bundle almost as well as he could. One day we were shocking wheat near the road, and a friend of the old man came by, driving a spring wagon. He stopped, and we went over to the fence to visit with him. In the back of the wagon was a basket of sugar pears. The man in the wagon asked me if I would like some pears. I was hot, thirsty, and hungry so I couldn't wait to get my hands on some of the sweet, juicy fruit. I had just finished eating two or three when I had a sudden pain in my stomach. I had to go to the bathroom, and I was a long way from the house or barn. I had three fences to climb before getting to the barn. Going over the last fence, I realized it was too late. If only there had been one less fence. I had learned the hard way that sugar pears were an excellent, fast-acting laxative.

Uncle Howard loved to hunt. He had excellent pedigreed bird dogs for tracking quail. During the winter months he also ran a trap line, collecting muskrat and coon pelts and an occasional weasel or mink pelt. The sale of these skins provided extra income.

I always looked forward to visiting my relatives at Christmas. There usually was a deep blanket of snow on the ground, which was just what was needed to track rabbits. Uncle Mark had a lever-action, repeating Winchester .22-calibre rifle that hung on brackets above the door in the kitchen. He taught me how to handle and shoot the rifle. We started out across the field in the morning, tramping through snow so deep that it almost came above the tops of our boots. Suddenly, a rabbit jumped from under a tuft of grass and started across the field, taking great leaps to elude the hunters. Uncle Mark brought his shotgun up and sighted along the barrel, and the dead rabbit went flying, end over end. Our agreement was that he would shoot all running rabbits and I would shoot all sitting ones. At the end of the day we skinned all of our bag and hung out the carcasses to freeze. The next day we took them to the local grocery store and were paid thirty-five cents for each one.

When I was twelve years old, I talked Dad into buying me a shotgun—the first and only gun I ever owned. It was a Stevens Single Shot 20-gauge. I could hardly wait until Christmas vacation and our trip to Uncle Mark's. The first day we went out to hunt I proudly carried my new shotgun under my arm. I had never tried to shoot a rabbit on the run, but we spied one hopping through a field. "He's yours," said Uncle Mark. I nervously brought the gun up and sighted along the barrel, trying to keep the swiftly moving rabbit in sight. Suddenly, the rabbit turned and headed straight down the corn row toward me. I waited and waited and finally pulled the trigger. Bang! went the gun, and I started yelling, "I got him! I got him!" "Yeah," answered Uncle Mark, "and you damned near shot off your foot." It was then I looked down to see the remains of the rabbit torn completely apart lying about two feet in front of me.

Hog butchering was done when the weather was very cold, so it was not unusual for Uncle Mark to butcher when we were there for Christmas vacation. Operations were started early in the morning. The big iron kettle was brought out to the barn lot and hung from a tripod. Nearby, posts were set in the ground and a big beam fastened to the top of the posts. Huge hooks were hung from the beam. The hog carcasses were hung on the hooks. Aunt Edith, with Mom helping her, got out the grinder and lard presses and gave them a good washing and scalding. The butchering knives were sharpened. Wood and kindling were laid under the kettle, which had been filled with water. The fire was started, and soon the flames were licking the underside of the kettle. It was not long before a cloud of steam was rising into the cold air from the boiling water.

The hogs to be butchered were brought out and killed with a shot from the .22-calibre rifle. Each hog was hauled up and hung to a hook by a hind leg. The belly was slit open from front to rear with a sharp butcher knife. The entrails were removed and the intestines carefully put aside to be used later. Scalding water from the kettle was poured over the carcass and brushes and scrapers used to remove the bristles from the hide. More water was used to thoroughly clean the inside of the carcass. After being scalded and cleaned, the carcass was laid on a table and cut up. The head was severed and saved to be used for head cheese. The feet were saved to be pickled. The hams and shoulders were carefully cut out, as were the slabs of side meat that were later to become bacon. The tenderloins and chops and spareribs were removed skillfully. The fat was carved out and placed in a big tub. The intestines were thoroughly cleaned and scalded again and again. (They were later used as sausage casing.)

Aunt Edith and Mom busily cut the scraps into chunks and ran them through the grinder. Then they mixed the ground meat with salt, pepper, and a touch of sage. After the ground sausage was prepared, the casing was fastened to a round pipe at the bottom of the sausage stuffer. The ground sausage in the stuffer was forced out through the pipe into the casing by turning a crank. Some of the sausage was kept aside to be used to make sausage cakes, which were stored outside in a big crock. Some sausage, in cakes or casing, was cold-packed in glass jars. The fat was heated on the stove in the house and placed in the lard press. A good part of the fat on the hog lay just under the skin, so when the fat was cut away, the skin came with it. As a result, the chunks of partially melted fat contained skin. When the plunger was screwed down, the white lard was forced out an opening at the bottom and collected in crocks. The lard was later used for frying meat and making pastries and cakes. The residue left in the press consisted mainly of the skin from the hog. Exposed to heat and pressure, it formed a crisp crunchy cake, called cracklings, which were very tasty. The hams, shoulders, and side meat were smoked, the side meat becoming bacon in the process.

After the butchering was completed, the cleanup began. All the utensils were washed and put away. The posts and beam were taken down, and the kettle and tripod were put back in the smokehouse to await the next butchering.

Grandpa and Grandma moved to a smaller farm of about twenty acres in Henry County, just two miles east of Uncle Mark and Aunt Edith. Once in a while I walked the two miles from the one place to the other. Grandpa still drove his horse and buggy, and we spent many pleasant hours together riding to town, either to Straughn to the south or New Lisbon to the north. Grandpa always had a small paper sack of peppermint lozenges in his pocket, and we shared them as we drove along. Grandpa was too old to do any farming, but he still had a few cows and raised a few acres of corn. After milking was done, I got the job of turning the cream separator. The milk came out one spout and the cream out the other.

Today Interstate Highway 70 runs across the north side of the old farm. When traveling that way, I always slow down, and the memories come rushing back. I look off to the south to see if Grandpa and Grandma might be standing in the barn lot waving. They're not. As I pass the interchange, my dream vanishes.

I WAS IN THE EIGHTH GRADE when we had the first death in the family. Uncle Tom, Mom's only brother, hadn't been well for some time, but still his death came as a terrible shock. Mom had gone over to be with him when his condition worsened, and she was with him when he died. She had left me at home with Dad, and I was very lonesome. I had never been separated from Mom before, and the house wasn't the same without her. Dad and I went to Uncle Clarence's for our meals. Finally, the message came that Uncle Tom was gone. Death was something I had never considered before, and I didn't quite know how to accept it. Dad and I drove over the day before the funeral. This was entirely different from our earlier trips. Dad and I didn't talk much, and when we arrived, we were greeted by solemn faces. There was no laughter, no jokes. Gloom was everywhere. What had to be done around the house was done quietly.

The day of the funeral, we went to the church and filed past the open casket. I had never seen a dead person. Uncle Tom looked to me as if he had just stretched out to sleep. His face looked so peaceful, and there was a hint of a smile on his lips. I sat quietly in the seat, listening to the sobbing and watching my mother and her sisters dab away the tears with their handkerchiefs. I wanted to run away, but I knew I couldn't. Finally, the organist began to play a solemn hymn, and the preacher got up and read from the Bible. He read verses selected to comfort the bereaved. He then said some nice things about Uncle Tom and gave a prayer. After that, the choir sang "Perfect Day." For a long time after that, I wanted to cry whenever I heard that song because it brought back memories of Uncle Tom lying so still in his casket.

A few months later, Grandma Trice took a severe cold. Again Mom left. The bad cold went on to pneumonia. The doctor came every day, but nothing he did could help Grandma and, finally, she died. I just couldn't believe that in less than one year two of my closest relatives had died. I guess I had always thought that the good times we had would always be. Suddenly I realized that death is inevitable. Never again would the white-haired lady bake my favorite pie. Never again would she let me feed the pet lamb. Never again would she play the organ for me. Never again would I sit on her lap while she read to me, and never again would she tuck me into bed.

OF ALL THE CHANGES machines made in our lives, none were more pervasive than those brought about by the automobile. In 1919 a major construction project was started to rebuild the National Road. The time had come to modernize the road—to transform it from a dirt and gravel road to a modern concrete-surfaced highway, with steel and reinforced concrete structures replacing the old wooden covered bridges. Although some curves were straightened and the grades over the hills were reduced somewhat, in general, the new road followed the original Cumberland Trail. The Hayworth Construction Company was the general contractor for the segment through the Marshall area. Large steam shovels were used in moving dirt from the cuts through the hills, but all of the grading was done by horse-drawn slip scrapers and graders. Gangs of men with picks and shovels put the finishing touches to the roadbed. Horse-drawn dump wagons carried the dirt from the steam shovels to the grade. Steam-powered piledrivers drove the piling for the bridge footings.

Progress toward completion of the project moved at a snail's pace because of the time consumed in getting the dirt dug and moved and the amount of hard work required to finish the roadbed. Farm families living along the National Road were inconvenienced for several years.

The construction company had an ingenious way of getting materials to the construction site. Narrow-gauge railroad tracks were laid from the supply yard near the Big Four Railroad. The tracks were in sections (similar to model railroad tracks). The sections could be easily taken up and moved. Tracks ran parallel to the highway roadbed. Small locomotives powered by gasoline engines pulled strings of small four-wheeled cars. Cement, sand, gravel, and steel reinforcing rods were carried on these little trains. Passing tracks were placed at strategic points along the way. Loaded trains moving to the construction site met and passed the empty trains returning to the supply yard. The sand and cement brought by the supply train were placed in the mixer. After being thoroughly mixed with water, the wet concrete was dumped on the roadbed. Men in rubber boots moved the concrete around, spreading it evenly over the surface and finally leveling it off with a machine set on wheels that ran on top of the concrete forms. The smooth finish was performed by hand. The road was opened to traffic about 1922. We now had a highway that could be traveled without any discomfort or inconvenience. No more big holes, no more dust in summer, no more mud in wet weather. We had moved into the twentieth century. The old double-lane covered bridge over Big Creek below Livingston was replaced by a modern steel truss bridge.

Soon after, State Route 1, which ran north and south through Marshall, was paved. We now had modern highways running east to Terre Haute and Indianapolis, west to St. Louis, north to Chicago, and south to Kentucky.

MY FATHER'S BROTHER, Uncle Earl, and Aunt Molly lived in Prairie Creek, Indiana, also known at that time as Middletown. Uncle Earl opened his office for the practice of medicine in Prairie Creek shortly after finishing his service in the Navy Medical Corps in World War I. He had met Molly Tucker, a true southern belle, while he was in port at Tampa, Florida. Aunt Molly never lost her soft southern accent.

Prairie Creek was a very small village, yet it boasted two doctors. Uncle Earl had his office in a building next to the house. Our families visited each other fairly frequently. The shortest route between Marshall and Prairie Creek was by way of Darwin on the Wabash River. We crossed the river on a ferry barge that held two cars or wagons. The ferry was attached to a cable that ran across the river from shore to shore. The cable prevented the barge from floating down river. A little flat-bottomed motorboat powered by an old automobile engine was chained to the side of the barge and furnished the motive power. At each end of the barge was a hinged gangplank that was lowered onto the riverbank when the boat was tied to the post on shore. After the vehicles and people were loaded, the gangplank was raised and the ferry pulled across to the other shore. After the boat was tied to the post on the shore, the gangplank at the opposite end was lowered and the cars driven off. The road leading down the riverbank was very steep and sometimes slippery so the driver had to be alert to stopping quickly before running off the end into the river.

On one occasion, Dad was driving Mom's Auburn Beauty Six, which had a gearshift and footfeed. I was lying on the floor between the seats half asleep when I heard Mom scream. I popped up just in time to see the car stop at the very edge of the gangplank on the far end. Dad had hit the accelerator instead of the brake, and we almost went into the river.

One day in 1927 Uncle Earl got in touch with Dad to tell him he had an urgent matter to discuss. The urgent matter was the news that an oil well was being drilled near Prairie Creek and the prospects looked very good. The company putting down the well had leased only a very small number of acres. If the well was a good producer, whoever held the leases for the surrounding area would be in a good position to make some money. Because he was in practice in Prairie Creek, Uncle Earl was well acquainted with all of the landowners in the area.

A group of five men joined together to finance the leasing operation. Included in the group were Dad, Uncle Clarence (the dentist), and Uncle Earl. It wasn't long until Uncle Earl had obtained a solid block of leases adjacent to the new well. Finally, oil pay sand was reached, and the nitroglycerin charge was placed. When the charge was set off, oil spurted high in the air. They had hit a gusher! There was a mad rush to lease the surrounding land to put down more wells, but Dad and his group held all the leases. They were "in the driver's seat," and they didn't know what to do. They knew nothing about the oil business. Pressure was being applied from the big oil companies to sell or to sign an agreement to let them develop the field. There were so many offers and counteroffers that they became more and more confused. Was a bird in the hand worth two in the bush or should they gamble for higher stakes? One of the best offers was for outright sales of the leases to a major oil company, with each man in the group receiving seventy-five thousand dollars.

In the meantime, though, bickering started between the three brothers. Dad wanted to sell, Uncle Earl wasn't quite sure, but Uncle Clarence wanted to make a deal with one of the companies. The company vice president lived in Marshall. Up until that time he had never had so much as the time of day for any of the brothers, but suddenly he became quite friendly with Uncle Clarence. The flattery Uncle Clarence received from the man went to his head. His new friend made frequent trips to the dental office to discuss each proposition. Finally, Uncle Clarence was persuaded to sign all leases over to the company, which would develop the field and share royalties with the three brothers and their two partners. After several stormy sessions, Uncle Clarence wore down the resistance of the others, and they agreed to sign over the leases. They soon realized, however, that there was nothing in the agreement that stated the company had to develop the field. It was a matter of time before the leases would run out; then the company would release the land for itself. The five men had been outsmarted by a professional.

The three brothers had a falling out over the deal. Dad and Uncle Earl blamed Uncle Clarence for talking them into the agreement with the oil company. Neither Dad nor Uncle Earl would have anything to do with their brother. The feud posed a serious problem because Dad and Uncle Clarence held their office building in partnership. It had always been their custom to come back to the office after supper to visit with their friends or see an occasional patient. In the summertime, they would line up chairs on the curb in front of the office. Uncle Clarence was always a member of that group, but after the feud began, he boycotted the meetings. He still came back at night, but he brought his own chair down from his upstairs waiting room, dragging the chair down the steps, bouncing the legs down step by step. He placed his chair next to the south corner of the building, ignoring the rest of the group along the curb, chewing and spitting his tobacco until 9:00 P.M., when he got up and dragged his chair back up the stairs, locked the office, and walked home, never speaking to anyone. The only communication between the two brothers was through their receptionists.

Aunt Alta and my cousin Frank visited us as if nothing had happened. Dad was friendly to them, and Uncle Clarence was friendly to Mom and me, but we never mentioned the feud between the two brothers. That went on for more than two years, until word was received that Uncle Henry had died. The three remaining brothers went to the funeral together and the feud was over.

4

A Boy's Education

THE LONG PERIODS of illness in my early childhood left me a little skinny boy who didn't have much endurance. I was the smallest boy in my class. I decided early on that my chief ambition was to take part in all sports and to get tough. I developed my own physical fitness program. I wanted a bicycle, but bicycles were expensive. One day I saw a small one, just the right size for me, standing in a rack outside the bicycle shop on Main Street. It was not new, but it had new tires and a fresh coat of red paint. The price was ten dollars. I ran to Dad's office immediately and started my sales pitch. Very reluctantly, he went with me to take a look. It took a lot of selling on my part, but finally I wore down his resistance.

"We'll take it," he said to the salesman. "Providing you put a new set of grips on the handlebars." This was quickly agreed to, and the sale was made. I'm sure no boy was ever any happier than I was with my new possession. I wheeled it all the way home because I didn't know how to ride.

Learning to ride was all trial and error. I went out to the big yard on the north side of our house, my idea being that falling on the grass was much better than piling up on hard concrete. After uncountable spills with the accompanying bruises and scrapes, I finally became quite adept at taking the turns at high speed, leaning way over to the side as in the pictures I had seen. One day I was riding leisurely down the street, both hands off the handlebar, reading a library book. There was a crash, and I found myself sitting on the seat of my pants on the pavement. I had hit a parked car.

As a part of my physical fitness program, I was out of bed at 5:00 or 6:00 A.M. summer and winter. Getting astride my bicycle, I took off down the highway south of town. I rode a mile or two into the country and back to town, ready for a big breakfast.

I was interested in all sports. After school Mom wanted me home, so our north yard became a baseball diamond in the spring and summer, a football gridiron in the early fall, and a basketball court in the late fall. All my buddies gathered there. After the baseball season was over, the base lines were erased, the bases removed, and the field was prepared for football. Miniature goalposts were erected at the east and west boundaries of the yard. Goal lines were the sidewalk at each end. Lime dust was sprinkled along to mark the side boundaries and the yard markers. When basketball season arrived, the goalposts were taken down and a basketball goal made from a barrel hoop was fastened to one of the maple trees. With all the feet running over the turf, soon the ground was bare, but Mom said she could grow grass after I had grown up. Dad was kept busy replacing broken windows, the result of an errant baseball or football.

Before school and at recess, we played ball in the school yard. The playground was not large and the surface was covered by cinders, so it was not particularly suitable for contact sports; nevertheless, we played tackle football. Even though I was the smallest boy in my class, I was determined to give it all I had. I gave no quarter and expected none.

When I was in the fourth grade, I played catcher on the baseball team. The pitcher probably weighed 150 pounds, and I weighed about 50 pounds. He had a terrific fast ball. The ball came blazing across the plate and, crouched down dangerously close to the hitter, I caught the ball in the pocket of my mitt. The force of the ball striking my outstretched glove would almost knock me down, but I seldom dropped one. For hours after a game my catching hand would sting and ache, but this was part of my plan. I was getting tough.

I gained the respect of classmates who were older and much better developed. They never excluded me from their games. I was one of the team because they knew I had guts. I was proud to be one of the group and was proud that I came from the so-called Bloody Third Ward, where the tough guys lived.

The section of town north of Main Street was where the elite lived; we common folks lived south of Main Street. A fierce rivalry developed between the north and the south. Any time a rival group crossed Main Street (no man's land) into the other's territory, a fight would develop. It was almost like the Civil War being fought over again. (I can proudly report that to my knowledge our side was never defeated.)

My cousin Frank lived on the north side, and when we had a family gathering, the first order of business was a fight between the two of us. As we grew older, we agreed to an uneasy truce so that we occasionally could visit each other without a fight. One memorable engagement involved BB guns—of course, the parents knew nothing about this or we would have had our bottoms blistered for even thinking of doing such a dangerous thing.

I never liked school, from my first day at the South Side School until I finished college years later. I could hardly wait for summer vacation. The last day of classes was the high point of the year. No studying, no teacher, no homework, and no tests for three months.

Of course, I wasn't as free as I thought I was because Mom still ran the house and issued the orders from time to time, giving me chores to do before I could do what I wanted to do. Chores still were better than school, however.

The creeks and woods around Marshall held a special fascination for me. I loved to roam alongside a creek, looking down into the water, and hoping to catch sight of a fish. I always had a fishline with a hook attached rolled up in my pocket. Before leaving home, I had dug some worms and had them snugly encased in an old Prince Albert tobacco tin full of dirt. This I carried in my hip pocket. Finding a likely looking fishing spot, I would cut a small branch from a tree with my pocket knife, attach the line to this makeshift pole, bait the hook, and toss it in the water. Sticking the butt of the pole in the soft dirt on the creek bank, I would lie back on the grass under a tree and wait for a bite. Lying on my back under a tree I could watch the white fluffy clouds floating across the blue sky. I relished the sight of birds wheeling and turning, a hawk gracefully soaring, swallows darting about, chasing flying insects, crows with their raucous cry. Perhaps a couple of squirrels would dart across the grass from one tree to another—rapidly climbing the trunk of the tree, running out along a branch, and then nimbly jumping to a lower limb while flipping their fluffy tails like fans in the breeze. This was the proper setting, all quiet and peaceful, for a boy to contemplate life and daydream about the future. Suddenly a jerk on the line would bring me to my feet. A bite. Grabbing the pole, I would bring a flopping fish out of the water. (If the fish weren't biting, it was all the better because fishing was just an excuse for being there. The real joy came from just being lazy, lying on the grass away from it all. Dreaming.)

Later on I acquired a fishing rod and reel. Sometimes I walked the two miles from town out to Blizzard's Ford on Big Creek. This creek crossing was about a quarter of a mile off the highway, down a dusty country road that crossed the creek through shallow water that flowed across a limestone formation and spilled over a little falls. Just above the crossing was a curve in the creek, and the water was deep enough for swimming. A sand and gravel beach ran down to the edge of the creek. This was a popular spot for swimming, and every Sunday afternoon a crowd could be found swimming or lying on the sand getting a suntan. Below the ford, around a bend, was another deep spot in the creek that we used as a swimming hole. The "Apple Trees," as this secluded spot was known, was off-limits to the girls. Only the boys swam here (without bathing suits). A long, thick grapevine served as a rope. Grasping the grapevine a boy could run down the bank, swing out over the creek, let go, and come flying down to splash into the water.

I had not learned to swim. Mom told me that getting in deep water was dangerous, and she didn't want me to take any chances because I might drown. I decided that as long as I was along the creek fishing, I had better learn to swim—and, besides, it looked like fun. Keeping it a secret from her, I took off with my rod and reel and as soon as I got to the creek, shed my clothes and jumped in the water. Starting in shallow water, I began to teach myself the art of swimming. As I became more proficient, I worked on out into the deeper water. By trial and error, I soon became a fair swimmer.

One day Mom took me to the creek and left me. After the car disappeared down the road, I laid my rod and reel on the bank down by the "Apple Trees," shucked off my clothes, and jumped in. I was having a great time swimming around in the deep water when suddenly I saw movement behind some bushes. The bushes parted, and there stood Mom. I was caught! "How long have you been swimming like this?" she asked. "Oh, for a long time," I answered. "Well, you're a good swimmer. Oh, I just came back to give you some money to get something to eat when you get hungry," she said, her voice almost a sigh of relief. She actually wanted me to be a good swimmer but didn't want me to go near the water. I had solved her problem in my own way.

Now I could go swimming with the rest without being afraid of a reprimand. I got a bathing suit and joined the others at the beach at Blizzard's Ford on Sunday afternoon. We sometimes worked along the edge of the creek, swimming very slowly and quietly, then diving down under the edge of the bank to catch a fish with our hands.

We didn't have a Boy Scout troop, but the Methodist minister, the Reverend Howard Leach, a short, heavyset man, loved boys and the outdoors. A wooden shack across the creek near Blizzard's Ford was used as a campsite. One fall when school was out for a couple of days, the minister arranged a camping trip at this shack. We all went out in his Model T. When we got to Blizzard's Ford, we found the creek had risen. We started across, and the car stalled in the middle of the creek. Our leader did not hesitate. Fully clothed, he climbed out into the swiftly running creek and carried each of us with our camping equipment to dry land. We made a fire, dried off, and enjoyed a big supper. We went happily to bed.

In the spring we headed into the woods to dig sassafras root. The roots were cut into short lengths and allowed to dry. After they were dried, a piece of the root was steeped in boiling water to make sassafras tea, supposedly a superb spring tonic to rejuvenate the body. I thought it tasted terrible but always took part in this spring ritual.

In the fall the woods furnished a bountiful supply of walnuts, hickory nuts, and hazelnuts. We reaped the harvest, bringing home gunnysacks full of these wonderful products of nature. Each day we went to school with our pockets stuffed full of nuts, and at recess there was a large group of boys lined up on the sidewalk cracking nuts by stomping on them with the heel of a shoe. A penknife or a nail was used to pick the nuts from the shell.

The official beginning of summer in Marshall was "Decoration Day," now known as Memorial Day. Decoration Day was a solemn occasion. The women of the town gathered the choicest peonies the day before and brought them to the firehouse, where they were eventually arranged in bouquets for the graves of veterans.

At 10:00 A.M., people gathered at the Courthouse Square. Veterans of the Spanish-American War and World War I were dressed in their old uniforms. Survivors of the Civil War were dressed in civilian clothes, but many wore campaign hats and medals. The City Band was assembled and, as the signal was given, stepped off smartly in rhythm to the beat of the drums. The old men of the Civil War, those who could stand the march, followed directly behind, their heads erect, eyes looking straight ahead, no doubt reliving memories of the victories and defeats of the War Between the States. Those who were too feeble rode in cars directly behind their marching comrades. Many of these men had long white beards. Next in line were the Spanish-American War veterans, followed closely by the veterans of World War I.

All the way to the Catholic Cemetery in the southwest part of town they marched. The band occasionally broke into a rousing march. Arriving at the cemetery, we all became quiet, and there was only the singing of the birds. Suitable remarks made by one of our leading citizens were followed by a prayer from the priest; then the firing squad fired three volleys over the grave of a departed comrade. There was a moment of quiet; then taps was played. As the last notes faded away, another trumpeter, who had gone to a distant corner of the cemetery, softly repeated taps as an echo. The parade re-formed and returned to the Courthouse Square. In the afternoon the ceremony was repeated at Marshall Cemetery. Again there would be an oration, a prayer, the firing squad, and taps.

The march back to town was almost an endurance contest. Because the day was usually hot, all the Civil War veterans and many of the Spanish-American War veterans chose to ride back. But this little boy, who was the smallest member of the band and had to carry and play his drum, stuck it out to the end. As the leader gave the order, "Dismissed," I ran directly to the Candy Kitchen to get that Coke I'd been dreaming of all afternoon.

The day before the first of May was spent gathering flowers: violets, Johnny-jump-ups, Dutchman's-breeches, lilacs, and lilies of the valley. That night Mom got out the scraps of wallpaper she had saved, and we made May baskets. Some were cone-shaped; others were square boxes with handles pasted on. Early the next day (May Day) before school or later in the evening, the baskets were filled with flowers and delivered around the neighborhood. Baskets were hung on doorknobs or placed in mailboxes. A knock on the door or ringing of the doorbell, and then the sound of little feet could be heard running down the walk. We generally hid behind a tree to watch neighbors open the door with smiles on their faces when they saw the baskets.

Every kid at one time or another wanted to have a lemonade stand, and I was no exception. But my ambition went further than setting up a table in the front yard for a day and selling lemonade to my friends at a penny a glass. I wanted a permanent business. I was about ten years old at the time, and when I approached my dad with the idea, he looked at me as if he thought I had lost all reason. I used my best salesmanship on him, and he reluctantly agreed to have a small building constructed in the corner of the front yard.

My folks really must have loved me to put up with such a thing. The building measured about eight by ten feet. A counter ran across the front. Screen wire extended from the counter up to the roof. A small door was placed at the middle of the counter to pass candy, ice cream cones, and pop through to the customer. At night, when I closed up shop for the day, I swung down a large hinged door and locked it from the inside. An ice cream cooler and a pop cooler were furnished free of charge by Mr. Rademaker, the ice cream and pop distributor. I carried a full line of candy bars and penny candy. A sign was erected out in front between the sidewalk and the street, and I was in business.

I was surprised by the immediate success of my venture. Sixth Street was also Illinois Highway 1 and carried a considerable amount of traffic. People traveling through our town on hot summer days saw my sign and stopped to get a drink or an ice cream cone. Soon I began to have requests for sandwiches, so I branched out into that business too. I began early in the morning and stayed open until the sun went down. When things got busy or when I had to leave, Mom helped. There were many children in the neighborhood, and my stand was a popular gathering place. Sales were brisk all summer long. The family who lived across the street to the north had five or six young ones who seemed to have an endless supply of money. The big day, though, was when their father, who was divorced from their mother, paid his monthly visit to the children. He had oil interests so he had plenty of money. He usually arrived about 6:00 A.M. in his red Buick touring car. As soon as he got out of the car, he started handing out the money to all of his children. The youngest, Donny, would immediately run across the street and ring our doorbell. I'd crawl out of bed and go to the door. There would be Donny, his pants halfway down to his knees, barefooted, with a dirty face, his hands full of money, wanting me to open up so he could spend it. I'd get my clothes on, go out, and unlock the stand, and Donny, a grin on his face, would be loaded down with goodies, and I'd have the money. Before the day was over, I had many visits from the others until they ran out of money.

South Side School was a block down the street. During the spring and fall, I opened up a half hour before school and caught the school traffic. Just before the last bell rang, I closed up and ran to school. At noon and after school I again did a brisk business. After two years I went out of business, the stand was dismantled, and the front yard returned to its original state. I had proved to myself that I could run a profitable business even at that early age. I had a nice bank account as proof.

DURING THE SUMMER MONTHS, Mom and I frequently went with Dad when he made a call in the country. We had too little time to spend together at home so these trips gave us the opportunity to be together, even if only for a short time. One evening we accompanied him on a call west of town. Driving home, we came in on West Main Street. Turning the corner onto Fifth Street, we saw a crowd standing in front of Dad's and Uncle Clarence's office. Dad sped to the building and worked his way through the crowd. The waiting room was full of people talking excitedly about a bank robber. In the examining room was a man stretched out on the table unconscious, with blood streaming from a hole in his head. It was obvious he was dying. "What happened?" asked Dad.

The state's attorney and the sheriff told him the story: A bank had been robbed in a town some seventy miles south of Marshall, and the bandits escaped. One of them was reported to have boarded a coal train heading north on the Big Four Railroad. The authorities called Marshall and asked the sheriff to stop and search the train. The man who was on the train was supposed to be carrying a small bottle of nitroglycerin. The sheriff and the state's attorney went to the railroad station and waited. As the train approached, the station agent set the signal to stop it. The state's attorney went down one side of the train, and the sheriff the other side. About halfway down the length of the train the state's attorney saw some movement between two of the cars.

It was getting dark and he couldn't be sure, so he cautiously approached the train. Suddenly a man stood upright with a gun in one hand and a small bottle in the other.

His gun drawn, the state's attorney shouted, "Put up your hands and come down." Instead of complying, the man fired a shot, widely missing his target, and jumped from the train, still carrying the gun and the small bottle. "Halt, or I'll shoot," yelled the state's attorney, but the man kept running. The one shot fired by the state's attorney hit the bandit squarely in the head, and he fell and rolled over. The bottle was retrieved gingerly, and, when examined later, was found to contain water. The station agent called Dad's office and Uncle Clarence, who was sitting out front visiting with his friends, answered the phone. When he found out what had happened, he jumped in his Sayer's Six touring car and went roaring to the depot. The bandit was loaded into the backseat and rushed back to the office. (He bled all over the backseat of the car, and Uncle Clarence was never able to remove the blood stains from the leather upholstery.) In those days there were no ambulances and no quick way to get a patient to a hospital. Since the patient was going to die very soon anyway, Dad applied a dressing to his head, and dispatched him to the county jail, where he died a few hours later.

FOR SEVERAL YEARS, with the help of a specialist, Dad held a one-day surgery clinic to remove the tonsils and adenoids of all the children and adults who "needed their tonsils out." Plans were made well in advance. Volunteers served as nurses, orderlies, and clerks for record keeping. The assembly line method was used. Each patient was brought into the surgery by an orderly. The ether mask was placed over the face, and the anesthetic administered. Quickly the surgery was performed, and the patient was removed to the back room to recover from the anesthetic. There was much blood and vomitus, but the efficient volunteers kept everything cleaned up and the patients as comfortable as they could be under the circumstances. After the patients were well awake and the bleeding was controlled, they were bundled up and taken home. As many as fifteen or twenty operations were performed in one day, and to my knowledge there was never a fatality or serious complication.

WHEN DAD decided to install central heating in our home, the basement had to be enlarged so that the furnace could be set up. There also had to be a large bin for coal storage, so the small cellar under the kitchen was extended under the rest of the house. This was a major undertaking. One wall of the existing basement was knocked down with sledgehammers, and the dirt was excavated under the rest of the house after the floor sills were jacked up. All of the dirt was dug out by pick and shovel and hauled outside by wheelbarrow. One of the best men with a pick and shovel was Raymond Vick, better known as "Esau." Raymond detested his nickname, and we boys loved to tease him by yelling, "Esau." We always stayed at a distance when we teased him because we knew he would start after us in a rage waving his shovel.

Abe Clouse did the concrete work. He was my hero, primarily because he always took time to talk to me and explain what he was doing. He was very patient and kind, and he always had a grin on his face. He seemed to enjoy every minute of his work. He wasn't handsome; in fact, when he grinned, he showed a gap in his front teeth where there were two missing. He had a very large family to support and didn't make much money, but he was proud and managed to support them all without any outside help. He didn't have a concrete mixer but mixed all of the concrete by hand. I loved to sit and watch him as he measured out the ingredients. So many shovels of gravel, so many of sand, and so many sacks of cement. He placed the sand, gravel, and cement in a big long mound, then started deftly turning over the pile with his shovel, working from one end to the other. This he did two or three times until the whole thing was thoroughly mixed. Then he made a long deep trench in the top of the pile. He poured water into the trench until it was full; then he folded in the sides of the trench with his shovel and again turned the whole thing from end to end. Occasionally, more water was needed to make the right consistency. After the concrete was thoroughly mixed, he shoveled it into his wheelbarrow and wheeled it up a ramp to the top of the forms. After dumping the concrete into the forms, he used a long-handled tool to push it into place so that the forms filled uniformly. He explained what he was doing step by step, giving the reasons why it was done just that way. I received a complete education in the craft of concrete construction from Old Abe.

The highlight of the whole operation was when Abe handed me a shovel and let me try my hand at turning concrete. I was so much an admirer of Abe that I asked my dad if I couldn't have two of my teeth pulled so that I could look "just like Abe." Abe liked people, and he enjoyed life to its fullest, even though he had to struggle to support his family. His one and only hobby was playing the fiddle at dances. He loved his fiddle and, after a long hard day working with concrete, he walked sometimes several miles—he had no car—to play at a dance. One night, while at a dance east of town, he got into an argument with another man. It was not a serious argument, and Abe thought nothing about it. After the dance he started home, his heart light, humming and singing as he walked along carrying his fiddle.

Just as he was crossing the railroad tracks, however, a man jumped out of the darkness, pulled a gun, and shot Abe, killing him instantly. My hero had been murdered. This was my first experience with violence, and I suddenly realized that the world was not all kindness and love. People could be cruel and did do terrible things to one another.

SOME OF MY fondest memories are of visiting the home of Grandpa Mitchell, who married Emma after the death of my beloved grandmother. Emma became one of the family instantly. She loved to have us come to her house on South Eighth Street, and I could always be sure of finding a plentiful supply of fresh-baked cookies.

Grandpa had quite a few cronies around town who, like himself, were veterans of the Civil War. They spent many hours sitting on the curb under the shade of the trees in the courthouse yard, their canes in their hands or at their sides, reliving the past. All the major battles of the war were fought and refought many times by these comrades in arms. When he wasn't sitting with his friends on the Courthouse Square, Grandpa could be found sitting in his favorite chair in the waiting room of Dad's office. He loved to visit with patients and never let anyone forget that these were his two successful sons, Roscoe and Clarence, the doctor and the dentist. Promptly at mealtime, he got up and went stepping down the street, cane in hand, on the way home for one of Emma's delicious meals.

As he grew older, Grandpa visited the office less frequently. He sat around the house and dozed. His mind became hazy about recent events, and at times he became confused, but when it came to the war, his memory was crystal clear. My cousin Frank and I visited him often. Grandpa seemed to brighten up when we arrived. Sitting in his rocking chair on the front porch with us sitting on the front steps, he would launch into a story about the Civil War. He seemed to never tire of reliving the history of the war.

His favorite story concerned the time he escaped from the Confederates. It seems he became separated from his cavalry unit. He was riding his horse through the trees, the enemy close on his trail. They opened fire, but by guiding his horse in and out between the trees, he outmaneuvered them and the shots went wide. Suddenly he found himself on a high bluff overlooking the Chickamauga River. Without hesitation, he jumped his horse off the high bluff into the deep, swiftly flowing river. Sliding out of the saddle, he grabbed the horse by the tail. Almost completely submerged, with just his face out of the water, he held tight to the tail of the horse. Its powerful legs moving rhythmically through the water, the horse pulled Grandpa to the far bank of the river. Half drowned, he pulled himself up on the bank. He lay quietly on the ground in a clump of bushes for quite a while. Looking back across the river, he saw the enemy finally turn their horses and ride away. They assumed he had drowned. Everything seemed peaceful, and there was no sign of the enemy. Finally, he mounted his horse and rode off through the trees, keeping a sharp lookout for enemy soldiers. It wasn't long until he came on some of his comrades. He was safe.

At the time, we didn't realize what a rare privilege it was to hear from the lips of this old soldier his own account of the battles of the Civil War, which we would later read in history books. I think that I had almost a direct link through Grandpa to the great President Lincoln. Finally in 1924, Grandpa died in his sleep. The old warrior had fought his final battle and lay down to rest.

AS MUCH AS I loved all my father's family, I dreaded the Mitchell-Blackman reunion, held at Harrisburg, which was the high point of the year for Dad. The weather was always hot, and the place we held the reunion was undoubtedly the hottest spot that could be found.

The location was on the grounds of the old one-room school most of the family had attended. The sun beat down unmercifully, and never even the slightest breeze stirred the leaves. Most of the people were total strangers to me, and I couldn't care less about getting acquainted with my distant relatives. Dad, however, planned for weeks in advance of the big day. He always insisted on leaving early in the morning (3:00 A.M.) for the 120-mile trip. We formed a caravan with Uncle Earl and Aunt Molly and their two children from Prairie Creek and Uncle Clarence and Aunt Alta and their two children. Heading south on Route 1, we never drove over thirty-five miles an hour, frequently stopping to add water to the radiator or to check the tires. The children slept most of the way. At Harrisburg we stopped at the home of Uncle Malin and Aunt Laura. Uncle Malin was a merchant policeman, a special officer hired by the merchants to keep an eye on their buildings at night. We would be joined by Uncle Henry, who was a deputy sheriff. The men would line up their chairs on the front porch, chewing tobacco or smoking cigars. We boys sat on the steps listening to all the talk, especially the stories about outlaws and bandits.

In those days, Harrisburg had quite a reputation for violence. There was a great deal of union unrest among the miners. Almost every man you saw was either carrying a gun under his arm or a revolver in a holster at his hip. Bootlegging whiskey was a way of life for many people. Harrisburg had two major gangs, the Birgers and the Sheltons, who controlled the flow of illicit whiskey.

These rival gangs operated out in the open and were engaged in a continuous feud. They had a well-organized, well-disciplined group of outlaws. Armored cars roamed up and down the roads. Whenever a rival group encountered the other, a gunfight broke out. Shotguns, rifles, pistols, and even machine guns were used. Cousin Lucian Blackman and his wife and another couple were once caught in a car during a blistering crossfire between the two gangs. Law enforcement agencies simply couldn't control the violence, so it was left to the gangs to try to kill each other off. The Birger Gang had its headquarters in a roadhouse called Shady Rest. One dark night the Sheltons resorted to aerial warfare. A couple of the Sheltons flew over Shady Rest at low altitude and dropped a dynamite bomb. The bombardier was an amateur. His aim was poor, and the bomb exploded harmlessly wide of the mark.

In the midst of one of these discussions, Dad recalled one of his childhood buddies from the farm. "Is old Charlie still around or is he dead?" he asked. "No, he isn't dead. He lives down in 'Shanty Town,'" said Uncle Malin. "I'd sure like to see him," Dad said. "Could we drive down there?" "Sure can," said Uncle Malin.

So we all piled in one of the cars—Dad, Uncle Henry, Uncle Malin, a cousin, and I. We drove down a dusty road through "Shanty Town," built years earlier by the mining company. Every house was the same size and the same architecture. When we arrived, it looked like Charlie's house was deserted. Dad knocked once, again, and then a third time. The door opened a crack, and the deeply wrinkled face of an old woman peered suspiciously out through the crack. "Where's Charlie?" Dad asked. "He ain't to home," was the answer. "Well, Aunt Sadie, I haven't seen you for a long, long time," said Dad. "Don't you know me? This is Roscoe, Roscoe Mitchell."

With that the door flew open wide, and the scowl on the old woman's face turned quickly to a wide grin. She threw her outstretched arms around Dad and yelled, "Charlie, Charlie, here's Roscoe." Charlie came cautiously out of the back of the house and, when he saw Dad, a wide grin spread across his face. He shook Dad's hand and said, "What a long time it's been since we've seen each other."

After a good visit we said good-by and went back to the car. As we drove away, Dad scratched his head and said, "Why did Aunt Sadie act so strange when she opened the door, and why did she lie about Charlie?" Uncle Henry chuckled and said, "Roscoe, you don't know about these things. You see, there is a lot of bootlegging going on around here, and Charlie is one of the biggest in the business. When they saw us drive up, they knew I was a deputy sheriff and Malin was a merchant policeman. You were the stranger, and they figured you were a federal agent and that we were going to raid the place."

Throughout my high school years, I continued to do everything I could to improve my physical fitness, but I was still small. I weighed only one hundred pounds when I entered high school but was determined I was going to participate in sports. Although Dad and Mom told me I was too small to play football, they never forbade me from doing so, and on the first day of practice I went down to the gym to get my name on the list. The coach took one look at me and shook his head, but he saw the determined look on my face and told the manager to fit me up with a uniform.

The budget for the Marshall High School athletic program was very modest. The same uniforms were used year in and year out, patched and repatched. Only a very small amount of new equipment was purchased each year. The varsity team was outfitted fairly well, but the "scrubs" got the leftovers. I was a scrub, in fact, the lowest scrub. My pants and jersey were too big, the pads didn't fit—the straps were worn and the elastic had lost its stretch. The shoes were badly worn, and the cleats were almost worn off. But I was happy, for I was going to play high school football. I didn't realize what was in store for me. Conditioning came first. I did pushups until I was exhausted, then jumping jacks, knee bends, wind sprints, and numerous laps around the field. This went on for an hour or more in the hot sun. I was like a man lost in the desert miles from a water hole. I was dying of thirst when I saw what I knew was a mirage over at the side of the field, but it wasn't. It was a real live boy with a bucket of cool water and a dipper, but the coach was right there watching.

"Wash out your mouth and spit it out, then just two gulps of water, no more so you don't get cramps" were his instructions.

Every muscle and bone ached in my body and I had yet to see a football. I began to wonder if I wanted to be a football player, but I remembered this was what I had been striving for all my life—striving to build my body, to get tough. The next morning I could hardly get out of bed, but that afternoon I rested up and ran back out with the rest of the squad. After a few days, all the exercises and running became easier to do, and I could see that the coach's conditioning plan worked. We were getting in good shape to withstand the tackling and blocking of football without serious injury.

There was a lot of work to do in a short time before the first game of the season. Plays had to be learned, and we all had to function as a team. Each man had to learn his assignment for each play. We had to learn to block and tackle. With the first scrimmage, I found out what the word *scrub* really meant. The scrubs were the "cannon fodder." Our group was the opposition for the varsity team. We were the enemy. The experienced boys of the varsity delighted in cracking through the line, inflicting mayhem on the scrawny, inexperienced freshmen like me. I was determined to give my all. I learned how to carry the ball and sidestep an onrushing lineman. I learned to catch a pass even when my opponent was right on my heels threatening to knock my head off. I learned to block and tackle without any fear. I still was far from being a candidate for the first team, but I knew that someday, if I kept at it, I would be in the starting lineup—not this year, or even next year, but maybe in three years. I never felt better in my life, in spite of the scrapes and bruises and black eyes. I had a ravenous appetite, and even though I was dead tired when I came home to supper, Mom could hardly fill me up. I began putting on weight, but my muscles were firm and there wasn't an ounce of excess fat.

As soon as the football season was over, I went out for basketball. Again I was a scrub, wearing a hand-me-down uniform. I knew I would never be a star athlete but was happy to be a part of the team, even if it was a very small part. I had the respect of the others because I had no fear and was willing to take the hard knocks without complaining. The friendships I made with the others on the squad have lasted all my life.

MY FAVORITE SUBJECT was manual training. I liked working with my hands even though I wasn't particularly skilled. Harry Findley, a fat little man, was the teacher. He had the natural ability of getting the best from each student. He liked people and loved his job. He was most patient. He was a philosopher without realizing it. He always had some story to tell that illustrated what he was trying to teach much better than what was in the book. He never lost his temper, even when a student pulled a "bonehead" trick. He didn't confine his teaching to showing a student how to handle tools or design and make a piece of furniture. He went much further. His discussions ranged over a broader scope, teaching us how to cope with living in a complicated society.

I eventually enjoyed English and math. Writing stories and learning to use proper grammar became most interesting to me. Algebra wasn't the easiest thing to learn, but I was determined to master the subject. I liked math so well that I decided to take all the courses that were offered: plane geometry, solid geometry, and trigonometry.

Mr. Hornbrook taught solid geometry. I had never seen a teacher before, nor have I seen one since, who had the natural ability he had in handling a classroom full of students. He went about the business of teaching with an air of quiet authority. He never raised his voice, yet he maintained perfect discipline. He had the respect and love of every one of his students. I vividly remember one example of the way he corrected a student. Sitting in the classroom one day right after lunch, I became drowsy. I wasn't listening to anything he was saying.

My mind had drifted far away from the schoolroom. I began to doodle with my pencil on the broad arm of my chair. Noticing what I was doing, Mr. Hornbrook stopped talking, picked up a sheet of paper from his desk, ambled down the aisle toward me, and carefully slipped the sheet of paper under the pencil. This maneuver snapped me back from daydreaming, and I looked up at him with a sheepish grin on my face. "Now isn't that better?" he asked. "The marks look better on the paper than on the wood." Then he turned around and went back to the front of the room and resumed his lecture.

We had no career counseling. Students were required to have a certain number of credits to graduate from high school, but there was little effort made to help them in selecting subjects that would prepare them for any particular field. I had decided I wanted to go on to an engineering school, so I thought I should follow the usual high school curriculum, with special emphasis on mathematics and manual training. No one advised me to take chemistry and physics. Neither of these courses appealed to me so I didn't take them. I did take Latin, which I disliked very much, because someone told me I'd have to have a foreign language to get into college.

Mabel Nowlin was our Latin teacher, and she took her job seriously. Our class met right after lunch, which wasn't the ideal time for a student like me to attempt to concentrate on the subject. My seat was next to the window, and I'm afraid I spent too much time gazing out the window and daydreaming. One day when we arrived for class, we found the door locked. Miss Nowlin came up the stairs on the run. She was late. She gave the key to one of the girls to unlock the door while she went to the teachers' cloakroom to hang up her coat. After the door was opened, we filed in to our seats. I had just sat down when I had the idea to lock the teacher out. I got up, went over to the door, and snapped the lock, and went back to my seat to look out the window. Almost immediately, the door handle turned and there was a jerk, but the door wouldn't open. The same thing happened again, but the door wouldn't budge. Then Miss Nowlin started yelling, "Open the door! Open the door!" but no one moved. Then she started beating on the door with her fists. Still no one moved.

"If this door isn't opened at once, you are all going to suffer." The girl with the key got slowly on her feet and timidly opened the door, and Miss Nowlin almost fell into the room. She was furious. "Who locked me out?" she asked, glaring about the room. I continued to gaze out the window with an innocent look on my face. I just knew that that girl would squeal on me, but she didn't and all the others remained silent.

"Well, since you won't tell," she said, "I'm going to give you a test." She couldn't have done anything that would hurt me more. I wasn't ever ready to take a test, even when forewarned and prepared. After the test, we filed quietly out of the room, my classmates all glaring at me. I knew they would like to kill me. All afternoon my conscience hurt me. After school I asked my best friend if he would go with me to confess my crime and take my punishment. When we walked into the room, Miss Nowlin was sitting at her desk grading the papers.

Looking up, she smiled and asked, "What can I do for you, Boys?" Looking down toward my feet, I said, "I just wondered how I did on the test." She grinned and said, "You did fine. You had a perfect paper." After a slight pause, I asked, "Do you know who locked you out?" Immediately her grin turned to a deep scowl. I wanted to turn and run, but I was too far committed. "No," she said, "but I'd sure like to find out." Gulping hard, I said in a very small voice, "I did."

Suddenly she broke into a big laugh, got up from her desk, came over and put an arm around my shoulder, and said, "You know, I thought that was a good joke on me." She was still chuckling as we left the room, the cold sweat trickling down my face.

5

The Town of Marshall in the 1920s

GROWING UP in Marshall was a wonderful experience. There were so many things to do. Yesterday was a pleasant memory, today was full of excitement, and tomorrow was something to be anticipated eagerly. Life in Marshall proceeded at a very leisurely pace. We did not need a calendar to tell us when spring arrived. The approach of spring was heralded by the days becoming slightly warmer and the gradual disappearance of the last patches of snow. The V-formations of ducks and geese high in the sky headed northward. Standing and watching the V, which seemed to waver from side to side in an undulating motion, a small boy could wonder where they came from and where they were going. How did they know when to head north? How did these birds pick a leader to follow, and how did the leader know where to go?

The crocuses peeking out as if hesitant to enter the scene were followed by grass turning green. The first March wind brought out the kites. We made our own kites from slivers of sticks taken from the waste pile at the lumberyard. Old newspapers and flour-and-water paste were used to cover the kite frame; string saved from grocery packages was tied together until enough was obtained to make a line to get the kite high in the sky. Strips of cloth from Mom's rag drawer were knotted together to make the tail. It was necessary to run "like mad" into the wind to get the kite into the air, but faulty balancing— too long or too short—or a capricious gust of wind from the wrong direction far too often would cause the kite launch to end in disaster. There is nothing that would cause a boy to want to sit down and cry more than to see the results of his efforts dashed into a treetop or wrapped around a wire. Regardless of the uncertainties of having a successful flight, every boy built a kite. One successful launch erased the memory of previous disasters. The crowning glory was attained when one's kite was at the end of a string longer than any belonging to one's friends.

The next two events that took place almost at the same time in the spring were marble shooting and roller-skating. It seemed as if boys had the same built-in sensory system as birds. With no other communication between boys—no planning—every boy would be shooting marbles and skating almost on the same day. Every boy had his favorite "aggie shooter." "Cat eyes" were special; "claybies"— made from clay that was covered with glaze and baked—were the cheapies. The game of marbles had its own terminology, including "knucks" and "lag." A cloth sack with a drawstring at the top was the container for the marbles. The winner kept the marbles he won from his opponent, and the champ would own several hundred.

Sidewalks served as a skating rink. The favorite place to skate was around Courthouse Square. This was the beginning of girl-boy relationships, and the boys could associate with girls without being ostracized by their friends. Boys who were especially skilled could show off without being too obvious. Most skating was done at night, but almost as if by magic everyone was home by 9:00 P.M. We did not worry about being molested because there was no crime—people did not even lock their doors. Automobiles were not a problem because there were so few on the streets, and people drove little after dark. Roller-skating continued on through the summer months, but the peak period of this activity was in the spring.

Jonquils, tulips, and lilies of the valley would appear, and we knew that it was time for wildflowers. Purple violets, white violets, jacks-in-the-pulpit, "Dutchman's-britches"—all grew in profusion just outside of town and even in vacant lots in town. It seemed every child, both boys and girls, wanted to pick wildflowers. My favorite spot was just west of town.

After getting permission from our mothers, my friends Sylvia and Alice and I walked west on Cherry Street past the Catholic Cemetery, past the old brickyard pond—the home of the frogs that croaked nightly—over several fences and across the Buser farm to a woods on a hill. Below the hill were two creeks: one came in from the east, the other from the south. Just before reaching the Old Stone Arch Bridge spanned by the National Road, the two creeks joined to form one that passed on under the bridge. The trees were filled with birds of all kinds, each making his own brand of music. At times it seemed as if they joined together in one giant chorus. There were variations with one and then another performing a solo.

Other than the songs of the birds, it was quiet and peaceful. Spread out below was a veritable carpet of wildflowers of all varieties. We wandered over the hill and along the quiet creeks below. The water trickling merrily over the rocks made another kind of music. Occasionally, a minnow would dart out from under a submerged rock. All of these wonders of nature were here to enjoy and that we did. After exploring awhile, we got down to the business of picking flowers. We gathered huge bouquets to take home to our mothers. There were so many flowers that after we had finished picking our bouquets it did not seem as if a single bloom was missing. Today, some sixty-five years later, I live in a house that we built on that hill. The flowers still grow here. The two little creeks still meander along, finally joining together and flowing under the Old Stone Arch Bridge (now on the National Register of Historic Places). The trees are still here, somewhat larger than when I was a boy, and the birds still join in their chorus each day. The wonders of nature never cease.

Marshall, as I remember it in the 1920s, was a sleepy town. It was said that it was a retired farmers' town. People who lived there wanted things simple. Any industry looking for a location in Marshall met with strong opposition. There was no active chamber of commerce working to entice newcomers. The town was a nice quiet place where people could move at a leisurely pace. The air was clean—no factory smoke. There was no clanging machinery and no trucks or wagons rushing around. The economy was totally dependent upon the people living in town and the farmers from the surrounding countryside.

Because it served as the county seat, Marshall had a handsome courthouse square in the center of town. The main business district surrounded the square, spilling east and west onto Main Street and north and south onto Sixth Street.

On the north side of the square, on the corner of Sixth and Main, was Grabenheimer's. The elderly Grabenheimer had emigrated from Germany, traveling across the Atlantic as a steerage passenger. When he arrived in Marshall, the old man carried all his belongings in a pack on his back. He decided to make this little town his home. Traveling across the wilderness from the port of New York, Mr. Grabenheimer made his living as a peddler, selling his wares to people living in the towns and on farmsteads.

He opened a small dry goods store in Marshall. Before long his business had grown until a larger building was needed so he secured a corner site in the middle of town. Mr. Grabenheimer built a three-story building, the highest structure in town, at the choice location. He stocked his emporium with ready-to-wear clothing for ladies and gentlemen. He had a children's department and a complete line of shoes. Mr. Grabenheimer married and had a son, Ben, a daughter, Amelia, and an adopted son, Joe. None of his children married. They lived in a large house on North Sixth Street and operated the store for many years. The Grabenheimers amassed a considerable fortune, which they later invested in acquiring farms in Clark County.

Behind their backs, the Grabenheimer boys were called "Beans." The nickname originated as a result of a business venture that their father became involved in years before. It seemed he purchased a large supply of beans at a very low price, with the certainty that he could resell them at a sizable profit. Unfortunately, the beans did not sell and became wormy and worthless. He dumped the whole mess in the gutter in front of his store. The town authorities forced him to clean up the beans and have them hauled to the town dump.

To the west of Grabenheimer's was Keifer's drugstore. Mr. Keifer lived in a large house in the south part of town. He was a fine gentleman who had a good stock of pills and elixirs as well as sundries. Keifer's boasted a beautiful marble soda fountain and snack bar, complete with wire chairs and tables for customers to enjoy their favorite sodas and sundaes. Mr. Keifer owned a small farm east of town where he raised pedigreed goats. One of the specialties of the soda fountain was goat's milk.

To the west of Keifer's was D. D. Doll's Grocery. Old Mr. Doll later was joined in his business by his only son, Louie. Doll's Grocery was the typical country store. There were high ceilings and wooden counters, glass showcases, rows and rows of shelves, an old coffee grinder, and wooden bins that swung out to reveal the contents. Sugar, salt, pepper, spices, and rolled oats were removed with a big scoop, placed in paper sacks, and weighed on scales with weights. About midway back in the store was a square office raised above the level of the floor. Miss Sarah Stewart sat in the office and kept the books. Mr. Doll also had his desk there and could sit and survey his domain, keeping an eye on the activity going on about him. In the rear was a large storeroom in which extra supplies were kept, along with large sacks of feed. Here also were the chicken coops. Farmers brought their produce of cream, butter, chickens, and eggs to be traded for groceries, feed, and other supplies. Fresh fruit and vegetables were for sale in season. I remember the smells of spices, coffee, chocolate, and bran all mixed together, a pleasant odor found only in an old-fashioned grocery store. The Doll home was an impressive three-story brick home of Italian Renaissance architecture, located on North Eighth Street.

Howell's Hardware Store was to the west of Doll's. Mr. Howell was a shrewd businessman and a director of the Dulaney Bank. He retired at a fairly early age and lived comfortably into his nineties.

Next to Howell's was the City Drug Store. Long before the advent of the now-popular coffee break, the City Drug Store was the meeting place at midmorning and midafternoon for merchants and small children to have a soda or cherry phosphate. All the latest gossip was discussed thoroughly, and sometimes heated arguments took place concerning politics, particularly near election time. My favorite concoction was a chocolate peanut stir, which I ate while sitting at a wire-legged table at the end of the soda fountain, near the front window. The heavenly mixture consisted of two scoops of vanilla ice cream in a Coke glass, covered with the best-tasting chocolate (I never have found any other chocolate with exactly the same flavor). The concoction was topped with a generous sprinkling of salted peanuts. I stirred this all together and sat with legs wrapped around the legs of the chair, leisurely savoring every bite, listening to the men talking, watching them sip their cold drinks and take a long draw from their cigars between sips.

Behind the soda fountain on either side of the store were showcases and counters backed by shelves along the walls. The shelves on one side had many little wooden built-in cabinets. Each cabinet had a door with a wooden knob, upon which were painted mysterious Latin words. The cabinets held the drugs used in compounding prescriptions. (This was before the days of modern, prepackaged pharmaceuticals.) Some of the shelves had old-fashioned apothecary jars with ornate ground glass tops, also labeled in Latin. Rows of brown glass gallon jugs, containing cough mixtures and elixirs, were lined up on the bottom shelves. Carl Taubeneck and John Davison were the owners. Mr. Taubeneck was the pharmacist. Mr. Davison, who always wore a bow tie and who never was seen without a cigar butt clutched between his teeth, took care of the general merchandise. In the back of the store was the former office of Dr. Prewitt, who had departed this life. The old office was left in its original state, perhaps as a memorial. There was a small waiting room plus two examining rooms with frosted glass doors.

Meehling's Grocery was next to the City Drug Store. Barter was fair trade here, too, and farmers received groceries and supplies in return for their products. Frank Meehling lived down the block from us on South Sixth Street. His son Bill worked in the store when he was a youngster and one day snuck off from work in the back room to explore a shed across the alley. Bubeck and Gallagher, the undertakers, stored their horse-drawn hearse in the shed. Bill's curiosity was aroused, and he timidly opened the back door of the hearse to take a peek inside. Unbeknown to Bill, this was the favorite siesta spot for one of the town's characters, "Buffalo" Anderson. Just as Bill got the door open, the huge bearded figure rose up as though he was arising from the grave. Bill tore out of the door, back across the alley and back to work, never to return to the shed across the alley.

Today Bill is a prominent attorney and serves on the board of the First National Bank, but he still has the propensity for becoming innocently involved in some caper and ending up the victim. After the regular dinner meeting of the Rotary Club one evening, Bill and Dr. Sam Deahl left the restaurant together. They were outside visiting when Bill spotted a new Cadillac sedan parked at the curb. "My, that is a beautiful car," said Bill. "You like it, do you?" answered Sam. "Well, get in and I'll drive you home." Just as Bill got in, Sam said, "Oh, I forgot something. I'll be right back." Bill settled down in the front seat, and Sam went back into the restaurant and out the back door. Bill patiently waited, but Sam never returned, and the owner soon walked up to get in the car. He was a total stranger, and Bill had to try to explain to him how he had been the victim of a practical joke.

To the west of Meehling's was Casteel's Dry Goods Store, with its yard goods and O.N.T. Thread Cabinet. Here women could obtain all the necessities to make a fine dress. Mr. Casteel at one time had been a pharmacist, but for some reason or other chose to go into the dry goods business. C. M. Sullins had his watchmaking and jewelry establishment next to Casteel's. In the back he ran the American Express Agency, quite a sizable business in itself. In the days before modern trucking, packages too large to be sent via parcel post and too small to be shipped by freight were sent via American Express on baggage cars of passenger trains. Arthur Wright made the deliveries. He had a large enclosed delivery wagon painted a dark green and emblazoned with an American Express emblem on either side. He sat on a high seat box at the front and drove the horse-drawn wagon.

Mr. Sullins was quite a kidder. He and my dad were very close friends. Like my dad, he had come from Pope County in southern Illinois. When they got together, the tall stories would flow continuously. Each would try to outdo the other. Mr. Sullins's favorite tale was how poor his family was and how his favorite treat was "dog fennel" pie. (Dog fennel is a bitter weed usually found in horse lots.)

On the corner of Fifth and Main was an old frame house. Mr. Jacobs, a roly-poly fellow, had his barber shop in the building. Later the old house fell, a victim of progress. One of the first filling stations in Marshall—the Ohio Oil Company, later Marathon—was built there. The pumps were of the old-fashioned, gravity-fed kind. A large cylindrical glass container holding ten gallons was attached to the top of the tall pump. These glass containers were marked in gallons and half gallons. First, a handle mounted on the side of the pump was worked back and forth by the attendant and the container was filled. Then, after the hose nozzle was placed in the gasoline tank, a valve on the nozzle was opened and the gasoline from the container flowed into the tank. The valve was closed when the desired amount of gasoline was in the tank. The attendant then figured the price of the sale.

On the corner of Fifth and Main across from the filling station stood Moye's Grocery, operated by James G. Moye. A short stocky man with red hair, Mr. Moye always seemed to be on the move. When I was about twelve or thirteen years old, I went to work for him on Saturdays. Although I wanted to work, it was not for Mr. Moye.

The Pennsylvania Railroad had started a major construction job relocating the right-of-way and building two new bridges. One bridge was over Big Creek, northeast of town, and the other was over Mill Creek, west of town. Four large work camps were constructed along the right-of-way, two on the west side and two on the northeast side of town. Several hundred men were employed. This was before the day of the bulldozer. The dirt had to be moved by hand shovels and spades, horse-drawn scoops and graders, and steam shovels.

Because of my long-standing love affair with railroads, I had determined that my ultimate ambition was to become a railroad engineer. I wanted to work on the railroad project and had almost talked one of the superintendents into giving me a job checking out tools. When Dad found out about my plans, however, he put a stop to them. Without my knowledge, he had a talk with Mr. Moye and announced that I had a job working in the grocery store. I attempted to talk Mr. Moye out of hiring me. I told him I knew nothing about that sort of business and would certainly get the orders mixed up. And besides, I could never learn to operate a cash register. Over my protests I was hired and reluctantly went to work.

I had to check in at 6:30 A.M. on Saturdays and work until all tasks were accomplished, usually about midnight or 1:00 A.M. on Sunday. My primary job was to replenish stock and keep the sack racks filled. Customers called in their orders early in the morning. The orders were taken from behind a tall desk with a sloping top. The order was written on a pad with a carbon copy attached. Most orders were put on charge accounts, and each charge customer had his own book. The order was filled and each item checked off as it was placed in a large metal basket. The items were totaled and the new balance written at the bottom of the page. The carbon copy was placed in the basket and the book filed in the cabinet at the back of the desk. The cabinet was called the McCaskey (the name of the manufacturer). All accounts were not good. Delinquent ones were marked with a red strip, indicating that the customer had no more credit.

Mr. Moye did not believe in any of his employees' taking breaks. If there was no customer to wait on or phone orders to fill, we were expected to find something to do—stuff more sacks in the rack, rearrange the sacks of feed in the back room, check the vegetables in the front window, climb up in the dark loft in the back room and bring down more sacks, sort potatoes, or fill the bins. I remember one time noticing the bin with rolled oats was about half full, so I went to the back room to get another sack. Full, the sack weighed one hundred pounds. I brought out the sack with a hand truck, set it down in front of the bin, ripped open the top, and tilted it into the open bin. To my horror I saw that I had the wrong sack—a torrent of steel cut oats was cascading into the rolled oats bin. I quickly set the sack back down and sneaked a look over my shoulder to see if the boss was around. Fortunately, he was absent. I took the scoop and started putting the oats back into the sack. Finally, I got close to the dividing line between the two kinds of oats. Again taking a look around, I thoroughly mixed together the steel cut oats and the rolled oats.

A grocery clerk named Flem, who had worked there a long time, used his seniority to avoid menial tasks. Any time he could, he passed along these jobs to the rest of us. When fashionable women appeared in the store, however, he always made the effort to wait on them—smiling and bowing and scraping. He usually came back from lunch in high spirits, with a smile on his face. The smell of wine on his breath made the reason for his smile obvious.

Hobe Nelson, one of my best friends, also worked at Moye's. He was about six feet tall and had large feet. Hobe thoroughly disliked Flem. Knowing that Flem had painful corns, Hobe enjoyed standing next to him at the high desk as he wrote an order. Eventually, Hobe would manage to set one of his large feet on Flem's pet corn. There would be a loud yell, with Flem hopping around on one foot, holding the other in his hand, all the while looking daggers at Hobe. With the innocent look of a babe, Hobe would mumble an apology and shuffle off.

Foster Blizzard and Fred Morgan were two other employees with years of experience. Fred drove the Model T delivery truck and tested all the cream that was brought in by farmers. When he wasn't doing this, he filled orders. Foster was in charge of the Dodge truck that hauled supplies to the four railroad camps. Mr. Moye had the exclusive contract to furnish all groceries and the ice for the camps, a very lucrative business. Foster made several trips a day in order to keep the crews well supplied.

Moye's carried a full line of fancy chocolates in bulk. One day a new shipment of chocolates arrived while the boss was at lunch. Hobe, Foster, and I decided to check the shipment. We pried the lid off the box and were down on our knees like crapshooters trying one of these and one of those, comparing the quality and flavor of each piece. Suddenly, we all had the feeling at the same time that we were not alone. We glanced up to the red-headed, red-faced boss glaring at us. Needless to say, our tasting party broke up.

Prohibition was in effect, and the most popular items in Moye's grocery were malt, sugar, yeast, bottles, caps, and bottle cappers—

everything that was needed for the complete home-brew artist.

Around the middle of each Saturday afternoon, the farm families began drifting into town. Most had baskets or perhaps a case of eggs. There would be cans of cream to be tested—and occasionally a bunch of old hens and roosters, their feet tied together with binder twine to keep them from getting loose.

Hobe also candled all the eggs. He had a small dark cubicle in the back room with a little box equipped with an electric bulb inside. Two round holes were cut in the front of the box. He took an egg in each hand and stuck the eggs in the hole. This was like a primitive X-ray. The light coming through the egg revealed whether a solid yolk was present. The eggs waiting to be candled were stacked in crates and baskets outside the cubicle.

Hobe loved bananas, and the stalks of bananas ripening on hooks just outside the egg room were tempting. He could reach out the door, hook onto a banana, and peel it almost without missing a stroke. He always threw the banana peel over his shoulder. One day the boss, in a hurry as usual, raced by the door and slipped on one of Hobe's discarded peels. His feet went up in the air, and down he came—seat first—on the concrete floor, just missing a full basket of eggs. The air was blue. Hobe just kept his head down, candling his eggs, never missing a stroke.

It was the custom for farmers to leave the eggs, cream, and chickens and take off to "do the town." This was the social event of the week. Men congregated on street corners to discuss the affairs of the day, to talk about crops and the weather. Children made a beeline to a drug store or the Candy Kitchen to get a soda or sundae. Women went to the dry goods or department stores to get some yard goods or maybe a new dress, for which money had been ferreted away. After a meal at a restaurant, if they had arrived in town before supper, most farm families went to the local theater to see the latest comedy and western show. Finally, after all of the visiting was done and the show was over, they came back to the store to do their grocery shopping for the week. The lull from six to nine suddenly became a storm. People were in a hurry to get the tally on the produce they had brought in and to get their orders filled. The place was a madhouse. By midnight the last baskets and boxes of groceries and sacks of feed had been loaded into the waiting wagons, buggies, and Model Ts, and it was time to clean. The front window, with its remnants of fruit and vegetables, was cleared. Produce was carried to the back room to keep over until Monday. Sweeping compound and brooms were brought out and the floor thoroughly swept from front to back. At long last the day was over. A sweat-soaked grimy boy would receive his pay of $1.50 and slowly walk the eight blocks down dark, quiet Sixth Street. Arriving home to a dark house where Mom and Dad had been asleep for hours, I would stumble up the steps to the bathroom, where I took a good warm bath, soaking off the grime gathered from a long day at the grocery store.

After working on Saturdays during the winter months, I was employed during the summer also, working six full days for ten dollars. After two years, at long last I was able to retire from the grocery business.

A BLOCK NORTH of Moye's Grocery on the corner of Fifth and Plum stood Randall's Mill. On a loading platform across the front of the structure, farmers could back up their wagons to unload sacks of grain to be ground into flour, meal, or feed. The mill had a huge coal-fired boiler with a tall smokestack. When the mill was running, the smoke poured from the stack, and the noise of hissing steam, whirling pulleys, flapping belts, and growling grinders could be heard up and down the block. The dust from the mill and the distinctive odor of freshly ground grain filled the air. In the early days of radio, Mr. Randall offered a prize of a new Atwater Kent radio as a promotion, and I obtained a free ticket and had high hopes of winning. There were only a few radios in town, and they were homemade. Atwater Kent was the Cadillac of radios. On the day of the drawing, I could hardly contain myself. The barrel was turned over and over to thoroughly mix the tickets, and a volunteer reached in and pulled out the winning tickets. I didn't win.

Across Plum Street on the corner was "Doc" Tingley's Blacksmith Shop. I spent many happy hours there watching Doc work at his forge and anvil. He was a short, stocky, bespectacled man with a bald head. His chest was broad, and his biceps were huge. He wore a skimpy undershirt and a leather apron. Farmers would bring their horses to be shod and the plowshares to be sharpened. Doc would stick the share into the white-hot coals of the forge and turn the crank of the blower. The flames would leap up and the fire would get hotter and hotter. Just at the right moment he would pull the share from the coals with large tongs. Laying it on the anvil, he pounded it with the hand sledge, shaping the cutting edge. White sparks flew and his huge biceps were covered with sweat, glistening in the light from the fire in the forge. Then Doc grasped the share with his tongs and plunged it into the tub of water, causing a huge cloud of steam to rise.

Before shoeing a horse, Doc always would get acquainted with the critter. He believed a formal introduction was important. After a pat on the head and a gentle stroking of the sides and flanks, Doc would lift the horse's foot gently, flexing the leg and straddling it with his back to the animal. Then he took a knife from the wooden toolbox and carefully trimmed the hooves. Next he took a big rasp from his box and smoothed the surface. Back to the forge he would go, turning the crank a bit and moving the shoe around in the fire. When the color was just right, he grasped the shoe from the fire with the tongs. Moving to the anvil, Doc deftly shaped a shoe to fit with his hand sledge. Frequently he would place the hot shoe to the hoof and then go back to shaping until it was just right. After cooling it in the water, he held the shoe to the hoof, placing one of the square horseshoe nails in the small hole in the shoe and nailing it to the hoof. The nail was clinched where it emerged through the side of the hoof.

Across the street to the north from the blacksmith shop was the county jail—the "Little Red Brick House." It was not large, as jails go, but with its barred windows and thick walls it stood as a formidable reminder to boys what might happen to them if they misbehaved.

Back on Main Street, west of Moye's store, was Spittler's Garage. Mr. Spittler was the dealer for Overland cars, which were much larger than Model Ts and sported a stick shift. The presence of a garage where the newfangled automobile was sold and serviced didn't scare the horse away because next door to the garage was the West Side Wagon Yard, which occupied almost a half block. The office was in the front, and out back was space for parking wagons and buggies and stalls for horses. The wagon yard was what the modern parking garage is today. The proprietor of a wagon yard ran a profitable business because travelers, whether in town for the day or staying overnight, needed a place to feed and shelter their horses. During the days of Prohibition, the wagon yard was said to be a favorite spot for bootleggers. Customers could easily transact business in an isolated stall, away from prying eyes.

Across the street from Moye's Grocery to the southwest corner at Fifth and Main streets stood a three-story building. On the ground floor was another grocery store, McDaniel's (later Sower's) Grocery. As was the case with the grocery stores, there was a storeroom to the rear. The second floor housed the Marshall Public Library. To gain access to the town's library, it was necessary to climb the stairs that ran up to the north side of the building on the outside. The top floor was unoccupied.

Claypool's Shoe Store, owned by Charles Claypool, was the next business south. The Allison sisters operated a millinery shop next to Claypool's. These two women created bonnets in the latest style, usually decorated with feathers and ribbons. To the south was Bert Robinson's harness shop.

Next was the Hurst monument shop. The front of the building was an office and display room with a large plate glass window facing the street. In the rear was the workroom where Mr. Hurst fashioned tombstones and monuments from Vermont granite and marble from Italy. Most of the work was done by hand with mallet and chisel. He also had a sandblast machine, a modern convenience that made it easier for him to cut letters into the stone. His supply yard was out back, where he kept the huge slabs of raw stone.

The office of Dr. L. J. Weir was located on the alley next to the monument works. In addition to an examining room and a consultation room in the rear, he maintained a drug room, where he kept bottles of powders, pills, elixirs, and cough medicines. Most of the medications of that day were dispensed by physicians. Dr. L. J. was a man of medium build who always seemed to be in a hurry. He carried one arm in a flexed position at all times. His elbow motion was permanently limited because of an accident that had occurred years earlier. I often watched him from Dad's office across the alley as he would scurry to his Model T parked in front, carrying his little bag, to make a house call. Frequently, even in the coldest weather, he would take the wooden oil stick with a notch cut in the end and, lying on his back on the pavement, crawl under to turn the top petcock in the crankcase to see if there was sufficient oil. (This was the way oil was checked before the advent of the dip stick.) If oil was needed, he would hurry back into the office and come out with a quart measure drawn from the supply kept in the office, lift the hood, and pour it down the oil pipe. No filling station for him: Dr. L. J. was a frugal man. His brother, Dr. John Weir, occupied another room in his office with a separate entrance. Dr. John had given up the practice of medicine years before and gone into the real estate and loan business. Dr. L. J. was always a good friend of Dad's, and frequently they acted as consultants for one another and would team up on difficult cases.

Across the alley was Dad's office. To the south was a large lot, one-half of it being vacant. On the south half stood a small two-story wooden building where Dr. Robert Bradley had his office. He was a highly respected physician who was getting on in years. His son Steve was also a doctor. Dr. Robert had passed on while Steve was in Siberia in the army of occupation following World War I. Dr. Robert really "died with his boots on." He was discovered head down at his desk in the waiting room. Dad was called for, and as he was waiting for the family to arrive, the outside door opened. Dad stepped out into the waiting room, and there stood a hulk of a man. "Where is Doc Bradley?" the man asked. "He just passed away," was the answer. "Humph, well, he was supposed to fix some medicine for me and I don't see it." With that the man turned and stalked out.

The next building, a two-story brick, was occupied by Walker's Laundry. Later, during the depression, after the laundry went out of business, the building was used as a soup kitchen and temporary sleeping quarters for those unfortunates who happened through town and were without money.

The *Herald* office was on the corner of Fifth and Locust streets. Harry Potter was the owner and editor of the *Marshall Herald,* a weekly newspaper. He was a short, roly-poly man who was completely bald. Potter always had a smile, and I never saw him without a corncob pipe. He was an ardent Republican and never missed a chance to roast the Democrats. At one time he was appointed postmaster and served in that capacity for many years. He always had something amusing to write about and frequently accompanied his articles with a picture of himself sitting on a chair, his back to the camera, with his pipe peeking out from the side of his face. If he could have been dressed in Santa's costume, he would have been the spitting image of Old Saint Nick himself. Mr. Potter was the national secretary of Alpha Gamma Rho agricultural fraternity. Because of his position, the national headquarters of the fraternity occupied the floor above the newspaper office. Often I would go past the office late at night and would see him through the front window, eyeshade in place, smoking his pipe and pecking out next week's stories on the typewriter. The linotype machine and printing press were in the back of the office.

On the southwest corner across the street was a feed store. On the opposite corner facing Locust Street was the Knights of Pythias building, a large three-story brick structure that also housed the Pythian Theatre. The building was the center of social activity for the town. On the second floor at the front of the building was a large clubroom. Many a fashionable dance was held there. Dressed in their finest, Marshall's elite attended these affairs. Their presence was well covered by the press and reported in the paper's society column. The K of P Lodge had its meeting room on the third floor at the front of the building. The entrance to the theater was at the middle of the front of the building. On the lower floor were two rooms, one to the west of the theater entrance and one to the east. The Christian Scientists had their meetings in the west room. Victor Janney and later Earl Finney operated an insurance office in the east room.

There was a fairly large lobby in the theater with a closed stairway leading up to the balcony. The seating capacity of the theater, including the balcony, was about three hundred. The main floor and balcony floor sloped so as to permit all patrons an unobstructed view of the stage. The only exceptions were those seats behind the posts supporting the balcony. A sizable stage with an impressive proscenium extended across the front of the auditorium. A large orchestra pit was located below the front apron of the stage. Before the advent of movies, some of the leading actors and actresses of the day performed on the stage. I can remember some of the old playbills with the pictures of these great artists pasted to the walls of the dressing room. The people of our town didn't suffer in those days for lack of quality entertainment. The first visual entertainment we had consisted of the magic lantern slide shows, which were projected on a screen hung on the stage. The first motion picture projectors were operated by turning a crank. It was impossible to turn the crank at a steady pace, so the images on the screen had a tendency to jump and jerk. Later the projectors were operated by an electric motor. There were two shows each night, Monday through Saturday. No shows were given on Sunday because Marshall strictly observed the Sabbath. Silent movies were accompanied by music from a pianist, who sat in the orchestra pit. The pianist had to be most adept because both music and tempo had to fit the action on screen. The pianist faced the stage, with her neck craned upwards, watching every movement on the screen. She had to react immediately to each scene, going from a march to a waltz or maybe a tender love ballad.

Each show began by a slow dimming of the lights until the theater was in total darkness except for the light over the music rack on the piano. The pianist would begin the overture, and then a series of slides were shown advertising various businesses in Marshall. The first film was a one-reel comedy—*Our Gang* or *Keystone Cops*. Next would come a short "trailer" of scenes from upcoming movies. Once the feature began, the pianist really got down to business. She worked away at the keyboard until the final embrace on the screen, fading into the words "The End." The pianists were truly versatile and innovative artists, yet they were probably paid no more than a dollar a night. Helen Coldren (Moore) started performing while still in school. I also remember Sylvia Ritter (Millhouse) sitting at the keyboard.

It was not uncommon to have a break in the film, when a slide would announce, "One Minute Please." Other slides were "Ladies, please remove your hats" and "No whistling or stomping." Western shows were popular. Tom Mix, Buck Jones, William S. Hart, and Clara Bow were a few of the featured players. (Buck Jones was to later die while trying to rescue some of the victims of the tragic fire at the Coconut Grove nightclub in Boston in the early 1940s.)

The great actors and actresses of the time appeared in the more dramatic shows. Most of these artists had earned accolades on Broadway. Probably the most prominent were the Barrymores—Ethel, John, and Lionel. Because there was no sound, it was necessary for the performers to communicate with the audiences by pantomime. Although abbreviated subtitles appeared at intervals, pantomime was still the main means of communication. As a result, the movement of the actors and their expressions were usually exaggerated and sometimes jerky. Stars of full-length comedies included Harold Lloyd, who performed impossible feats—jumping from buildings, being caught by a cable, hanging from a cliff, or missing an onrushing train at the last second. Charlie Chaplin was the master of mime, with his black mustache, derby hat, baggy pants, big shoes, and cane. Although he was a comic, his acting often evoked tears that would quickly turn to laughter when he was caught in some impossible situation. In my opinion, his greatest performance was in *The Tramp*. Fatty Arbuckle was another popular comic who was able to provoke laughter. However, his career went into eclipse when he became involved in a major scandal.

One movie that made a lasting impression on me was *The Four Horsemen of the Apocalypse*, a major production, with a full orchestra employed to furnish the musical accompaniment. As far as I was concerned, it was a horror picture. What could happen to us in this world as depicted in this movie scared the daylights out of me. I was unable to sleep that night, and the movie haunted me for weeks. Another great picture was *Ben Hur*, with chariot races and a huge cast. *The Ten Commandments* required a cast of thousands; as I remember, the script closely followed the words of the Bible.

When I was small, admission for a show was a nickel and later was raised to a dime. I had no allowance but depended on my parents to give me a nickel or dime from time to time to pay for the luxuries of life. As a result, I didn't often get to the show. I decided to try to get some sort of job with the owner, Leon Cox, that would entitle me to a free pass. No cash ever exchanged hands for any of these extra jobs around the theater. Each week Mr. Cox printed a small folder giving the title and a brief description of the movie to be shown during the week. The movie bill changed three or four times weekly. He divided the town in fourths and had a boy distribute the folders early Monday morning to each household in his assigned quadrant of the town. When there was a vacancy, I got the job. My territory was from Main Street south and from Sixth Street west, constituting the southwest quarter of Marshall. Each Saturday I picked up my stack of folders and took them home, where I folded them into a small square that could be flipped from the sidewalk to the doorstep. I got quite adept at hitting the target. Of course, if it was raining or snowing, I had to walk up and put the folder inside the screen door or in the mailbox. About 5:00 A.M. Monday I took off to cover my route, walking all the way. This took at least two hours. I felt like the mailman—neither rain, sleet, nor snow kept me from my appointed rounds. In exchange I could walk by the ticket taker any time I wanted to see a movie. Later I graduated to the exalted position of janitor. This meant that I had to sweep the entire floor of the theater each day. There was a popcorn and roasted peanut machine, so I swept up plenty of peanut shells and spilled popcorn.

In the late 1920s we began to hear about "sound movies." Mr. Cox, being a progressive man, purchased a new sound projector. This was quite exciting, and people could hardly wait to get a sampling of what it was like to hear as well as see the action. The new machine had a large, side-mounted turntable, which was operated by the same motor that moved the film through the projector. An extra large phonograph recording was placed on the turntable and carefully synchronized with the film. Large speakers were installed backstage behind the screen. Most of the recording consisted of orchestra music, a technological improvement that did away with the need for a pianist. Dialogue on the record was minimal. It often happened that the operator failed to synchronize the picture and the recording properly, and the result created a hilarious situation: perhaps a man's voice speaking when the screen showed a woman, or a loud march being played when the scene was that of two lovers. The first sound pictures were not great successes. Shortly thereafter, however, the true "talkies" appeared, with the new process of the soundtrack being an integral part of the picture film. The new talking pictures by Vitaphone were an instant success. I believe the first full-length production was *The Jazz Singer*, starring Al Jolson. That classic was followed by another great production, *Show Boat*. The day of the silent movie, with the dedicated and talented pianist in the pit, was gone forever.

Occasionally, there was live entertainment. A vaudeville show traveling our way might be booked for a performance or two. This was a treat—just like in the city—vaudeville acts followed by the movie. Every year there was at least one "home talent show," sometimes two. The always popular "minstrel show" featured local talent, as did the school operettas. Sometimes we were quite surprised to find someone in the community who was rather shy but on stage became a surprisingly accomplished actor or actress. Acting sometimes revealed hidden talents. Usually, however, these productions evoked laughter, even when they were supposed to be serious drama. An entrance would be made at the wrong time, an actor would forget lines, stage fright would take over, a door would slam at the wrong time, or some scenery would fall over. However, this was show business in a small town and people loved it. There never was an empty seat.

Minstrel shows were the highlight of the season. All the men were in blackface, and Mr. Interlocutor was decked out in white tie and tails. I remember one particular performance, when several of the cast had imbibed too much of the "fruit of the vine." All of the performers were standing in line on a raised platform. One prominent businessman near the middle of the line began to turn pale, his eyes became glassy, and he began to weave. The man to his left, who was a strict prohibitionist, grabbed him by the arm and held on. In spite of that action, the businessman continued to weave. Finally, his knees buckled, and the inebriate fell backwards, disappearing through a crack in the back curtain. The cast continued with their song, never missing a note. Next the star vocalist began to sing "Melancholy Baby." He was standing downstage next to the piano. He was well known for his drinking but nevertheless was a fine singer. He, too, began to weave. His tongue became thick, he mumbled the words, lost his pitch and timing, and finally his knees buckled. He lost his grip on the piano and collapsed on the floor. He was dragged off, and the show continued as if nothing had happened. In spite of these mishaps, the audience enjoyed every minute. The show was a great success.

I remember appearing in *The Gypsy Rover*, an operetta produced by the high school music department. I was in the first grade and played one of the gypsy children. My mother made my costume (there were no rented costumes then). None of the children had any lines, but we thought we were important. We were in show business. Our entire time on stage was spent sitting around the campfire, while the actors sang and spoke their lines. My next appearance on stage was in an eighth grade operetta titled *Bits of Blarney*. Miss Allison, the grade school music teacher, picked me to play one of the leads. I had decided that performing in a show was "sissy stuff," however, and I wanted no part of it. I told her I couldn't sing and I couldn't act and would do the show no good. She insisted, and I was told to attend rehearsals each day. Then I found out that in one scene I had to dress up like a girl. That did it. I refused to attend rehearsals. Each day after school I went straight home. After two weeks, Miss Luckhaupt, my eighth grade teacher (who was also principal), told me I was wanted in her office. Being called to the office was the one thing that every student abhorred. This meant the worst had happened and you could expect to be punished severely. Miss Luckhaupt was a very kind person, loved by all students. I slowly walked to her office, feeling like a man walking to the gallows. When I entered, there sat Mr. Colbert, the school superintendent (who was hated by all the students). I did feel at ease, though, because Miss Luckhaupt was also in the room. Mr. Colbert wasted no time on pleasantries. With a fierce scowl on his face, he came directly to the point. "I understand you refuse to take part in the play," he said.

"That's right," I answered. "Why?" he demanded. "Because I don't want to."

"You haven't been going to rehearsals. "Where do you go? Uptown to run the streets?" "I do not. I go home to help my mother with the work."

"You're going to be in the play, and that's that." "I am not," I exploded. "I'm not going to be in any old play where I have to dress up like a girl." "You're nothing but a smart aleck," yelled Mr. Colbert. At that point, Miss Luckhaupt quietly said, "George, will you be in the play for me?" "Yes, I will," I answered. Then turning toward the superintendent, I pointed my finger toward him and yelled, "But I wouldn't do anything for him."

I returned to the classroom mad as a hornet. The performance went on. My mother furnished me with a dress, long silk stockings, and high-heeled shoes. I also had to wear a wig. The whole thing was most humiliating, but I had promised my principal I would do it, and she knew that I was doing it just for her. I refused to take my clothes off, but instead put the dress on over my clothes and rolled my pants up before putting on the silk stockings. Of course, I had to be made up with lipstick and rouge. I didn't think I could stand such an outrageous thing but gritted my teeth and went on. When I made my entrance, I refused to walk like a girl. Instead, I took long strides, which resulted in splitting the dress. I almost wrecked the whole show. That was my final appearance in a theatrical production.

The old Pythian Theatre served our town for many more years, but with the advent of good roads that allowed easy access to the large cities, the old movie theater went into decline. Finally, there was a show on only two or three nights a week. One dark foggy night in the 1950s, as I was returning home from the hospital in Terre Haute after delivering a baby, I noticed a dull glow in the sky. I was still about six miles from Marshall, driving on Route 40. I continued to watch the glow, and the closer I got to Marshall the brighter it became. I realized as I neared the city limits that it was a fire near the center of town. I just knew it was my office. With my heart in my throat I drove faster. When I arrived on the Courthouse Square, there it was. Not my office, but close by, the old Pythian was completely ablaze, with flames shooting high in the sky and hot sparks falling everywhere. All the fire trucks were there, and the courthouse lawn was filled with spectators. The building was gone. An old friend was gone. There would never be another Pythian Theatre. No more "home talent shows." No more minstrels. No more operettas. An era had passed.

NEXT ON Locust Street to the east, separated from the theater by a vacant lot, was the Cole and Cole Building and Loan Association. That very lucrative business was operated by Lou, Frank, and Vern Cole. Loans were made to furnish capital to build homes or to buy farmland. The Coles also had the only abstract office in this part of the county, and its proximity to the courthouse afforded easy access to county records.

I can still see Miss Alma or her sister Miss Hester Shipe walking across the street to the courthouse to search the records for an abstract. These two women ran the office with the help of Miss Elizabeth Hagist. The interior of the office was something out of the past century. Nothing had been changed. The lighting was furnished by a naked light bulb suspended from the high ceiling.

The office personnel sat on high stools, working at a tall desk with a slanted top. All entries were made by hand in the huge ledgers, using a steel pen that was dipped frequently in the nearby inkwell. They used an old typewriter for abstracts. A safe occupied a spot along one wall. Heat was furnished by a coal stove. Lou and Vern lived side by side in large, two-story houses on North Sixth Street. Frank never married but resided in a smaller house nearby. Frank had a good tenor voice and sang in the choir at the Congregational Church. He was in great demand to sing at funerals.

Next to the Cole and Cole building was another grocery store, Lichtenberger's. As the name indicates, Harry Lichtenberger was German. He was most thrifty and never wasted anything. He had a good business and was a member of the board of directors of the Marshall State Bank. Since his whole family worked in the store, he had no overhead for hired help. He carried a full line of groceries and meats. His wife worked along with the four daughters, Selma, Joy, Mae, and Helen, the youngest, who was about my age. Harry believed in everyone working hard all the time. The girls stocked the shelves, put up the orders, and then made deliveries in the Model T truck. No time was allowed for visiting around town. They were expected to deliver the groceries quickly and get back to work in the store. The girls attended school, but when they weren't in school, they were in the store working. After graduation from high school, they were required to continue in the store, and they worked there until they were married. One time Harry splurged and bought a new Studebaker touring car. It was a fine machine, and he kept it spotless. It was driven only on special occasions and then only for short distances. In the wintertime he put it up on blocks, and it remained there until summer. Even after the car was many years old, it had only two or three thousand miles on the odometer. Mr. Lichtenberger lived to a ripe old age of nearly one hundred years. His grandson is now our son-in-law, and our grandson is named Mitchell Keith Lichtenberger Miller.

The next business establishment to the east was a large furniture store owned and operated by H. M. Dewey, who was also an undertaker. He carried an extensive inventory of fine furniture, floor coverings, and paint. In the back was a large workshop where he did some furniture repair and picture framing. Across the alley to the rear was a large warehouse for furniture storage. His caskets were kept upstairs on the second floor of the furniture store. He also had a room upstairs where embalming was performed. There was an elevator, operated by ropes and pulleys, used to transport the caskets from one floor to the other. Funeral homes were just coming into vogue, but Mr. Dewey managed his business out of the upper floor of the furniture store. The custom was to have the funeral either at the church or in the home. Upon the death of a family member, a wreath of mourning was placed next to or on the front door of the home of the deceased. If the head of the family was a businessman, another wreath was placed on the front door of that office. Mr. Dewey had a motorized hearse, but he also had a horse-drawn hearse in the shed. The hearse was brought out and used when the streets and roads were in bad shape. Mr. Dewey and Dad were very close friends and spent many happy hours conversing in Dad's waiting room after office hours.

On the corner of Sixth and Locust streets, next to Dewey's, was the Marshall House Hotel, a three-story building containing approximately fifty guest rooms. Some of the owners were J. W. Lewis, who also served in the state legislature, the Waldons, and the Ridgleys. Mr. and Mrs. Ridgley operated the hotel during the late 1920s and early 1930s. Their grandson Jake was one of my closest friends. Mrs. Ridgley managed a fine dining room on the first floor, just off the lobby. She was very particular about its operation. The Marshall Rotary Club, founded in the 1920s, had weekly meetings at the hotel, with Charles Clapp leading the singing and Helen Coldren playing the piano.

An old man by the name of Tip O'Grady resided in the hotel. He came from a good family but had taken to drink and had become an outcast. He and a number of cronies got together frequently—riding to Terre Haute on the bus to sample the good life or going fishing around Marshall. Of course, Tip needed fresh, live minnows for bass fishing. My cousin Frank and I knew this, so we made a deal to furnish the minnows for a nominal price. We would take a minnow seine to one of the nearby creeks, seine out a bunch of minnows and put them in Tip's minnow bucket. Tip paid us in advance and instructed us to leave the bucket on the sidewalk alongside the hotel, where a water spigot was located. We delivered the minnows and turned the spigot so fresh water trickled into the bucket. The following day the bucket was still there and the next day and the next. By that time the minnows were all floating belly up. Finally, the bucket disappeared. In a few days Tip would contact us, and the cycle began once more.

Later, when I was in college, Wilbur Clark, better known as "Tub," worked as a night clerk in the hotel. (He was very intelligent as well as a prolific writer who later became editor of a trade journal.) Dean Findley, Leland Baker, and I, all students at Purdue University, spent many evenings while home on vacation in the lobby discussing the various issues of the day. One New Year's Eve the discussion got around to the field of science. Leland was majoring in science, Dean was in pharmacy, and engineering was my field. The subject at hand was the question of how much alcohol it would take to get a cockroach drunk. Although the hotel dining room had not been in service for several years, the old kitchen was still there and it was home to a large group of cockroaches. Leland had some 100 proof alcohol purloined from the lab at Purdue. We took the bottle of alcohol and a medicine dropper and proceeded to the kitchen. Down on our hands and knees we went catching cockroaches. After gathering a large assortment in a box, we took them one at a time, carefully dropping alcohol, drop by drop, from the medicine dropper into what we took to be each roach's mouth. The number of drops administered to each subject of the experiment was carefully recorded. The roach was released and again it was carefully noted if the subject staggered and, if so, how much. I still chuckle when I think of that New Year's Eve—four embryonic scientists kneeling on the floor of the kitchen of the old hotel, solemnly conducting an experiment with cockroaches when the new year arrived.

Harlan's Hall was located directly across the street east of the Marshall House, a two-story building that extended from the sidewalk in front to the alley in the rear. On the ground level were the stalls where Jud Harlan bought and sold horses. Many of these animals were brought in from the western ranges and some were still untamed. Harlan was an expert who really knew his horseflesh. He was a shrewd trader and accumulated considerable wealth from the business. The entire upper level of the building was occupied by a huge auditorium reached by a wide stairway from below. At the south end of the auditorium was a stage, and there were balconies above both sides of the main floor. The auditorium was used for dances, plays, and musical and athletic events. When the Marshall High School gymnasium became too small to accommodate the spectators at basketball games, all home games were played in Harlan's Hall.

During the 1920s and early 1930s, a patent medicine called "Crazy Crystals" took the country by storm. It was a saline cathartic, but all kinds of claims were made for the therapeutic miracles that would occur from ingestion of the wonderful medicine. Some shrewd promoters persuaded Dr. Edward Pearce to join them in producing a competing "Dr. Pearce's Sane Crystals." The group located in the lower level of Harlan's Hall. The horse stalls were removed and in their place were installed elements of a "pharmaceutical" laboratory, bustling with workers producing boxes of "Dr. Pearce's Sane Crystals." A huge sign informing the public that this was the "home of Sane Crystals" was painted on the side of the building.

North across Locust Street was Cane's Department Store, formerly Foster Martin's. On the upper floor of the building were two offices. Dr. Walter Turman practiced dentistry in one of the offices. I remember particularly his old-fashioned equipment. The drill handle was attached to a large upright metal stand by a small belt, which ran over a series of pulleys. The contraption was powered by a large wheel driven by a foot pedal. Dr. Turman stood at his chair with the drill in one hand and a dental mirror in the other. The small mirror on its long thin handle was thrust into the patient's mouth and used to press the cheek back, thus giving a view of the back side of the tooth. The drill, which was held in the other hand, was placed against the tooth, and the dentist fiercely rocked the pedal up and down with his foot, spinning the wheel and driving the drill. He had to be quite skilled to do all those things at one time.

The other office on the upper floor of the building was the location of the Citizens' Telephone Company. The switchboard extended along one wall. The telephone girls, as they were called, were seated in front of the switchboard on high stools equipped with back supports. They wore headsets with small receivers over both ears and a curved mouthpiece into which they spoke. This piece of equipment left both hands free. The switchboard was full of little metal holes (the jacks). The flat horizontal surface in front of the operator contained plugs that were attached to the insulated wires. The plugs, row on row, stood upright in front of the operator. When a light flashed on the board, the operator inserted a plug into the jack. The plug was connected to her headset. After she had been given the number, she disconnected her plug from her jack and with great dexterity selected the plug that corresponded to the number being called. Then she plugged into the jack from which she had just disconnected her plug. Having accomplished that in a twinkling of an eye, she pushed a small switch on, then off, on, then off. The procedure caused a bell to ring on the phone of the person being called. When the conversation was finished, a light went off above the jack, indicating both parties had hung up. The operator then removed the plug from the jack, allowing the plug to drop back in the upright position in front of her.

The telephone office also served as an unofficial information center. The telephone women knew about everything that was going on in town, and they loved to visit with their customers when business was slow. It was common to hear snippets of gossip: "Did you know that Mr. Johnson just died?" or "Mrs. Sullivan just got word that her children are coming to visit," or "Little Jenny Selleman is very low with pneumonia. They've had the doctor out there twice today."

The telephone office also served as an answering service, "You want Doc Mitchell? He's not at the office or home. He is out to see John

Semple. I'll ring out there for you." "You're looking for Sally Jamison? She's not at home. She went down to Widow Lowe's to spend the day and help her can tomatoes. I'll connect you there."

The telephone women also called the fire department, the police, and the sheriff when they were needed. For all of their service to the community, these women were paid the grand sum of ten cents an hour.

At Cane's Department Store, the lower floor had the latest ladies' fashions in beautiful dresses, skirts, and blouses. Down the line were the unmentionables—chemises, the underwear that reached to the knees, and, of course, the corsets with whalebone stays, to pull in the tummy and accentuate curves. There was a long, low counter along one side of the store with a row of revolving stools. Women sat on the stools facing the counter and examined the yard goods. Bolts of fine silks, linens, and woolens were stacked on the shelves back of the counter. Nearby was the big Clark's O.N.T. Thread Cabinet, its drawers full of spools of silk, cotton, and linen thread in all colors. An elderly woman who used to clerk in that store once confided that she always viewed with apprehension my mother's visit to the store because I was always in tow. Every time I came into the store, I had to inspect all the spools of thread. Afterwards, the clerk rearranged the entire contents of the thread cabinet, placing each spool back in its proper place.

To the back of the store was a balcony office, occupied by the bookkeeper, who handled all the cash and charges. A network of wires ran from the office to all points in the store, forming a miniature trolley system high above the floor. Each trolley wire had a carrier that ran on wheels. The wheels ran on top of the wire, and the carrier was slung below the wire. A wire basket was attached by a coupling to the bottom of the carrier. At each end of the wire the propulsion unit was mounted. The unit contained a strong spring. The carrier was set in motion by pulling a rope that hung from the propulsion unit. That action released the compressed spring, which kicked the carrier with its attached basket along the wire. When the basket reached the end of the wire above the head of the clerk, the bookkeeper pulled another rope that released the basket from the carrier permitting it to lower down to the counter. After putting the money and sales slip in the basket, the clerk pulled the rope, bringing the basket back up and latching it to the carrier. Then a pull on the other rope sent the carrier and its basket up to the office on the balcony. It was always a treat to visit the store to see the little baskets rolling along the trolley wire.

To the north, next to Cane's, was Booth and Handy's, an establishment featuring men's and boys' clothing. True Booth was tall and gangly, with a droll sense of humor. He loved to tease boys, but he did it in such a way that it was always a pleasure to go to his store. His partner, Sol Handy, wasn't in the store too much because he was too busy as the postmaster. There was an excellent selection of the best brands of dress clothing, as well as Oshkosh overalls and Big Yank blue denim shirts. I remember getting my first pair of long pants here—bell-bottom flannels.

Going on up Sixth Street was the post office, where Mr. Handy was the postmaster. The building had a fine facade of iron posts, with cast-iron decorative work across the top and down alongside the plate glass windows. The lobby was L-shaped. Across the front were the postal windows with fancy metal grillwork, behind which the postal workers stood wearing their green eyeshades. These consisted of a band that fit around the head with a green isinglass visor. Along the other side of the ell were rows and rows of numbered post office boxes. Each box had a door that was opened with a key. The doors were embellished with fancy scrollwork. In the center of each door was a square window through which the patron could check the contents.

Marshall had two mail carriers. Elmer Stover carried mail to the homes and businesses on the north side of Main Street, and Arthur Deaner (and later Tom Clark) covered the south side. They made two deliveries each weekday and one on Saturday. I've always wondered how many thousand miles they walked through all kinds of weather. It was noted that they had very flat feet encased in heavy black shoes, and they always walked as if their feet hurt. The mail for rural areas also was dispatched early each morning from the post office. Each carrier was responsible for sorting his mail and getting it ready to deliver. The city carriers had a big leather bag with a strap attached that was slung over the shoulder. The letters were placed in small stacks held together by a leather strap. Packages were also placed in the bag, and if there were more than could be carried in the bag, they were strapped to the outside of the bag. It was not unusual to see the postman walking along with a bag full of mail with a number of packages dangling from straps. In the winter the rural carrier was like the doctor. Each had to go by horse and buggy or in some cases horseback. Each had a road cart, a two-wheeled lightweight vehicle pulled by one horse. The driver sat on a board seat out in the open. There was no wood floor to set his feet on, but instead a loose canvas that was draped down like a hammock. Bundled up in a big coat, fur cap and gloves, his feet and legs encased in felt boots, a heavy robe across his lap and around his legs and feet, the driver bounced along with his mailbag between his knees.

Dr. Duncan's Drug Store was next in line. The doctor came from Kentucky. He was a true gentleman of the South. His wife, a gentle southern lady, was an artist. Dr. Duncan practiced medicine but also operated his drugstore. His sodas were among the best in town.

John Rademaker operated Rademaker and Sons Bottling and Ice Cream Plant, north of Duncan's Drug Store on the alley. Mr. Rademaker made fine ice cream and bottled all varieties of soft drinks. In the front he had a few tables and chairs where a hot, thirsty boy could sit to eat a big ice cream cone or drink a bottle of ice-cold pop—each cost a nickel. In the back was a large room with ice cream freezers and mixing and bottling equipment; the concrete floor was always wet. There was a constant clanking as the motors of the ice cream freezer hummed amid rows of bottles marching along on the conveyer. The capper moved up and down, firmly setting the cap on each bottle. At the end of the line a man stood taking the bottles off and placing them in wooden cases, twenty-four bottles to a case. The products of the business were distributed by truck all over Clark County and into the neighboring counties.

Clem and Gunder's Barber Shop was across the alley. Carrol Clem had a beautiful bass voice. He sang in the Chamber of Commerce men's chorus and in the Methodist Church choir. He also played the big bass horn in the Marshall Band every Thursday night during the summer. A little boy who was scared to death was taken by his mother to visit the barbershop one day. Mr. Clem sat him up on a board laid across the arms of the barber chair, placing first a towel and then a big sheet tightly around his neck. The sheet was so large that the only thing showing was the tiny head of the little boy. He then took the hand clippers, which were operated by squeezing the handles together. The boy twisted and squirmed as the barber clipped. He tried to look behind to see what was making that noise. Then the clippers caught some hair and pulled. That did it! There was a loud scream and a struggle. How was he going to get away from the thing? He was wrapped up in the sheet. Mom and the barber finally got the situation in hand and things settled down again. Finally came the scissors, which weren't so bad. After a few final snips, the sheet and towel were removed. Then out came a big brush with soft bristles. With a shake of the talcum powder can over the brush and then the soft bristles brushing lightly over the neck and face, it was all over. I'd had my first haircut.

Later, when I began to have fuzz on my face, I went to see Mr. Clem for my first shave. Along one wall was a big cabinet with shelves. Arranged on the shelves were shaving mugs, each with a brush. Each mug was individually identified with the name of the owner emblazoned on it in gold leaf. The owners of the shaving mugs made up the "Who's Who" of Marshall. Each morning early, these men came in for their shave. The barber took down from the shelf the mug belonging to that customer. In the bottom of the mug was a round cake of shaving soap. The soap and warm water from the spigot of the tin container on the top of the stove was made into the lather by vigorous stirring with a shaving brush. The chair was adjusted to a horizontal position by pulling the lever at the side. The customer lay comfortably with his head on a small headrest and his feet stretched out onto the footrest. After a generous application of lather to the face, a steaming hot towel was applied. Again the hot water came from the container on top of the stove. The barber then leisurely stropped the straight razor on the broad leather strap attached to the side of the chair. After the towel had cooled, it was removed and fresh lather was applied to the face. Then, with deft strokes and no wasted motion, the barber shaved with nary a nick. Again a hot towel was applied followed by a generous sprinkle of spicy hot shaving lotion. All but the hardiest let out a gasp when the lotion hit the face. Then the barber patted the lotion over the face, finishing the job with a dry cotton towel. Mr. Gunder seldom engaged in conversation unless the customer had something to say. He went about his work in a leisurely, relaxed fashion. Both barbers chewed tobacco, and they each had a spittoon into which they could direct a stream of tobacco juice without missing a stroke with scissors or razor.

The Marshall State Bank occupied the next location to the north of the barbershop. It was one of the ten oldest banks in Illinois and looked it. The front was of about the same architecture as the post office with iron posts, decorative ironwork, and big plate glass windows. The lobby was covered in linoleum; several teller windows extended from the big front window to the back. The counters were of oak with iron grillwork separating the customers from the banking personnel. Along the north wall was a row of high oaken desks with sloping tops. Several additional oak tables and chairs were placed about the work area. The vault with the thick steel door was located to the rear. There were no private offices. The only other room was the boardroom, which extended off to the south from the lobby at the rear of the building. Large oak double doors closed off the room from the lobby. For years a Colt .45-calibre revolver, which was probably of Civil War vintage, encased in a leather holster, was fastened to the door on the inside of the boardroom. In case of a holdup, someone had the responsibility of running to the boardroom, grabbing the gun, and firing at the holdup man. The odds were two to one the thing was so rusty it couldn't have been fired. A rash of holdups in the area during the days of the Dillinger gang and others caused all banks to become skittish. The Marshall State Bank was no exception, so a special electric lock was placed on the front door. The door was kept locked at all times, even during business hours. A customer approaching the door was identified by one of the tellers who reached under the counter to press a button that released the lock. The customer then could enter. It was practically impossible for any stranger to enter the building.

The board of directors met on the last Friday of each month, and it was the custom to pay the directors with silver dollars. The directors' fee for years was two dollars per meeting. Dad was a director who later became president of the bank. I looked forward to these meetings because I knew I would get one of those silver dollars when Dad came home. The other he gave to Mom.

In the early 1920s Bobby Brown was president of the bank. A frail man who always appeared to be in ill health, he didn't spend much time in the bank, but he did visit the office each day, even if only briefly. I often saw the big sedan driven by his daughter Mary pull up in front of the bank. The door would open and this little bit of a man would step out with cane in hand and totter through the door of the bank.

Bert Hogue, a bachelor who lived down the block from us, also worked in the bank. He lived alone in a two-story frame house on the corner with a small barn out back where he kept his car. He had a mane of snow-white flowing hair. Each morning at precisely the same time he backed his Dodge Roadster out of the barn and turned out on Sixth Street heading north to the bank uptown. He always wore a dark suit. Set square on his head was a dark hat. I can still picture Bert, both hands gripping the steering wheel firmly, eyes straight ahead, put-putting up the street, his beautiful white hair flowing out from under the broad hat brim. His speed never varied—a sedate fifteen miles an hour.

Others who worked in the bank during the 1920s were Drew Casteel, Robert Geisert, George Robertson (president for a period of time), E. D. ("Uncle Dick") Morton, and W. E. Morris. Mr. Morris had been in the banking business in Kinmundy, Illinois, his hometown. He accepted a position at the Marshall State Bank and continued on for many years as cashier, later vice president, president, and finally, as chairman of the board. "Uncle Dick" Morton, a portly man with a multitude of friends, was the cashier for many years.

The upper floor of the bank was occupied by the law firm Snavely and Miller. H. R. Snavely was a stout man with a bald head rimmed by a fringe of hair. He was very active in community affairs and the Methodist Church. He later acquired considerable oil interests in Texas and devoted a good part of his time to overseeing his investments. His young partner, Victor Miller, was a skilled attorney. Although active in community affairs, he carried a good part of the load of the law practice. He was also elected state's attorney.

Prohibition was the law of the land during Vic's term in office, and he was kept busy prosecuting bootleggers.

Bert Kaiser had a poolroom on the corner of Sixth and Main, just north of the bank. He was also a distributor for newspapers and magazines. Bert served as mayor of Marshall at one time. Later he sold out to John Cole and retired.

We have now made a complete circuit of the Courthouse Square.

Turning right (east) on Main Street next to Bert Kaiser's poolroom was Leasure's Shoe Store. Emanuel Leasure was a stooped man with white hair and wire-rimmed spectacles. Mr. Leasure was of French ancestry. His son Harry helped him in the business, and his daughter Jessie worked at the Marshall State Bank. He stocked shoes for all the family plus rubber boots and overshoes. Each morning Mr. Leasure walked from his home several blocks away on South Eighth Street, carrying the lunch his wife prepared for him in a tin lunch pail.

Going on east, the next building housed the Marshall Candy Kitchen. The business was operated by the Hilakos brothers, George and Pete. The brothers had immigrated to Marshall from Greece by way of New York and St. Louis. Entering the Candy Kitchen on one side, a customer immediately saw a cigar case and then a long soda fountain made of beautiful marble. Behind the soda fountain was a back bar also of marble. Mounted above the bar was a huge mirror. Opposite the soda fountain was a row of glass cases filled with the tasty products of the kitchen, homemade candy. In the rear of the building were tables and booths where the customers sat to drink their sodas and eat the delicious sundaes created by Pete and George. In the back stood a big electric piano (later a jukebox). A nickel in the slot caused the piano to go into action. The Candy Kitchen was the "hangout" for all the high school kids. Many a love affair came into full bloom with boy and girl snuggled close together in a booth sipping a Coke.

Waitress Edna Cunningham was a good friend to every youngster who came in. She had a quick smile and always had a new joke to tell: "Say, kids, have you heard this one?" Then she would lower her voice almost to a whisper, and we would hear the latest. These weren't dirty jokes, just cute ones. Edna always had a sympathetic ear and patiently listened to every tale of woe. The victim of "fickle dame" love always felt much better after telling the story to Edna.

Hornbrook's Restaurant, better known as the "Busy Bee," was next to the Candy Kitchen. Cleo Hornbrook and his father operated the business. It was typical of small-town restaurants—a big plate glass window in the front and a large room with a high ceiling. The ceiling was metal with a design stamped into the metal. Unshielded lightbulbs hung from long electric cords suspended from the ceiling.

Along one side of the room was a long counter with stools. A heavy shelf ran along the wall back of the counter. On the shelf stood the coffee urn and extra supplies. Plates, dishes, cups, and saucers were stored beneath. Delicious home-cooked meals were prepared in the kitchen. Plate lunches often included such fare as roast pork or roast beef, mashed potatoes and gravy, bread and butter, and coffee, all for a quarter. No one was left hungry. For a nickel extra one could have a huge slab of homemade pie. When I was in high school, I went to town nearly every evening after supper to play pool. About 8:30 P.M. I left the poolroom, went to the Busy Bee, and got a huge bowl of homemade chili for a dime. After finishing this off, I walked the six blocks home and was in bed by 9:00 P.M.

Harold Luse's jewelry store was next to the Busy Bee. Harold was a dapper man with a small black moustache. He was a fine watchmaker and did a good business repairing watches and clocks. The upper level of the building was occupied by a dry-cleaning firm owned by Basil Moore, who later became a funeral director. He also became an expert on Abraham Lincoln and Will Rogers. Awareness of his story-telling ability spread outside of Marshall so that now he is in great demand to appear before audiences all over the country. He has a pleasant voice and excellent delivery and can go on for hours telling the stories of Abraham Lincoln and Will Rogers.

Rademaker, the same Rademaker who operated the ice cream and bottling plant, owned a poolroom next to the jewelry store. Many a small boy, including me, learned, or attempted to learn, the game of pool here. Frank Tingley operated the business for Mr. Rademaker and saw to it that there was no roughneck activity.

Albert Sockler, and later Bill Buehler, operated the large garage next to Rademaker's. Mr. Sockler sold Overland cars and operated an automobile repair shop to the rear of the showroom. He was a short stocky man who always moved at a fast walk, almost a run. He was a rabid sports fan, particularly of high school football. His son Harry was the star quarterback and later played at Millikin University. After college he went into coaching. Mr. Sockler never missed a game at home or away, and he could be seen constantly running up and down the sidelines as the Marshall team moved forward or retreated. When Harry did something spectacular, Mr. Sockler always puffed out his chest and yelled, "That's my boy!"

During the 1920s Mr. Lichtenberger moved his grocery store from the south side of the Courthouse Square to the building east of Sockler's Garage. The Royal Neighbor Lodge had their meeting rooms above the grocery. Next to the grocery was the Bloodworth and Buckle Barber Shop. Emory Bloodworth was a man of few words. He was a tobacco chewer like Carrol Clem and Joe Gunder, the barbers over on

South Sixth Street. Emory was also a cigar smoker, and I believe the cigar was really his favorite. He stood at the chair, cigar stub clenched between his teeth, wearing his green eyeshade pulled low over his forehead, with the waist of his pants well below his drooping belly, clipping hair and listening to his customer, occasionally interjecting a low grunt into the conversation. Emory at one time was mayor of Marshall.

Mr. Buckle was a pleasant man who liked to visit with his patrons. He wasn't talkative but would carry on a conversation about baseball and other topics of the day as he clipped hair. Occasionally, he had a new joke to tell. Early each morning after breakfast, he walked from his house in the south end of town to the poolroom, where he picked up the morning paper. He and the proprietor of the poolroom engaged in small talk for a few minutes and then "Buck" went to the barbershop. He took off his coat and proceeded to have his morning shave. Standing in front of the mirror with a towel around his neck, he put a thick coat of lather on his face and with deft strokes of the straight razor soon was clean shaven. A hot towel and lotion completed the job. He then sat in his barber chair leisurely reading the morning paper until his first customer appeared.

Marshall was an early-to-bed, early-to-rise town. All places of business were open very early in the morning and remained open until 6:00 P.M. On Saturdays they stayed open until late at night, closing only after the last customer had been served.

The Wallace brothers operated the meat shop on the corner next to the barbershop. All of the fresh meat and some of the smoked products were home produced and processed. The Wallaces had a slaughterhouse at the edge of town. Cattle and hogs were purchased from the farmers and were fed and watered until they were needed. There were fields of grass for the cattle and feedlots for the hogs. After slaughter, the animals were hung on hooks. The hides were removed from the cattle and the bristles scraped from the hogs. The entrails were removed and the carcasses thoroughly cleaned with scalding water from huge iron kettles suspended over an open fire. The carcasses were then transported in a wagon to the butcher shop where processing of meat took place. Hams, shoulders, and sides of bacon were smoked and cured in the smokehouse to the rear of the shop. Fresh sausage was ground from the scraps of pork, seasoned by a blend of spices. The entire floor of the shop was covered with a thick layer of sawdust obtained from the local sawmill. The fresh sawdust had a pleasant odor that blended well with the smell of the fresh smoked meat.

The butcher shop was a pleasant place to visit. A huge walk-in refrigerator stood back of the counter. It reached almost to the ceiling.

The door to the refrigerator compartment, where the sides of beef and pork hung, was entered by a heavy door to the side. The front of the refrigerator had several large doors with glass mirror fronts. These compartments contained processed meat that was ready for sale. There was no mechanical refrigeration, so huge cakes of ice in compartments at the top of the big box furnished refrigeration. As much as one thousand pounds of ice could be placed in the box at one time. Since the bigger the chunk of ice, the slower it melted, the largest cake, that weighing three hundred pounds, naturally was the one the butcher wanted. In order to get the ice into the top of the refrigerator, a block and pulley arrangement was suspended from a beam in the ceiling. The iceman dragged the huge cake of ice inside, hooked the rope around it, hoisted it to the level of the ice compartment, and pushed it inside.

When the supply of steaks, chops, and roasts in the front compartments was running low or if a good customer wanted a special cut, the butcher would drag out a carcass from the walk-in compartment. The carcass was flung on the top of a big round cutting block. These wood blocks measured some two feet in thickness and were worn and scarred from use over the years. The butcher took a big knife and deftly gave it a super edge by rapid strokes of the butcher's steel (a long, round piece of steel attached to a wooden handle). I watched, fascinated by the way the butcher did his job, the knife in one hand and the steel in the other, stroking the knife up one side of the steel and down the other, back and forth until the knife was sharp as a razor. I could never understand how he could do this, with the knife flashing up and down, without occasionally slipping and cutting his hand. With the skill of long years of experience, he quickly had a nice roast or stack of chops or steaks all the same thickness stacked on the table. The thickness was measured by the butcher's eye, not a ruler. If a bone got in the way, he reached up, took the meat saw from the hook, and sawed the bone in two. He had a huge meat cleaver that came into use when extra trimming was needed. The meat was weighed on the big scales, wrapped in brown butcher's paper, and tied with string pulled down from the ball in the string holder. Phone orders were taken, and the deliveries were made to the house by a delivery boy (the "meat boy") driving a horse and wagon.

An iron ledge about a foot wide and about a foot from ground level ran around the butcher shop on the north and east sides. The ledge on the east side was the favorite spot for loafing for one of the town characters. On most any day in warm weather, "Dolly Peert" could be found sitting there. Whether that was his real name I don't think anyone knew. Dolly was a short, skinny fellow who always wore threadbare "cast offs." His pants were baggy, and the frayed sleeves of his coat hung down almost to his fingertips. Dolly was blind; he had no apparent means of support except for a blind pension, but he never seemed to worry. He always had his cane at his side, and after so long he got up and went up the street, tapping the tip of the cane on the sidewalk. Coming to a curb, he slowly and carefully stepped into the street. He knew every crack and crevice in the sidewalk and must have completely memorized the entire town because he never fell and never was involved in an accident. He was always greeted in the same way, "Hi, Dolly!"—"Hi, Peert!" his response. In discussing a female, his comment was always the same, "She's a mere, mere girl from Meretensville." I was never able to find out the significance of Dolly's statement. He received a certain amount of good-natured teasing, which he accepted without rancor. In fact, I think he thought it was the way people showed affection for him.

One time some of the boys carefully pushed one parked car forward until it was in contact with the car in front. Then they walked up to Dolly and said, "Boy, we want you to see the car that just came into town." Guiding Dolly to the back of the rear car they turned him loose to feel his way around. Slowly, he worked his way forward to the front, feeling the side of the car all the way, alongside the rear car and on forward till he came to the front of the second car. With that he exploded, "Damn, that's the biggest car I ever seen."

Dolly did some bootlegging on the side. No one seemed to know the source of his supply, but he usually had some squirreled away. Because he was blind, he could not accurately determine how much was poured into a bottle. He had a unique way of measuring and dispensing his corn squeezings. Taking an empty bottle, he filled his mouth from the full bottle and then squirted the mouthful into the empty, repeating his process until he had the bottle filled with the proper amount. (Apparently, he charged by the mouthful.)

Across Seventh Street from the butcher shop was a harness shop operated by two brothers, John and Charley Brandenstein. Inside the large musty room were workbenches and machines where new harnesses were made and old harnesses repaired. Plows, discs, harrows, corn planters, cultivators, reapers, and wagons were all pulled by horses. Sometimes as many as four to six horses were hitched to a single piece of equipment. This was a thriving business and kept Charley and John busy long hours cutting, stitching, and riveting leather straps.

The leather material arrived in their shop in the form of huge tanned hides. As they had need for straps, a hide was laid out on the large cutting table, and a sharp knife was used to cut out the strap of proper width and length.

At the front of the shop stood a full-size model of a horse, a handsome creature, wearing a set of harness produced by the brothers. Brother John played the bass drum in the city band. As a boy of seven or eight years, I sat proudly beside him playing my snare drum.

On down Main Street was Charlie Blundell's restaurant (in later years Tom's Cafe). Beyond the restaurant was Henry Bryant's Garage and Battery Shop. In a small building next to Bryant's was Grant Pritchard's Jewelry and Watch Repair Store.

On the southwest corner of Main Street and Michigan Avenue was the National Dixie Hotel (the name later was changed back to the original, the Archer House). The building recently has been restored. It is one of the oldest hotels in Illinois, built in 1854. Charlie McMorris owned and operated the hotel, which stood at the intersection of the National Road and the Dixie Highway, hence the name. Mr. McMorris was rather distinguished, large and portly and partially bald. He always walked with his head held high. He had a "mincing walk" and took shorter steps than a man of his size normally would. He was always well dressed—the perfect image of an innkeeper. His other interests were horse racing (trotters and pacers) and politics. At one time or another, he held positions by political appointment. The one I remember best was his appointment by the governor to the Board of Trustees of Eastern Illinois Teachers' College (now Eastern Illinois University) at Charleston.

The building that housed the National Dixie was one of the oldest buildings in Marshall. There was an ample lobby. The parlor was used for private entertaining. Guest rooms were located on both the ground floor and the upper floors. The structure was extremely well built, with large floor and ceiling joists. The walls were solid brick measuring some two and one-half feet in thickness. It was reported to be an important stagecoach stop for travelers along the old National Road and the Dixie Highway. Both Abraham Lincoln and President Grover Cleveland had sampled its hospitality. The original name, the Archer House, was in honor of Colonel William B. Archer, who laid out the original town of Marshall.

Across Michigan Avenue, at the apex of a triangular lot lying between Michigan Avenue and Eighth and Locust streets, was a filling station of unique architecture. It was a small, two-story, Chinese pagoda owned by Lloyd Pulver. The filling station was operated from the lower level, and Lloyd had an office on the upper level. He was the area distributor for one of the major oil companies.

Directly south of the filling station on the same plot of ground was the old grain elevator, the Clark County Coal and Feed Company, operated by John Newberry and his son Harold. The Newberrys bought grain from the farmers and sold feed and coal.

Directly east on the corner of South Eighth and East Main was Black's Hotel, a large two-story frame building. The owner, Mr. Black, who was also a preacher, was in great demand to officiate at weddings. Frequently, couples came from nearby Indiana to have the knot tied by Mr. Black, who then registered them as guests. Many a couple spent their nuptial night in one of the guest rooms at the Black Hotel. Directly east of the hotel was Simpson's Chevrolet; the modern, fireproof garage was erected during the 1920s by Dan Spittler.

Leaving Simpson's Garage and walking across Main Street, one continued up along the north side, returning again to the intersection of Michigan and Main. Crossing Michigan, observing the stop-and-go signal that stood on a post embedded in a large round block of concrete exactly in the middle of the intersection, one came to O'Hair's filling station. Next to O'Hair's, a one-story, triangular-shaped building stood facing Main Street. A restaurant owned and operated by John Mullens was in the building. Located at the intersection of two highways, the restaurant had a good business. Tom Koutsoumpas was the night cook. Just like the Hilakos brothers, Tom had emigrated from Greece to Marshall by way of New York and St. Louis. In fact, he came to Marshall because of the Hilakoses. Tom was a short, stocky man of swarthy complexion, partially bald, but with considerable black hair. When he arrived in this country with his brothers and sisters, he had nothing, not even a pair of shoes. He was full of energy and always seemed to be in a hurry. He had married a local girl, Audrey Davis, shortly after arriving in Marshall.

As night cook, Tom was responsible for the entire operation. It was amazing to see him work. He had no help. He waited on customers at the tables and counter, rushed back to the kitchen after taking the order, prepared the food, laid out the silverware, served the food, rang up the sale, cleared and cleaned the tables and counters, and washed the dishes. He worked from 6:00 P.M. to 6:00 A.M., seven days a week. For all of his work, he received fifteen dollars per week. Meanwhile, Tom and his wife began a family that finally totaled five children.

Tom's ability as a chef became known up and down the highway. The National Road, now known as U.S. 40, was a major east-west highway. Trucks began to appear on the road, and their numbers increased each year. The truck was becoming a major mover of interstate freight. With Tom at the stove preparing delicious, wholesome food, the restaurant was crowded with hungry truckers. The parked trucks up and down Main Street became a traffic problem for the one policeman on duty.

Dad and Tom had been friends since Tom first came to town. Dad was his family doctor and officiated at the birth of all the children. The building that housed Charlie Blundell's restaurant on the opposite side of Main Street was owned by Dad and my uncle. When Charlie was planning to retire, Dad attempted to persuade Tom to take over Charlie's operation.

"Oh, no, Doc, I couldn't do that," said Tom. "Why not?" was Dad's reply. "Because I don't have any money, and I don't know anything about running a business." "Nonsense," said Dad. "What have you been doing all these years but running a restaurant and doing a fine job of it. As for money, I'll help you get a loan at the bank."

Finally, after a lot of arm-twisting, Tom agreed to take the plunge. He changed the name to Tom's Cafe. Next, he purchased a big walk-in refrigerator, which he stocked with sides of beef, hams, and other meats purchased at wholesale prices. He had a meat block at the rear where he did his own cutting. Tom immediately showed that he was wrong when he said he knew nothing about business. The crowds began coming. The truckers also followed Tom to his new location. He couldn't ask for more. At the end of the first year, he paid off his loan. The meek immigrant who came here in complete poverty in a relatively short time had become very successful.

Going on west from John Mullen's restaurant, one passed the Big Four Wagon Yard. This was similar to the West Side Wagon Yard described earlier. The Big Four Yard had about seen its days. It was still being used some by farmers who came to town, but it wasn't many years before it was torn down.

Tom Crump operated a restaurant in the next building west. His was the Owl Cafe. Tom was a man of medium build whose clothes always looked like he had slept in them. He seldom smiled, and if one didn't know him, one might think he was mad at the world. He had a very low, gruff voice and usually drawled his words. Never in a hurry, just ambling along taking his own sweet time, he always wore an old crumpled fedora hat. I never saw him without a well-chewed stogie. Tom's looks and manner were very deceiving because he was a practical joker beyond comparison. He had a whole glass showcase full of practical joke material at the front of the restaurant. The exploding cigar was one of the most popular items. Tom loved to turpentine cats. He would catch a cat, lift its tail, pour on some turpentine, and turn it loose. Then all hell would break loose. The cat, screaming and clawing, would run up the alley and down the street and finally disappear from sight. The city hall and fire station building were just up the street. One day a screaming cat burst through the rear door of the city hall and ran out the front. Shortly afterwards, Tom ambled in the back door and asked the startled office worker, "Where'd the son of a gooooh?"

Pat Smith's tire repair shop was next to the Owl Cafe. Pat had a twisted leg that required the use of a crutch. His disability didn't keep him from being successful. It was something to see Pat wrestle the tires around the shop. Slipping a roller jack beneath the axle, he would prop his crutch nearby and flop to the floor. With tire iron and mallet, he soon had the tire from the rim, a hot patch on a damaged inner tube, the inner tube back into the tire, and the tire onto the rim—and the customer was ready to go. Pat didn't seem to mind the long hours or the hard work.

City Hall and the fire station were next to Pat's shop. The seat of our city government was a two-story building. The police station and calaboose, collector's office, and mayor's office occupied the main floor. The city collector was in charge of billing and collecting all water and electric accounts. There were only two city policemen—one day and one night patrolman—and no police cars. The day policeman walked about the business district, visiting merchants and the shoppers. The night policeman checked the front and rear door of stores and offices. If an unlocked door was found, he checked out the premises. If no intruder was found, he called the store owner. Once in a great while, there was evidence of a break-in. In that case the policeman called for help, and an attempt was made to track down the intruder. The sheriff was available to join in the investigation.

When there was a problem in the residential area, the policeman had to make the trip on foot. Fortunately, there was very little crime. No one locked the doors of their homes in those days. The calaboose consisted of two small cells in the rear of the police station. They stood empty most of the time and were used to lock up the occasional drunk or participant in a fist fight. The prisoner was usually held only long enough to sleep off the effects of his overindulgence or until he was brought before the justice of the peace and fined. If the seriousness of the crime justified longer incarceration, the prisoner was transferred to the county jail.

One night a man living south of town heard someone walking about in the house. He got out of bed, tiptoed to the bedroom door, and peeked out. He saw a man ransacking the silverware drawer in the sideboard in the dining room. He recognized the intruder as the new hired hand. Not being the bravest man in the world, he decided not to confront the intruder. After gathering up his loot, the hired man left the house and started walking up the road toward town. The victim of the burglary had a brother-in-law named Pat who lived up the road, so he called him out of bed and asked him to watch for the burglar and to follow him at a safe distance. The victim then called the sheriff and the city night policeman. It was raining, so Pat put on his rubber raincoat and watched for the burglar. After he passed by, Pat mounted his bicycle and followed. The burglar was just passing our house on South Sixth Street when Pat caught up to him and asked for a light for his cigarette. Just at that time the sheriff and the night policeman arrived walking from the opposite direction. When the burglar saw he was trapped, he started to run. The sheriff pulled his gun and shot, missed the burglar and hit Pat in the thigh, driving a piece of the rubber deep into the flesh. The night policeman was an old man, but he continued chasing the burglar, yelling, "Stop or I'll shoot." The burglar ignored the command, and the old policeman pulled the trigger repeatedly, but the gun was rusty and wouldn't fire. I was sleeping in a downstairs bedroom and the noise woke me. About that time I heard a banging on the front door and the sheriff yelling, "Doc, Doc, hurry. My God, I shot a man." The burglar was never found. The piece of the rubber raincoat that had been driven into Pat's leg caused an infection. Recovery was slow, and he was left with a permanent limp.

My bedroom was at the front of the house, and Mom and Dad slept in a bedroom at the rear of the house. A door from the back porch opened into their room. About 5:00 A.M. late in May, I was awakened by my mother yelling, "Scat, scat." I was only half awake and couldn't figure out what was going on. My first thought was that a cat had jumped in bed with her. Then I heard her scream, "That man got my purse." Wide awake now, I jumped out of bed, looked out the south window, and saw Dad in his "long johns" streaking around the house. When I got to Mom, she was just coming back into her bedroom from the back porch. She was really upset. "I had him by the belt as he went out the door; then I realized I had on only a thin nightgown and it was broad daylight, so I let go." Dad came stumbling back in out of breath. The burglar outran him and made it to the car where his accomplice was waiting down the street. The sheriff was called, and he took off down the highway, but the burglar had too great a head start. Mom had her purse on the top of the dresser, and it was stuffed with receipts for bills she had just paid, but only a couple of dollars in cash. She awoke as he crept in through the open door from the porch, and it was just as he grabbed the purse that she yelled, "Scat." A few days later, I happened to look under her bed, and on the floor where she could easily reach it was my baseball bat.

"What's that doing there?" I asked. "The next time the guy won't get away," was her answer. "I'll see to that." Mom was small, but she wasn't afraid of the devil himself. Tramps were quite plentiful then. A knock at the back door was often that of a man down on his luck asking for a bite to eat. Mom was big-hearted and never refused a man a meal. She fixed a plate heaped high with good home-cooked food, and the man then sat on the back steps and ate. One day the neighbor next door had a tramp at her door who was very belligerent. She refused his demand for food and locked her door. She watched as he left and saw him go to our back door. She couldn't see if my mother fed him or not, but when she looked again, she thought he might have gone into the house. The neighbor decided she had better call Dad at the office. In a few minutes Dad walked into Mom's kitchen.

"What are you doing here?" she asked. He told her about the tramp and that he just came home to check up. Seeing that everything was all right, Dad went back to the office. After he had gone, Mom got to thinking the man could have slipped in and might be hiding. She went to the cabinet drawer and took out a big butcher knife. Starting in the basement, she searched the entire house clear to the attic.

THE COUNCIL CHAMBER was on the second floor of City Hall. The room was quite large and was used for other meetings; one night each week in the summertime it served as the rehearsal hall for the City Band. Harold Bright was the band director and County Superintendent of Schools. Old Professor Wallace was the director of the band prior to Mr. Bright's taking over the responsibility. The band was composed primarily of men, with a very few young people. Starting at the age of four or five years, I wanted to play the drum. I started by tapping a tin plate with sticks and finally talked my dad into getting me a drum. I played the phonograph and beat on the drum sometimes two or three hours a day, torturing my mother and, in the summer when the windows were open, the neighbors. When I was about six years old, Mom and Dad decided I was serious so they talked to Mr. Bright. He gave me a tryout with the Sunday School orchestra at the Methodist Church. He thought I had the makings of a drummer so he taught me to read drum music. The Sunday School had a set of drums—a snare drum and a bass drum with a foot pedal. The only problem was that I couldn't sit on a regular chair and reach the foot pedal so I sat on a red Sunday School chair. I could work the foot pedal all right then but could just barely see over the top of the bass drum. Mr. Bright told Mom that if I was really going to become a good drummer I had to learn piano, so those lessons began. Only my love for the drum kept me at the piano, which I detested and never did learn to play. By the time I was seven or eight years old, I had become proficient enough to join the City Band. Mr. Bright was a strict taskmaster. We rehearsed and rehearsed until we were perfect. Mr. Bright screamed, stomped the floor, and cajoled until everyone was almost exhausted, but no one talked back. On those hot, sultry nights in the council room with no fans and no air-conditioning, he had the druggist, the automobile salesman, the harness maker, the school teacher, the barber, the county clerk, and this little boy and others sweating until we were soaked through; but each Thursday night, when we appeared in concert on the courthouse lawn, it all seemed worthwhile.

The fire department was housed in a long narrow bay next to the police station. In earlier days the fire apparatus was pulled by the firemen. It consisted of a two-wheeled hose cart. The wheels were quite large, and suspended between them was a hose reel. All the firemen were volunteers. Most of them worked in the various stores around the business district. When a fire call came to the telephone office, the operator called the police station. The policeman then rang the fire bell that hung in a cupola above City Hall. If the policeman couldn't be reached, the operator called one of the volunteers, who ran to City Hall to ring the bell. The noise summoned the other volunteers, and when enough had arrived, they ran down the street pulling the hose cart to the scene of the fire.

In the early 1920s the firemen acquired their first motorized fire engine, a Model T truck, which carried long lengths of hose stacked neatly in the rear compartment. There also was a tank with chemicals that had a smaller gauge rubber hose attached. It was possible to unreel the hose and use it on the fire until the larger hose could be attached to the fire hydrant. Because there was no pump, the only pressure available was the pressure in the water main. If the water level in the watertower was low, the pressure in the hose was low. The Model T had a step on the rear and running boards on either side where the firemen rode.

I was away attending Epworth League Camp for a week one summer. I came home to find that our house had almost burned down in my absence. Mom had fixed up an apartment in three rooms upstairs and rented it out. The small kitchen was outfitted with a three-burner gasoline cookstove. One day the occupant of the apartment ran out of fuel in the midst of preparing dinner. She filled the gasoline container that fit to one end of the stove. She failed to turn off the burners while she was filling the tank, and when the flow of gasoline from the tank hit the hot burners, there was an explosion. The tenant screamed, "Fire!" Mom went running upstairs and found the whole apartment ablaze. She ran back downstairs, got the garden hose, and brought it back to the upstairs bathroom and hooked it to a spigot.

While Mom battled the blaze, the tenant called the fire department. Seeing that the fire was out of control, Mom backed out and closed all the doors to the apartment. She went downstairs and out on the front porch and sat in the porch swing to wait for the fire truck. Looking up the street, she finally saw the Model T putting down the street at all of fifteen miles an hour. One man was running along behind almost keeping pace with the truck. She heaved a sigh of relief. They were arriving before the whole house was ablaze, but the truck didn't stop.

Instead, it putted on by and around the block and back toward town. Eventually, back it came and stopped. Then an argument ensued between the firemen as to which fireplug they were going to hook to. The decision was made finally, and they got to work. Because Mom kept her head and had the forethought to close all the doors and seal off the flames, the fire was confined to the apartment, and the rest of the house was saved. Later she learned the reason for the trip back to town after they had arrived at the fire the first time: they had forgotten the wrench needed to turn the water on.

Going down Main Street to the west, one came to the corner of Seventh and Main. Around the corner to the north on Seventh Street was Nelson's Shoe Repair Shop. On the north at the corner of Seventh and Locust was Rector's Livery Stable. Mr. William Rector was the proprietor. He was a short, heavyset man who wore glasses with thick lenses. Mr. Rector also played cornet in the Marshall Band. The building was constructed of brick with offices in the front and stables to the rear. Mr. Rector operated the jitney service and had the contract to carry mail from the post office to the two railroad stations, the Pennsylvania on the north side and the Big Four out at the east edge of town. He picked up the incoming mail and delivered it to the post office. There was frequent train service, and each passenger train carried a post office car. The postal crew aboard the car sorted the mail and had it ready to dispatch to the proper town or city as the train rolled along. The jitney service served the public by providing transportation for the train passengers to and from the railroad station. Regular stops were made at the local hotels, but in addition to that service, individuals could call the livery stable and have the jitney come to their home to pick them up. Mr. Rector kept close contact with the railroads, so that if a train was late, he didn't deliver his passengers too early—a truly deluxe service. In the winter and spring, when the streets were almost impassable, he used the horse-drawn jitney with Jake Godden driving the team from his seat box high up in front on the outside. In good weather he used the Model T Ford jitney.

Coming back down Seventh Street to Main Street and turning west, one came to Lloyd Hanley's Grocery Store. Just west of Hanley's was Jim Hooper's Plumbing and Tinsmith Shop. Just west of Hooper's was the bakery. It was operated for many years by C. R. Johnson. Here "Golden Crust" bread was produced. In addition, all sorts of cakes, cookies, donuts, crullers, and sweet rolls were made fresh early every day. Mr. Johnson had a big business and shipped out large quantities of fresh bread each morning to surrounding towns. This was before the day of truck delivery. The bread was shipped in large containers by passenger train. He started his day at 3:00 A.M. when he placed some of these containers in his Model T touring car and took them to the Big Four station to go south on the early morning train.

The Johnsons lived next door to the south of our house. Early one morning Dad received a call concerning a patient in the north part of town. He had to make a house call to see a man who was quite ill. Crawling out of bed, he dressed and went to crank up the Ford. It wouldn't start. Giving up on the Model T, he went next door and borrowed Mr. Johnson's car. Cars had no keys then, only a switch on the dash. Not wanting to wake up his neighbor, he started the car and crawled in, backed out of the driveway and took off up the street. Mr. Johnson was just getting out of bed to go out to make his usual early morning bread delivery when he heard his car start. Running to the door, he got a glimpse of the car before it disappeared up the street. He ran outside and made such an uproar that Mom raced out to see what was wrong. Mr. Johnson told her that his car had been stolen. He quickly summoned the sheriff. Mom, meanwhile, began worrying about Dad. Had a thug lying in wait knocked him in the head and made a getaway in the Johnson car? She decided our garage should be checked. Mr. and Mrs. George Farris had the apartment upstairs so Mom called upstairs and asked George if he would go out to check the garage. George, who was a large, portly man, was a bit of a coward. He finally said he would watch outside if Mom would go inside. She did and found the car, but Dad wasn't there, and there was no evidence of a struggle. She told Mr. Johnson that Dad was gone but his car was still there. Finally, they all came to the conclusion that Dad had borrowed the car. "He was going up to Clint Clatfelter's," Mom said. Mr. Johnson called the sheriff again and told him where he might find the car, then mounting his bicycle, he pedaled up the street. The sheriff and Mr. Johnson on his bicycle both arrived at Clatfelter's at the same time, and there was the "stolen car" sitting at the curb. About that time Dad came out. When he saw the sheriff and neighbor Johnson standing there, he lost his temper. "What in the hell is all this about?" he stormed. "All I did was borrow your damned old car when mine wouldn't start, and, besides, it's a noisy old thing full of rattles and those side curtains are loose and flopped all the way up here."

I loved to visit the bakery, especially when the dough was being mixed. Afterwards, the smell of baking bread permeating the air was more pleasing to my nostrils than anything in the world. I could almost eat my weight in raw dough, and there was nothing tastier than a slice of fresh hot bread with rich country butter. Early each morning I rode my bicycle up to the bakery and got fresh hot buns and cinnamon rolls for breakfast. Minnie Kleinman ran the store located in the front of the bakery. For twenty-five cents I got a bag of those goodies and rode as fast as my legs could pedal. I ordered hot cinnamon rolls and several cups of cocoa, and Dad had egg sandwiches (a fried egg placed between the halves of a hot bun). This was truly living in paradise. Later, the bakery was sold to Glen Davis and his brother-in-law Bob Wilson. They continued the tradition of producing delicious breads and pastries.

Archie Hornbrook, who had been a good friend of mine since we were kids, became the chief baker. I spent many delightful evenings loafing in the back, watching Archie perform his magic—mixing the dough, forming the loaves, and popping them into the big oven using a long-handled paddle. (The night before I started college, I dropped by the bakery to say good-by. Archie was short-handed that night: one of the men hadn't made it to work so I volunteered to fill in. I worked all night helping to get the bread baked. At about five o'clock the next morning I finished, went home, cleaned up, and took off to start my college career at Purdue University.)

On down the street west from the bakery was Nell's Cafe. Nell Boesiger operated the restaurant. West of the restaurant was the Marshall Auto Sales, the Ford agency. Originally the firm was operated by Perry Lewis and Sam Prevo. Later, Mr. Lewis sold out his interest to Mr. Prevo. Theirs was a large two-story building of more modern style than the Victorian architecture of most of the other buildings in the business district. A long ramp extended from just inside the vehicle entrance at the east side of the building up to the second floor. Automobiles were stored on the second floor. The large showroom was to the front of the lower floor, and a large repair shop was in the rear. Frank ("Hunk") Archer was the manager and general overseer. Miss Gilbert took care of the bookkeeping. Clift Saiter was in charge of the parts department, and "Lou" Siverly was chief salesman.

C. A. ("Cant") Dixon had a wagon and farm implement business to the west of the garage. Coles Hardware Store was on the west of Dixon's. Cant Dixon, Sam Prevo, Hunk Archer, and Lou Siverly always had the time to play a joke. More often than not, one of the group would be the target of the others. Cant had a big English bulldog that divided its time between his home and the store. One day Hunk and Sam went down to Doll's Grocery and picked up a few handfuls of feathers from an empty chicken coop. Then they purloined Cant's old bulldog. Using glue they proceeded to stick feathers on the patient old dog's jaws and nose. Quietly they took the dog to Cant's house, where he lay down on the porch and went to sleep. Back at the garage, Hunk called Cant at the store, disguising his voice, and said, "This is Mirandy Fossnagel, and you're going to have to pay me." (Mirandy was a colorful person who walked her poodle every day down Main Street. We believed that she always looked to see if men were watching.) "What do I have to pay you for?" asked Cant.

"For all my chickens that your dog killed," was the angry reply. "Aw, my dog didn't kill any of your chickens," said Cant. "You go look at him. He has feathers all over his mouth, and you owe me five dollars and I want it now!" "I'll check it out," said Cant, "and if what you say is true, I'll pay you." "Just leave the money with Mr. Archer at the garage, and I'll get it later," said Hunk, in a falsetto voice. Cant made a beeline for home and, sure enough, there was the old bulldog lying peacefully asleep on the porch with chicken feathers all over his jaws. A little later a very meek Cant walked into the garage and threw down a five-dollar bill on the counter in front of Hunk. "What's this for?" asked Hunk. "It's for those damned chickens my dog killed that belonged to Mirandy. She told me to leave the money with you." He turned and stalked out. It wasn't long before the story was out, and poor old Cant suffered along until he could think of a trick he could play on Hunk.

Life in Marshall in those days was leisurely. Men in business were not so wrapped up in competing that they didn't have time for a joke.

West of the hardware store was Oakley's Grocery Store. The Dulaney National Bank was located between Oakley's and Whitlock's Variety Store at the corner of Sixth and Main. The Masonic Lodge was located on the second floor of the building. The Dulaney Bank was founded years before by the Dulaney family. Robert Dulaney was president; his brother-in-law Dr. J. R. Burnett was vice president; and Dr. Burnett's son Woodford was cashier. The bank was housed in a Victorian-style building.

Turning the corner and going up North Sixth Street, one came to Bubeck and Gallagher's Furniture Store and undertaking establishment, owned by Charles Bubeck and Joe Gallagher. A stairway to the north of Bubeck and Gallagher's went up to the photography studio of John Merrick. Mr. Merrick was kept busy taking wedding pictures, family portraits, and graduation pictures. He also functioned as a news photographer. Any event of importance had to be photographed by Merrick. Before flashbulbs, taking pictures involved considerable preparation and equipment. First, Mr. Merrick, who walked with a limp, positioned the subjects. Then he hobbled back to the big camera mounted on a tripod, threw a big black cloth over his head, and squinted through the lens, twisting knobs and turning cranks until he had his subjects in perfect focus. He pulled the slide out from the side of the camera, and he took the little bulb that was attached to the shutter by rubber tubing in one hand and the flash in the other. Saying "Watch the birdie," he squeezed the bulb and triggered the flash simultaneously. The train of black flash powder in the tray at the end of the stick ignited with a loud bang and a bright flash. Smoke filled the room from the burned powder, and everyone would have a wide-eyed look of surprise on his or her face. More often than not, the subject would move or blink, and the whole process had to be repeated.

Back downstairs on Sixth Street and on north was Spotts's Meat Market. The butcher shop, like Wallace's on Main Street, had sawdust on the floor and essentially the same equipment—big refrigerator, meat block, scales, knives, and cleavers. Mr. Spotts was short and heavy with a big belly. His son Gene was my best friend, and Dad and Mr. Spotts were also very close friends. They had an arrangement whereby all the meat we bought was charged, and all charges for professional services Dad performed for the Spotts family were put on the books. Once each year they got together and compared bills, canceling out the charges. Occasionally, a small balance was owed to one or the other, and this might be paid in cash at the time or let run on into next year and "taken out in trade."

Mr. Spotts made the best homemade bologna I ever ate. I could never get enough. I devised a way of getting an occasional chunk of the delicacy without having to pay. I had my own barter system. I would come into the shop to visit with Mr. Spotts a while and then ask him if he wasn't having a little stomach trouble. Of course he always did, so I would say, "You need some soda mints." "Is that what I need? Do you suppose you could get me some?" he would reply solemnly. "Yep, I'll be right back."

I'd scamper out down the street and over to Dad's office. I'd go into the drug room, get a pill box from the drawer, and fill it with soda mints. Back to the butcher shop I'd go, hand the box of pills to Mr. Spotts, who would then hand me a generous hunk of bologna. The game was played many times.

Next to Spotts's Market on the north was the *Clark County Democrat,* a weekly paper. Norman Bennett was the owner and publisher. He had taught country school for a number of years before going into journalism. He was an ardent Democrat. At election time and sometimes between elections, the barbs would fly between the *Clark County Democrat* on North Sixth Street and the *Marshall Herald* on South Fifth. Mr. Potter, the editor of the *Herald,* was just as strong a Republican as Mr. Bennett was a Democrat. These jousts between the two papers provided good entertainment for the readers. Everyone took politics seriously.

Coming back down Sixth Street to Main we have arrived at Grabenheimer's Corner, where our tour began. This has been a description of downtown Marshall in the 1920s as seen through the eyes of a boy who spent many happy hours there.

6

The Making of a Young Man

DAD HAD BEEN A STOCKHOLDER and director of the Marshall State Bank for many years. In 1929 he was elected president. A local man came in one day to discuss a loan. He had the opportunity to buy a 116-acre farm and needed the loan to finance the deal. Dad decided that the bank could not loan him the amount he needed, but he offered him an alternative. The bank would loan him one-half the required amount, and Dad would become an equal partner by putting up the other half. This was agreeable, so the two of them bought the farm, which was located about five miles northwest of Marshall. There was an old brick house, a barn, and a few outbuildings located on the farm. The land was run-down because it had been farmed for years without any effort being made to replace the soil components so necessary to good crop yields.

They decided to stop cultivation and let the land rest. Sheep were purchased and put on pasture. In the spring there was a goodly number of new lambs, and when they were ready for market, we trucked them to the stockyards in Indianapolis, stopping every few miles to check our load. We traveled at night to avoid overheating the animals. About halfway to our destination, we stopped for sandwiches and coffee. It was difficult to stay awake—I wasn't used to being up so late. We arrived at the stockyards about 4:00 A.M. I had never seen stockyards before. The yards were huge, and even though it was the middle of the night, there was a lot of traffic. Trucks were arriving from all directions, filled with bawling cattle, squealing pigs, and sheep and lambs crying a pitiful "baa."

The pungent odors from the stockpens penetrated the air. The markets didn't open until 8:00 A.M., so there was nothing to do but wait. The commission offices were open, however, and we went to the one Dad had selected. A man came out to inspect our load of lambs. We backed up to the unloading chute, and the lambs went scampering down the runway into a pen.

Then we parked the truck and pulled out a canvas tarpaulin, spreading it on the cobblestones under the truck. We lay down on our hard bed to rest before the markets opened. I had never tried to sleep under such trying conditions before—the cobblestones poking me in the back, the odor from the pens, and the bellowing and squealing of the animals. When I awakened, the hot sun was beating down. Our commission man sold our lambs, and we almost topped the market.

Dad's partner wanted to sell out so Dad purchased his interest. The farm now was all ours. A hired hand was employed to live on the farm and do the work. He and his wife and two daughters moved into the old brick house. We had no modern machinery. The plows, cultivators, mower, discs, harrows, binders, and wagons were pulled by teams of horses.

Dad was still building up the soil so he rented acreage to produce crops. The place he rented contained one hundred acres and was about one and one-half miles south of our farm. All the farming equipment either was pulled down the road or loaded on the wagon to be taken to the fields to be tilled. The tenant was furnished a couple of cows to provide milk and two or three hogs for meat. Otherwise, we were engaged in grain farming.

During summer vacation from school I was put to work. I was routed out of bed early, and Dad would take me out to the farm. Usually I dozed all the way.

There was hay to rake, corn to hoe, brush to cut, gravel to haul, or stables to clean. There was a lot of brush to cut back in the bottom and on the slopes of the hills; also, the fencerows always needed clearing. The brush seemed to grow back as fast as I cut it. I usually carried my lunch, but occasionally Dad brought out a basketful of warm food from Mom's kitchen at noon. Toward sundown he drove back to get me.

The maintenance of the roads was essentially the responsibility of the farmers who used them. Therefore, when the crops were in, we hauled gravel from the creek behind the barn and spread it on the road. The gravel was of very poor quality, containing more dirt than gravel.

The wagon was fitted up with dump boards. These were two-by-fours that had the ends whittled down to form handles. The dump boards were laid lengthwise to form the bottom of the wagon bed. A side board was placed on each side and the end gates inserted in the slots of the side boards. About halfway between the front and back of the wagon a two-by-four, with a cleat on each end, was laid across the top to keep the side boards from buckling when the wagon was loaded.

The wagon was driven to the creek bed and loaded, using long-handled shovels. The load was taken to the road and dumped in one of the many low spots always there. To dump the wagon, the end gates were pried out, the cleated two-by-four removed from across the top, and each side board brought up and laid on the ground. Then the man at each end turned each dump board over, dumping the gravel to the ground. The wagon bed then was reassembled and the wagon pulled forward so the gravel could be spread.

Another job that had to be done periodically was the repair of the telephone lines. The telephone system was owned by the local subscribers. The switchboard was located in the house of a family named Clark, so the system was known as Clark's Switchboard. All the telephones were hand-crank models. Connection to points outside the local system was through the switchboard. The rates—or dues, as they were known—were quite nominal, and no provision was made for professional maintenance. If a pole came down, it had to be replaced by one of the subscribers. Frequently, the replacement was the trunk of a tree from a nearby woods. If the wires were down or an insulator was broken, a farmer put his ladder and tools in his wagon and drove down the road to fix it.

The days of the Model T were past. The new Model A had a much more powerful engine and a gearshift transmission. We still did not have a tractor to pull the farm machinery, but Dad and I devised a way of pulling the hay rake with the car. The hay could be raked up into windrows in about half the time it took using a plodding team of horses. Dad was convinced that we needed a tractor. He purchased a secondhand McCormick Deering Model 10-20. The big drive wheels were made of steel with "spade lugs" bolted to the rim. These lugs gave increased traction. To start the engine required turning the starter crank, just as it had with the Model T. However, cranking the tractor was more difficult because the engine was much bigger and in the early morning the oil in the crankcase was cold. Cold oil is like sorghum molasses.

I wanted to drive the tractor, so Dad gave me the job. Wheeling the giant machine around, pulling the disc or rotary hoe, was exciting. I could move up and down the field churning the earth, the engine roaring and the exhaust spewing black smoke. The glamour soon wore off, however. That which had been fun quickly turned into a monotonous, hot, dirty job. The seat was made of steel and after an hour or so of bumping over uneven ground, my bottom became bruised and sore. Later it became numb. I found a sheepskin and placed it on the seat. The cushion helped some, but after several hours of pounding, even this didn't prevent my bottom from becoming sore.

I was at the age when I didn't like to go to bed early. My friends and I got together in the evening downtown and visited or maybe drove around in a car, just talking or singing. Regardless of the hour I got to bed, I still was routed out at 4:00 A.M. My working clothes consisted of a pair of heavy shoes and socks, a pair of jeans, and a felt hat with the rim cut off. The sun was hot and, after a few days' exposure, my skin turned a deep brown color. I rode along up and down the field, continuously engulfed in a cloud of dust. The fumes from the exhaust, mixed with the dust, made breathing difficult most of the time, and the heat from the engine, combined with the sun's hot rays, made me feel as though I were sitting on top of a stove. The terrific heat caused me to work up a thirst in a short time, so I carried a jug of water with me. The jug was hooked to the fender over one of the drive wheels by a leather strap. Of course, the water soon got warm, but at least it quenched my thirst. Perspiration flowed freely all the time. The dust mixed with sweat formed mud. The hot sun dried the mud and, by the end of the day, I had a thick layer of mud caked from my waist up.

There was an abandoned house on the land we rented, and I always got my water from a well near the old house. One day I turned the jug up to get a refreshing drink. The water had a strange odor, similar to kerosene, but I kept on drinking. After work that night I took my bath and put on my good pants and shirt and went uptown to attend the weekly band concert. It was a hot, humid night, and I began to sweat profusely. I noticed a strange odor—where was it coming from? It was me. The sweat pouring from my skin smelled like skunk. It dawned on me. The strange-tasting water I had been drinking all day had been contaminated by skunk oil. The old well contained the carcass of a dead skunk.

One year Dad decided that all one hundred acres of corn was to be hoed by hand. Hobe and I were assigned the job. The long rows stretched out almost as far as the eye could see. It was slow work walking down each row, hoe in hand, chopping away at the weeds. The ground had been baked hard by the hot sun, and each time the blade of the hoe struck the ground, it sent a jar through our arms. After going down the row and back to the starting point, we had to sit a while under a shade tree. Dad had the habit of dropping by to see if we were busy, so when we sat in the shade, we filed our hoes in order to look busy. It seemed an eternity, but finally we finished the job—one hundred acres of corn hoed by hand.

I had always wanted a log cabin, so after the crops were in, Hobe and I, along with my cousin Frank and one or two others, started in on the project.

The site was on a bluff overlooking the creek below. We went back into the woods and began felling trees. We used the team and wagon to haul the logs to the building site. None of us had ever had any experience in building, but we did have a Boy Scout manual, which contained sketches of a log cabin.

We hauled loads of rock up from the creek. The logs were notched at the ends and put in place just like the picture in the book. We dug a pit and carried water from the creek to mix up the clay mud to chink the spaces between the logs. A stone chimney was constructed at one end of the cabin with a fireplace inside. We were very surprised to find that our fireplace worked perfectly. The roof was covered by tin, and a wide plank floor was put in. We then built in two double-deck bunks. The door at the front end from the fireplace was made from planks. A small window was located on each side of the cabin. When it was completed, it looked like the cabin that Abe Lincoln lived in when he was a boy. We had to have a name for our masterpiece. After much discussion, we christened it "Lazy Ranch." We carved the name into a wooden plank and hung it over the door.

When we started the project, I think most of us thought our enthusiasm would cool and it would never be completed, but that was not the case. After the cabin was completed, Hobe and I decided to stay out there all week long, coming into town only on the weekends. We constructed a cooler for perishable items down in the creek. Our refrigerator was a stone jar sunk in the creek bed. The cool water flowing around the jar kept things fresh. We cut steps into the side of the bluff down to the creek so that making a trip to the refrigerator was no chore. We cooked all our meals over the fire in the fireplace. After supper we cleaned up the table and washed and dried the dishes. Later, we sat in front of our cabin like two pioneers of a century earlier—he smoking his pipe and me chewing my tobacco—looking down toward the creek, listening to the sounds of the evening. Sometimes we engaged in conversation, but more often we sat in silence until it was time for bed.

One evening I was frying meat over the fire. I had just thrown more wood on the fire and was down on my haunches, holding the frying pan over the fire with one hand and holding the big fork in my other hand, when suddenly a red-hot coal popped out from the fire. It struck me directly in the center of my right eye. I screamed and almost dropped the pan. The pain was excruciating. I had never before had a pain so severe. Our only source of light was an oil lamp and the light from the fireplace. Hobe tried to look in my eye, but he was unable to get the lid open because of the spasm from the pain. We had no transportation, and it was six miles to town. There was no telephone, so I suffered it out until morning. Sleep was impossible. The only relief I could get was from cold packs made by soaking cloths in cold water. That was the longest night in my life.

Dad always came out early in the morning, and when he arrived the next morning, he found me pacing up and down holding a cold cloth over my eye. By that time, even with the cold packs, my eye had become quite swollen. He wasted no time in getting me in the car and taking me to an eye specialist. His examination revealed that I had a severe conjunctivitis with a large, deep ulcer already forming in the cornea. I was told that, due to the length of time the eye had gone untreated, there was great danger of a severe infection and that the prognosis was not good. I might even lose the eye. I wore a patch and had to go for daily treatments for six weeks. I was most fortunate, though. I recovered completely and had no loss of vision.

During the winter months when snow lay deep on the ground, Hobe and I spent many weekends in our cabin. During the day we went hunting and at night, snugly buttoned up in our cabin, we sat by the fire and talked while the cold winds blew hard outside. This was adventure.

One day in August I was busy cutting brush out of the fencerows when my cousin Frank drove out to the farm. He was going squirrel hunting. Although I did not consider myself a hunter, I decided to go along. Walking in the cool woods was a great improvement over working in the sun cutting brush. There was an old double-barrel 12-gauge shotgun, almost an antique, at the house. The gun had hammers on both barrels. We walked into the woods looking for signs of squirrels. We came to a group of hickory trees with nuts lying thick on the ground. Some of the nuts were broken into pieces, giving evidence that squirrels had been working on them. I decided I was going to sit down and wait for a squirrel. Frank, who was an experienced hunter, told me that was not the way to get a squirrel.

"You have to keep walking and looking for squirrels up high in the trees," he said. "Well, I'm tired from working all day and I'm going to sit here under a tree and wait for the squirrels to come to me," I answered. He tramped off through the woods, leaving me sitting on the ground. I had propped my gun against the tree trunk and soon began to get drowsy. It wasn't long until I had stretched out on the ground and gone to sleep. When I awoke, the sun was setting. I opened my eyes when I heard a noise and, lying there on my back, I saw movement on a high limb of a tree. I kept watching and soon I saw a squirrel running along the limb. About that time he was joined by a second squirrel. They were having fun chasing one another from limb to limb. Very carefully and quietly I got up and got the gun. I brought the gun up and steadied it against the tree. I waited patiently until the two squirrels were almost side by side, then I pulled the trigger. Down dropped one squirrel, and I quickly aimed at the second squirrel and squeezed the trigger. Down dropped the other squirrel. I picked up the two squirrels and walked back to the house. I got back before Frank did. It was almost dark when he came walking in empty-handed. Then he saw my two squirrels.

"Where did you get those?" he asked. "Right where you left me," I answered. "Let me tell you how to hunt squirrels," I added. "Find a likely spot, lie down and take a nap, then get up and shoot the critters and come home." I got no answer from Frank, only a dirty look.

Dad loved his farm. As a boy he had worked hard plowing, harvesting crops, milking cows—helping his father scratch out a living for a large family. All that time he was dreaming of the day when he could escape from the life of hardship on the farm to become a successful doctor. Now that he had accomplished his dream he was drawn back to the soil. The love of the soil, deep in his heart, was still there. He was a boy again, reliving the days when he was growing up.

He rose early every morning to go to the farm. He checked on the livestock and talked with the hired hand concerning the plans for the day. He walked through the fields, the early morning dew leaving its wetness on his shoes and pant legs. He saw the green corn and beans laid out in a panorama across the landscape. He listened to the birds, their happy songs joined by the sounds of crickets and the humming of bees, forming a melodious chorus. The sweet scent of newly mown hay and the smell of freshly turned earth combined to form an unequaled perfume. Here was peace, just the relaxation he needed. After an hour or two at the farm, Dad was ready to return to town, passing by the bakery to pick up freshly baked rolls before heading home for a big breakfast. He was then ready to start on his rounds seeing patients, dealing with the multitude of problems of the sick and injured.

Dad operated the farm to suit himself, and it was not a particularly profitable operation. It was his hobby. He knew that the farm was run down. No attempt had been made by the former owners to rebuild the soil. Production had decreased steadily over the years until it was impossible to get a decent yield. Instead of planting corn, wheat, and beans, he sowed sweet clover. From the Department of Agriculture, Dad had learned that sweet clover replenished the nitrogen in the soil and nitrogen was necessary for good crop production. It wasn't long before the entire tillable acreage was covered by a lush stand of sweet clover. As the clover matured and fell, it reseeded itself.

After a few years Dad decided the time had come to put in a crop of corn and wheat. The heavy clover sod was plowed and seeded. That year a bumper crop was harvested. The corn made one hundred bushels per acre—an unheard of feat on that type of soil. My father was engaged in soil conservation and soil building long before it became a common practice.

One day Dad announced he had purchased a carload of wild horses from Wyoming. He had a circus the day the horses arrived. They were brought in on the railroad and transported to the farm by truck. It took several men to handle these wild animals, each with a brand on its flanks. He had two young men living on the farm who were almost as wild as the horses. I can still see Dad sitting on the top rail of the fence watching those hired hands trying to break the rearing, screaming horses. He was like a boy watching his first rodeo.

After finishing the horse project, my father decided to go into the dairy business. It was necessary to build an addition onto the barn to house the dairy herd. The Pennsylvania Railroad car shops in Terre Haute were busy renovating and rebuilding boxcars and had a large supply of old boxcar siding for sale for next to nothing. Dad decided that the old boxcar siding was just what he needed to build the cow shed. I was pressed into service as a carpenter and spent the summer sawing and hammering and getting my hands full of splinters from the old wood. Finally the project was finished, and Dad started assembling a dairy herd. Eventually he had a herd of thirty-five milk cows. Twice each day these cows were milked by hand—there was no milking machine. The milk was put into sterilized cans, which were placed in a large cooling tank in the milk house. The cooling tank was a large concrete vat filled with water from the well. The water was pumped into the tank by a gasoline engine. My father acquired an old Dodge touring car, and he had the body back of the front seat cut away and a flatbed was built behind. Each morning when I arrived at the farm, my first job was to load the full milk cans on the truck and tie them down for the trip to the Kraft cheese plant in Marshall. As much as 150 gallons of milk were taken into the plant, where the milk was dumped into a large weighing pan. After the milk was weighed and dumped, I drove to the back of the plant, where I filled a number of rusty old milk cans I had brought along with whey. Back at the farm the whey was poured into troughs for the hogs. Nothing was wasted.

Dad always sought better ways to work the farm. He corresponded with the various agricultural schools in the area. One day he received a pamphlet from Purdue University describing a new type of silo that could be constructed at practically no cost. Silage was good feed for the dairy cattle and could supplement the hay and grain that he had been feeding, so we built the silo. This was a trench silo. No one in the whole area had ever heard of such a thing. Silos were huge cylindrical structures that stretched thirty to fifty feet in the air. All the farmers were skeptical. They argued: "Putting silage in the ground and covering it with dirt will make it rot." The argument did not deter Dad. A site was selected on a slope behind the barn. Using slip scrapers pulled by teams of horses, we began slicing the dirt out of the slope. When we finished, we had a huge trench measuring about twenty feet wide, ten feet deep, and fifty feet long. The end down the slope was open. We brought in an ensilage cutter and set it up next to the trench. Next we cut the green corn out of the field and hauled it to the cutter on wagon racks. After the ensilage had been blown into the trench, a layer of dirt about two feet thick was laid over the top and the open end was sealed by a wall of wooden planks with a door placed in the middle of the wall. To the surprise of the skeptics, the ensilage was well preserved and was fed to the cattle.

As a boy, Dad had always wanted a goat, but Grandpa had better things to do with his meager funds than to indulge the whim of a youngster. One day Dad proudly announced he had found a goat for sale. It was a huge "Billy" with long whiskers. No sooner was Billy turned loose than mayhem ensued. Billy ruled the place, walking around with a haughty air, head raised high, chin whiskers moving up and down with the movement of his jaws as he munched on some recently acquired goody. He ate everything in sight and was always on the alert for some unsuspecting person bent over tying a shoe or picking up something from the ground. Butting people was his favorite pastime. Billy was wild with a bad temper. One day he decided to explore the inside of a house, diving through a window, charging through the bedroom, snatching a red necktie from the bedpost, and exiting through the bedroom window. The owner chased Billy but was unsuccessful in catching him. That was the final straw. The goat had to go, but no one could catch him. A few days later the problem was solved. Billy had disappeared. We were all relieved, but our relief was short-lived.

A call was received from Clarksville several miles away. "Did you lose a goat?" Reluctantly, Dad gave an affirmative answer. "What color?" the caller asked. Hoping against hope, Dad described the animal. "Well, it's your goat all right," the man said. "He showed up here a day or so ago and is out in my barn lot. Please get him as soon as you can. I want to get rid of the darned thing. He's tearing up everything on the place." Turning to me, Dad said, "Son, take my car and go up to Reely's at Clarksville. Get the goat and take it back to Cary Miller's down by Spiketown and give it back to him."

HARD WORK on the farm during the summer was good conditioning for a boy who played football in the fall. My junior year I had gained until I weighed a good solid 145 pounds and had increased my height to above five feet eight inches.

That year I was one of twenty-two boys who reported for football. We had some terrific talent and the competition was stiff. The school had meager funds to buy equipment, but the coach was able to scrounge enough money to buy about fifteen new jerseys. He let it be known that the fifteen best members of the squad would be given the jerseys. When the day arrived on which the new jerseys would be doled out, I was overwhelmed when I was given one to wear.

Although I was not a starter, I knew I would get to play a lot. It wasn't long before I got into my first game. What a thrill! The little, skinny guy who had started out two years ago as a scrub was finally in a big game. The quarterback called my number on the first play. The center snapped the ball, and I took off like a rocket. The line in front of me opened a hole. I slid through and directly in front of me was a fullback ready to smash me to the ground. I executed a smart side step and kept running at full speed. Next were the opposing halfbacks running toward me, ready to tie me in knots. Again a side step and a twist of the hips and I was free. The defending quarterback was the last man between me and the goal line. No one could catch me. I was now in high gear. What exhilaration I felt as I streaked across the goal line! A touchdown! My first time in a high school football game—the first time I carried the ball—and I had made a touchdown.

Our team kept rolling along Saturday after Saturday—Gerstmeyer of Terre Haute; Wiley of Terre Haute (we beat them by more points than they had ever been beaten); Martinsville with their galloping ghost; Robinson, Paris, Charleston; and finally our arch rival, Casey, on Thanksgiving Day. We won two games by a score of eighty to zero and had only twelve points scored against us during the season. The next-to-the-last game on the schedule was to be played at Effingham the Saturday before Thanksgiving. Because of a teachers' institute meeting we had no school on the Friday before the game. Our last practice was on Thursday, and we each took our equipment home after practice. I felt unwell and ate much less for supper than usual. I decided to go to bed. My usual routine of eating a big supper, walking uptown to play pool, having a bowl of soup at the restaurant before returning home to bed at nine o'clock, was not followed that night.

Mom knew I was sick. She got a flashlight and looked down my throat. My tonsils were red and swollen and covered by white spots, and my temperature was nearly 104 degrees. I had follicular tonsillitis. When Dad came home, the examination was repeated. He got out his cotton swab and gave my tonsils a good swabbing, then loaded me with aspirin. "Son, you have a badly infected throat, and you will stay in bed until you are well," he said.

Tonsillitis was very serious before penicillin. Complications of scarlet fever or nephritis were common, and the death rate was significant. That fact didn't bother me. I had only one thought in mind. I was going to play in that game Saturday. I dutifully stayed in bed all day Friday, taking aspirin and submitting to frequent throat swabbings.

On Saturday morning, a cold, gray day of rain, sleet, snow, and then rain again, I jumped out of bed and got my clothes on. "Where are you going?" asked Mom. "To Effingham to play ball," I answered. "You are not!" she said, her jaw set firmly. "Well, I feel fine, and I know Dad will let me go," I retorted. "We'll see," she said. Dad then appeared, asking what was going on. "I feel great, Dad, and I've just got to play today," I pleaded. "Well, you do look better, and your throat has improved," he said as he took a look at my tonsils. "I guess it will be all right," he said. Mom didn't argue, but the look on her face was one of complete disapproval.

I grabbed my equipment and took off through the cold rain to the Candy Kitchen, where the bus was waiting. I played a good part of the game, sliding into the icy mud puddles that dotted the playing field. A long, hot shower after the game failed to warm me. I sat huddled up on the bus, wrapped in my overcoat, shivering. I had chills all the way home. My body burned with fever. When I walked in the house, I went straight to bed and stayed there until the following Wednesday. I was feeling much better. The biggest game of the year was on Thanksgiving, the next day. We had been undefeated until now, winning by big scores against the best teams, but the grudge match each year was the Marshall-Casey game played each Thanksgiving. I just had to play in that game. As I had done the Saturday before, I crawled out of bed on Thanksgiving and talked my folks into letting me play.

The day was even colder than the Saturday before. The ground was frozen and covered by a layer of ice. We slid around all afternoon, falling or being knocked to the frozen surface, but we came away from Casey with a six-to-two victory. We were delirious. We had won the Wabash Valley Championship (the first time in the history of our school), this ill-equipped squad of only twenty-two boys.

A victory dinner took place that night at a local restaurant, but I was too sick to attend. My throat was almost swollen shut. It burned as if it was on fire. I was unable to swallow. It was then I made my decision. I wanted my tonsils out, and I didn't want to wait.

"Dad, I want my tonsils out tomorrow," I announced. "What's wrong with you, are you crazy?" he answered. "Don't you know with all that infection it would kill you?" "I don't care. If it isn't done tomorrow, I'll never have it done." The argument went on for some time. Finally, he called the surgeon at Paris Hospital, and they had a long discussion. He came back from the phone with a grave look on his weary face.

"Son, the doctor agrees with me. You may not survive the operation, but he finally agreed it might be worth a try, since you seem so determined," he said. Early the next morning before daylight we went to the hospital. The temperature was almost zero. I was tired and sleepy, and my throat was killing me. I didn't much care what happened. The sore throat I had before was merely a minor scratching sensation compared to how I felt after surgery. I knew the knife had slipped and the surgeon had slit my throat. A cot had been placed in the room for Mom. She was going to stay by me all night long. I didn't know why because I certainly didn't feel like going anywhere. I had slept all day so I wasn't in the mood to sleep that night. About every fifteen minutes I asked what time it was. Poor Mom didn't get any sleep, either. I did manage to doze off about 4:30 A.M., but promptly at 5:00 A.M., a cute, bright-eyed student nurse entered the room with a basin of warm water, washcloths, and towels.

"What's your act?" I managed to squeak. "I'm going to give you a nice warm bath," she announced with a smile. "Like heck you are," I said. "No woman is going to give me a bath. Now get out of here before I dump that water on you."

With that she made a fast exit. Later she tiptoed back in to ask me what I'd like for breakfast. "A pitcher of cocoa I'll take," I said. It wasn't long before I had my hot cocoa. It tasted good and I was hungry. I belted down a glassful and then it happened. All the ether I had taken didn't go into my lungs. Some of it had mixed with the blood I had swallowed and had landed in my stomach. It had just been lying there quietly awaiting the proper catalyst to cause an explosion. That cocoa was the proper catalyst. As soon as it hit my stomach, the explosion came. I threw up all over myself, the bed, and half the room. Old blood mixed with cocoa, gastric juices, and bile, and bearing the fragrance of ether, was plastered everywhere. Mom pushed the call button, and the nurses came running in; what they saw didn't make them happy at all.

"Where's my clothes? I want to get out of this place," I yelled. Remarkably, I felt good. All the bad stuff was out of my stomach. By 6:30 A.M. I was checked out of the hospital and on my way home. As I walked down the hall, the nurses had nothing to say, nothing but heads shaking in a negative way.

When I arrived home, Dad had a serious talk with me. He told me how lucky I was to be alive and that I was going to stay home until I was fully recuperated. "No school for at least a week," he told me. That was great. I was in full agreement. A week's vacation on top of the regular Thanksgiving was wonderful. All week my friends came to visit after school and in the evening. By the end of the week my throat was no longer sore and I could eat anything. Dad told me I could return to school on Monday.

"But you're not going out for basketball," he said. "So far you have been most lucky, and I'm not going to let you stretch your luck any further. If you go into that cold gym wearing that skimpy basketball uniform, you'll end up with pneumonia and I'm not going to have that."

I got a hearty welcome back to school, and the coach told me he had my basketball uniform ready for me. That evening after school I went to the gym, dressed out, and was on the floor shooting baskets when I looked over at the entrance to the gym. There stood Dad in his overcoat with a cigar stub sticking out of the corner of his mouth. He didn't say a word, just glared at me, shook his head, and stalked out. When I came home to supper nothing was said. The folks had given up on me.

During the summer before my senior year, I spent a week at the Methodist Church Epworth League Camp near Springfield. One of the Ellington twins from Martinsville was also there. Martinsville was an arch rival of Marshall, and the Ellington twins were stars for Martinsville. Naturally, Ellington and I discussed the prospects of our two teams for the football season. He confided that he would be playing, but his brother would not because he was ineligible.

Martinsville opened its season with a home game against Shelburn, Indiana. Because our season did not open until a week later, the coach took us with him to Martinsville to "scout" their team. They had an excellent team, the best in years, and they beat Shelburn easily. As I stood watching the game, I saw both Ellingtons in the game. I asked the coach if both boys were playing, or was I seeing double. "No, you're not seeing double. They're both out here," he said. "Why did you ask?" Then I told him about my conversation the previous summer. On the basis of the information I gave the coach, our school investigated and, sure enough, Martinsville had played an ineligible man and, as a result, had to forfeit the game they had won! Thus began the feud between Marshall and Martinsville.

Bill Deahl, a restaurateur of Martinsville, was one of the most rabid fans I have ever seen. He was livid with rage and began a campaign to get even with Marshall. His target became Charley ("Cocky") Bush, our quarterback, a natural athlete. Charley was a star in every sport, and during summer vacation he had spent several weeks visiting relatives and playing baseball in Missouri. Deahl made a trip to Missouri to see if he could dig up some dirt. Upon his return he filed charges against Charley, claiming that he had played professional baseball and therefore was ineligible to play high school football. The state commissioner of athletics conducted a hearing. After examining all the evidence, he ruled that Charley had done nothing that would affect his eligibility.

The entire Martinsville community was furious. Martinsville played at Marshall that year, and I never played in a game that was dirtier. Martinsville punched, slugged, piled on, and kicked. Any Marshall head exposed from under a pileup was jumped on with both feet by a Martinsville player. The officials were kept busy all afternoon ejecting members of the Martinsville team from the game. Finally, they had the last eleven players (the third team) in the game. We won by a big score.

When the basketball season started, the feud continued. The night we played them at Marshall, two boys from our school decided they would have some fun and agitate the people from Martinsville a little more. While the game was in progress, they went to the local chicken hatchery and got a case of eggs that had failed to hatch. As the Martinsville fans left the game, they were met by a barrage of overripe eggs. The Marshall boys made a fast getaway and drove on to Martinsville, where they dumped the remaining eggs on the front porch of the superintendent of schools.

The Martinsville superintendent had lived in Marshall at one time and recognized both boys. The next day he appeared at the courthouse and swore out a warrant for their arrest. They pleaded guilty and were sentenced to sweeping the streets of Marshall for a period of several weeks. That punishment didn't bother either of the boys. They managed to be sweeping the gutters in front of the school each day when school was dismissed.

Marshall had never won the championship of the Eastern Illinois Conference in basketball. The conference was made up of sixteen eastern Illinois high schools. The tournament was played over a span of three days at Casey. We advanced through the preliminaries to the semifinals on Saturday afternoon. Our arch rival, Martinsville, had been eliminated earlier, but the Martinsville fans returned for the games that Marshall played. They were not interested in cheering us on but rather in harassing us. The principal target of their harassment was Charley Bush. The Martinsville people continuously chanted "Boo Bush! Boo Bush!" throughout each game we played. Charley, in spite of his quick temper, maintained his poise and seemed oblivious to the chant. He completely immersed himself in the game.

Saturday night's game was the championship. Our opponent was powerful Robinson, a team that consistently won. The gymnasium was packed. We came out to warm up before the game and were greeted by our faithful hecklers from Martinsville. The referee finally tossed the ball up at center court, and the game was on. The Robinson team, with its power, speed, and good shooting began to work on us. The butterflies in our stomachs were flying about, but soon we scored. As the game progressed, our confidence increased. Bush, with his quickness, ran circles around the defenders. Strohm, with his accurate outside shot, scored, then scored again. Our defense tightened, and we began to force turnovers. At the half the score had evened up. The second half was back and forth all the way.

As a guard I seldom took a shot; in fact, I wasn't particularly accurate. We managed to stay out of foul trouble, and the entire first five played the whole game. The game was nearing the end, and the lead had changed hands many times but was now tied. I was bringing the ball down court and, when I reached center court, I saw that Robinson had everyone covered. I didn't want to cause a turnover now with only a minute or so left to play. Looking down court to the basket, I felt a surge of confidence that I hadn't felt before. I could make that shot. I stopped, carefully pushed off a high archer, and straight to the basket it went, swishing through the net. That was the only basket I made, but we returned to the lead, winning the championship.

Here we were, number one—lined up in the center of the court for the presentation of the huge trophy. Pandemonium prevailed as we proudly carried the trophy to the locker room. Finally, we showered, dressed, and started for Marshall, where a victory dinner at a local restaurant had been prepared. Strohm and I were riding with Mr. Geddes, the principal, with the trophy safely stowed in the trunk of the car. We were discussing the game when we came into Martinsville, and we couldn't believe our eyes. Main Street was lined with people, perhaps as many as two hundred, as we slowly approached.

Mr. Geddes, a mild-mannered man, exclaimed, "My, my, Boys, what is this?" I knew exactly what was going to happen. "Roll up the windows!" I yelled. I had barely gotten the words out when the first eggs hit. Down Main Street we went, running the gauntlet through an enraged mob, eggs flying from both sides of the street. We finally came out on the far side of town. Our caravan went on to Marshall. We had decided that when we got to Marshall we would put our trophy on display in the window of the student hangout—the Candy Kitchen. Just as we stopped in front of the Candy Kitchen, people came pouring out the door as if the place was on fire. We were puzzled. What was wrong? We finally got inside, and it looked like something out of a barroom brawl in a western movie. The two Greeks who owned the place were standing on top of the soda fountain jumping up and down, and broken glass covered the floor. Finally, we were able to calm the proprietors down enough to find out what happened.

Bush had walked in and found a Martinsville boy sitting with his girlfriend, one of our classmates. Bush had restrained himself as long as he could. All of the bottled-up fury caused by the taunting by the Martinsville people throughout the tournament finally exploded. He tapped the boy on the shoulder and quietly told him he had best get out of town. The fellow was six feet tall and weighed a good 170 pounds. Bush was about five feet six inches and weighed 135 pounds. Slowly the boy stood up and said, "I don't know who's going to make me." The bomb went off. Witnesses stated that Bush hit him about six times squarely in the face before he got all the way to his feet and he went down flat on the floor, blood gushing from cuts on his face. Bush turned and walked out. He was perfectly calm—all his anger was gone.

The Martinsville boy was hauled over to Dad's office for repairs. We suddenly realized that Bush might be in deep trouble. The girlfriend of the boy he beat up was the sheriff's daughter. We had a conference and discussed measures we would take to get Bush out of trouble. If he was arrested, we would all chip in to pay the fine. We received a progress report from Dad's office. Dad had to do considerable suturing to repair the damage, and the sheriff was there to watch.

As Dad worked on the poor, beat-up guy, he kept telling him, "You had no business here. You should have stayed in Martinsville. You knew what would happen. It serves you right." Everything Dad said was echoed by the sheriff, who would someday be the father-in-law of this poor guy.

About two weeks later, on a cold night, the main street of Marshall was deserted. The only person in the Candy Kitchen, which was about to close for the night, was Barney Millhouse, one of our football players. As Barney walked out the door, he saw a truck loaded with boys coming down Main Street from the west. He realized immediately these were Martinsville people looking for a fight. He ducked back into the Candy Kitchen and got on the phone calling for reinforcements. Soon boys arrived, coming from all directions. There wasn't much of a fight because the Martinsville boys were outnumbered. They turned around and beat it back home. It was discovered later that some of the Martinsville boys had guns, but, fortunately, there was no bloodshed. The officials of both schools realized things had gotten completely out of control, so they agreed to cease all athletic contests between the two schools for an indefinite period until all emotions were brought back to normal.

Arriving at school one morning, I learned there had been a break-in the night before. There was a large hole in the ceiling of the home economics room. It was assumed the burglars were looking for the silverware stored in the cabinets in the room. It was speculated that the burglar had climbed the fire escape alongside the gym, crossed the roof, and come down through a trap door into the space between the roof and the ceiling of the classroom.

During the noon hour, while I was in the parking lot, I ran into Hobe. He had a worried look on his face, and I knew something was wrong. As soon as we were alone, he said, "I'm going to tell you something, but you must keep it a secret."

There wasn't any break-in last night. It was Jimmie Tingley and me trying to catch some pigeons. I had noticed pigeons flying into an opening under the roof of the building, so we figured we could catch a lot of these birds after they had gone to roost. We came out about 9:00 P.M. and went up the fire escape by the gym. We walked across the roof and went down through the trap door into that space between the roof and the ceilings of the rooms below. I warned Jimmie to be very quiet because I thought there was a meeting going on in one of the rooms below. I also told him to be careful and not step into an open air shaft I knew was there somewhere. This shaft leads to the manual training room in the basement. There isn't any floor in the attic so we had to step on the joists that supported the ceilings of the rooms below. We had flashlights, but we thought we had better not use them. I was stepping carefully from one joist to the next when I missed and went through the ceiling with both feet. I threw out my arms and caught the joists, or I would have fallen clear through to the room below. There I was, hanging by my arms, with the rest of me swinging through the ceiling into the room below, and I could see there was a light on. Jimmie thought I had fallen down the air shaft, but he soon found me and helped me get back up into the attic. We made a fast getaway back out on the roof and down the fire escape. No one came out of the building after us, so we jumped into the car and got away.

After a few days, things got back to normal. The ceiling was patched, an inventory was taken, and nothing was missing. The mystery of the hole in the ceiling was never solved.

One morning, the early risers coming up to the town square were shocked to see what appeared to be a man hanging from the top of the flagpole in the courthouse yard. Closer inspection revealed the "man" was a dummy with a sign attached. On the sign was some sort of symbol—a numeral three with an "M" in the upper part of the numeral and the letter "H" in the lower half. How did that dummy get there and who hung it there? It was a mystery. A few weeks later, another dummy was hung from the parapet of the high school. The same sign was attached. Again, no one knew how it had gotten there. Several weeks later the same symbol appeared, this time painted on the side of the town water tower. For months afterwards, that symbol mysteriously appeared around town. No one could explain the reason, and no one could even come close to guessing who was responsible.

One morning we arrived at the high school and were waiting for the first bell to ring. Suddenly, instead of the bell ringing, we heard the loud noise of an automobile horn. Of course, this brought an uproar of laughter from all the students. The bell system was controlled by the main clock mechanism that automatically rang the bells. All day long, the end of each class period was signaled by the loud squall of the auto horn. The school officials were frantically trying to find the horn, but it was very well hidden somewhere in the building. Finally, the clock mechanism was disconnected, and the bells were rung manually.

The superintendent called a special assembly and questioned the students, trying to find the culprit. He threatened, then he begged, but no one knew a thing. All the rest of the year the class bell was rung manually. The night of graduation arrived, and the seniors in their caps and gowns marched into the gymnasium. The commencement address was given, the diplomas awarded, and the class marched out. Then Jim Stephens, Dean Findley, and Rex Cork walked up to the superintendent.

"Now that we have our diplomas, we have a confession to make. We are responsible for connecting the bell system to a horn, and we will show you where it is," said Jim. They took the superintendent to a remote corner of the attic over the assembly room and there was the horn. Jim was an honor student, almost a genius. He and the other two had made a key that would open the lock on the front door of the school. Late at night, when the building was empty, they came in and connected the horn. Because of the complexity of the bell system, they had to run a separate circuit and splice it into the existing system. This required many hours of work. The superintendent was so relieved that the mystery was solved that he just laughed and congratulated the boys on their ingenuity. "One other thing," said Jim, "we are also known as the Three Marshall Half-Wits." At last, the mystery of the 3MH symbol was solved!

Jim entered Louisiana State University the next year and was a top student. The summer after his freshman year he drowned while swimming. Dean graduated from Purdue with a degree in pharmacy, and Rex had a very successful career with Marathon Oil Company.

7

Off to Purdue

DAD AND MOM hadn't talked to me much about what I was going to do with my life. So far I had enjoyed doing the things I wanted to do—working in the summer, going to school in the winter, having fun with my friends. I had given no serious thought to my future. I had some vague idea that I wanted to be an engineer, but I had not sought any information concerning schools, curricula, or entrance requirements. Since I thought mathematics probably would be one of the more important subjects, I took all the math courses offered. Also, I thought an engineer would be required to know about machinery and the use of tools, so I took all the courses offered in Manual Training along with a course in Farm Mechanics. The school had no such thing as a guidance counselor, so I just floated along. Finally, in my senior year I made up my mind to study engineering and decided on Purdue University. I knew nothing about the school, but I definitely knew that it was my choice.

About this time Dad began to discuss my studying medicine. He was a doctor. Mom was a nurse. I was the only child. It seemed natural to him that I should be in medicine. Besides, I had uncles and cousins who were either doctors or dentists. I didn't want to be a doctor. I definitely wanted to be an engineer. I had made up my mind, and I wasn't going to change it.

Occasionally, I drove for Dad when he made a house call in the country. As we drove along, Dad, puffing on his cigar, would casually bring up the subject of college.

"Well, Son, it's time we get things arranged for you to go to college. We'll drive down to Indiana University at Bloomington and get you set up to start on your premed course," he'd say. "I don't want to go to med school. I want to be an engineer, and I want to go to Purdue. Besides, I don't like being around sick people, and I can't stand the sight of blood," was my answer.

The discussion would get more lively and finally turn into a heated argument. Finally, both of us stopped talking and drove on in silence. Sometimes we wouldn't speak to one another for several days. Finally one day Dad admitted: "I did what I wanted to do, and I guess you have as much right to do what you want to. You go to engineering school and I'll back you." There was never another argument.

I contacted Purdue University and received a catalog and admission forms. After studying the catalog, I decided I wanted to be a mechanical engineer. I forwarded my application with the letters of reference and, after what seemed like an eternity, received a letter of acceptance. My roommate would be Jim Stover, who had been a star halfback on the Marshall football team. Jim attended Purdue on a football scholarship arranged by the Marshall coach, Don Ping.

Mom, Dad, Jim, and I made our first trip to West Lafayette in late summer. Jim and I found a suitable room in a private home on South Grant Street. The rent was set at ten dollars per month for each of us.

Freshman orientation consisted of test-taking. The examinations went on for three days. We were subjected to exams in chemistry, mathematics, English, and even a psychological test (matching up funny-looking squares and triangles, trying to keep from putting square pegs in round holes, looking at ink blotches and trying to imagine what they resembled—a bird, a bug, a man?).

I was confident that the math exam would be a snap because I had taken numerous math courses in high school—algebra, plane geometry, advanced algebra, trigonometry, and solid geometry—and had made excellent grades. Unfortunately, the exam had me baffled. I finally muddled my way through, but I knew I had done badly.

The English exam also caught me in a depressed state. The exam sheet contained one sentence: Write a theme, not to exceed one thousand words, on any subject. I hadn't been particularly fond of English in high school but had managed to get through. What could I write in one thousand words or less that would be interesting and might catch the eye of an English professor? Suddenly an idea popped into my mind. Mom had told me once about Grandpa's trying to learn to drive an automobile. He had always driven horses and had nothing but contempt for the automobile, in his opinion a newfangled invention that would never be a success. Uncle Tom had finally prevailed on him to at least give it a try. With that plot for a story, I proceeded to fashion an account of Grandpa's encounter with the automobile, combining a mixture of fact and fiction. My final effort was not bad, but not particularly good either.

Finally, we had a thorough physical examination. We were told that if we flunked the physical we wouldn't have to take ROTC military training. I had no desire to participate in such activities. Marching had no appeal for me and, besides, I considered myself a lover, not a fighter. I knew that flat feet would disqualify me so when I stepped barefoot on the glass-topped box with the mirror slanted at an angle below, I wiggled my feet and tried to flatten them out. The doctor, seated in a chair, looked in the open end of the box where he could get a good look at the bottom of my feet reflected in the mirror. "Feet perfect," he told the recorder. I had failed in my attempt to flunk. I was a perfect physical specimen. I was a prime candidate for the military.

A few days later I got the results of all the testing. Chemistry was a complete bust, as I had expected—I made a total grade of ten out of a possible hundred. Math I flunked. I was informed I would be required to take a noncredit math course, which actually was a review of high school math. The score in psychological testing was satisfactory and, of course, my physical exam qualified me to take military training. My score in English, however, was very high. Grandpa's story had made me a winner in this category. I was excused from taking freshman English, given credit for the course, and placed in a sophomore course in writing. After looking over my scores, I didn't consider myself a winner. In fact, I wondered if I would be permitted to register. This was the depression era, and perhaps the university was hard up for the fifty-dollar tuition paid by out-of-state students.

Registration was a mob scene in the armory. There were more people in that building than twice the population of Marshall. I was lost and confused. It took me almost two hours to work through the mob and complete my registration, finally coming to the area for military registration. To my surprise, I was handed a paper sack and told to get in line.

First, I was given a cap and then told to remove my shirt and tie and put them in the sack. The soldier threw me a khaki shirt. Again the order was "Put it on." Then came the khaki wool coat (or "blouse," as I later learned was the proper name). Next, off came my pants and into the sack they went. A pair of wool khaki riding pants was thrown in my direction. These I put on and was surprised that they almost fit. Next came the leggings, canvas on the outer side of my calves and leather on the inner side. I decided the leather was there to cut down on the wear and tear when I straddled a horse. The leggings had a long, heavy lace that ran through the eyelets on one side and over hooks on the other side. I began to thread the lace tediously through the eyelets and over the hooks. If I had to do that every day, I would need to get out of bed an hour earlier than usual in order to get to class on time. (It never dawned on me that once the eyelets were threaded it was a simple matter to pull a loop through and hook it over the hook, finally pulling the upper free end of the lace tight and tying it snugly.) After my encounter, I was dressed in full uniform except for shoes.

"We don't fit you with shoes," I was told. "Take this order slip to the local shoe store. They will fit you with army shoes, and the cost will be ten dollars." I'd never had a ten-dollar pair of shoes in my life, and now my first expensive shoes were to be army shoes, which I didn't want in the first place. As I turned to leave, the sergeant barked: "Get those shoes pronto. You must be in full uniform when you report for your first class."

As I walked slowly down the street to my room carrying my paper sack full of civilian clothes, wearing a uniform that did not fit, my white shoes a sharp contrast to the drab army khaki, the words of the sarge, "You're in the army now. You're in the army now," kept going through my mind. I wondered what terrible crime I had committed during my relatively few years on this earth that would cause me to be subjected to that kind of treatment.

My noncredit math course was like nothing I had ever experienced before. It was taught by Dr. Hazard, whose name accurately described the man. There were about twenty-five hapless souls in the class, and Dr. Hazard saw to it that he made life miserable for each of us. He was a large man with a florid face and appeared to be in a permanent state of rage. His daily routine was to call the class to order and then begin a tirade. Walking slowly up and down the aisle, he told us how dumb we were and that we shouldn't be there in the first place. At times his voice would rise to a crescendo, nearly to a scream, his face would be livid, and his heavy jowls would quiver. When it appeared a stroke was imminent, he would let out a big sigh like air escaping from a punctured tire, then slowly walk back to his desk shaking his head. In between these tirades he taught us math. Each day he gave us an impossible amount of homework that had to be completed and placed on his desk the next day. Even though the problem had been worked properly and the answer was correct, it was marked wrong if the line between the numerator and denominator was a fraction too long or too short or if the equal sign was not made to his satisfaction. He never told students what their mistakes were.

"Why don't you go back to the farm, where you belong," was his stock statement. One day, when he had been particularly obnoxious, just as he passed my seat, he made a snide remark that burned me to the quick. Under my breath I said, "Go to hell!" His sharp ears caught my remark and he whirled around, face red, eyes blazing. I thought he was going to hit me, but he regained control of himself. "What did you say?" he bellowed. "Nothing, not a thing," I meekly replied in a very small voice.

Chemistry was a whole new experience. I was completely baffled by the formulas, symbols, and terminology. The chemistry laboratory was a disaster. All the fragile equipment and glassware brought me nothing but grief. I believe I set a new school record for equipment breakage. I soon used up the fee required from each student and had to put more money in the till. I spent long hours studying. I memorized formulas, conducted experiments in spite of my clumsiness, and finally was able to bring some order out of chaos.

In English I fared better. I had Professor Cordell, the perfect image of an Ivy League professor. He had a closely cropped mustache, black hair with a trace of gray, and he usually wore a slightly wrinkled tweed suit. His tiny office off the landing at the top of the stairs in Old University Hall was always cluttered with books and papers. The musty smell of old books, mixed with the odor of pipe tobacco, permeated the room. When not in the classroom, Professor Cordell could usually be found at his desk writing or comfortably lounging in an old chair reading, completely relaxed, his pipe emitting an occasional puff of smoke. His office door was always open, and a visit from one of his students was always welcome.

The machine shop—with row after row of lathes, drill presses, and milling machines—was a new experience. Power for the machinery came from an elaborate overhead system of pulleys and belts. Each student learned the basics in the operation of each machine. We were required to cut a set of gears to within exact tolerances and to mount the gears on a base so that they would mesh and operate perfectly. We learned to read blueprints and became skilled in the use of calipers and the micrometer. In the pattern-making shop we constructed wooden patterns to scale. These patterns were used in the foundry to make the molds. I especially liked working in the foundry. The instructor was an old man named Wendt with a thick German accent. It was obvious his education had been attained not through the formality of a university but through practical experience, first as an apprentice and then as a journeyman. He was a master of the craft, and he taught us a great deal.

My roommate had come to Purdue to play football. Although I was no star like Jim, I loved the game, so I went over to the gym to see if I could go out for the freshman team. I wasn't very big—only five feet eight and 140 pounds—but I wanted to play. I was issued a set of equipment and told to report to the freshman coach. Practice began each afternoon at 3:00 P.M. and continued until nearly 8:00 P.M. The first hour was spent in conditioning calisthenics and wind sprints. I had never worked so hard in my life. There were nearly a hundred freshmen out for practice each day. (More than four times as many as we had on the entire squad in high school.) I was one of the smallest on the squad. Most were on football scholarships and had been superstars in high school.

I soon found out what part the freshman played in the entire scheme. We were the "gun fodder." We were given the plays of next week's opponent. We learned the plays and ran them repeatedly until we thought we had them perfect; then several teams would be sent up to the varsity practice field. The members of the varsity squad were giants. I had never seen a college football game in my life and I couldn't believe the size of these men—180, 200, 225, even 250 pounds. Not anyone even close to my weight and height. Several of the members of the varsity had received all-American recognition. Although we were expected to give these supermen competition, it didn't take me long to see why so many freshmen were needed. The varsity chewed us up like a dog would a rabbit. (A fractured hand interrupted my football career first semester.) Jim and I dragged ourselves home each night, stopping at Mom Campbell's boardinghouse for supper. Mr. Campbell worked in a large butcher shop in Lafayette but had only one or two days' work a week because of the depression. However, because he was a longtime employee, the owner gave him a discount on meat.

"Mom" had several children of her own and was most generous to us. The table was loaded with all the good food imaginable, and there were no restrictions on the amount one could eat. The price was right, too—thirty dollars a month for thirteen big meals each week. Jim and I got by for breakfast on a pint of milk each, which was left on the doorstep every morning by the milk deliveryman. I detested milk, but it was cheap and I had to have something in my stomach before going to class. His mother and my mother alternated in sending us homemade cookies to supplement the milk diet.

We had little time for social activities. Occasionally, we dropped over to visit some friends who were from Marshall. Dean Findley and Leland Baker were good friends who were finishing their last year at Purdue. Dean was in the School of Pharmacy, and Leland was in the School of Science. They had a ground-floor, rear apartment over on State Street. Roger Mann lived with them. He was a graduate student and instructor in the biology department. Roger was a rather quiet, studious type.

The bull sessions we had were a welcome break in the routine of study. Some of our discussions reached great philosophical heights, thanks to the presence of Roger. One night when we arrived for a visit with our three friends, we were surprised to see Roger sitting on the back of the sofa with a faraway expression on his face. Dean and Leland motioned us to a seat on the floor across the room. What was going on here? What was our quiet, reserved Roger doing sitting on the back of the sofa? Then we noticed he had a wadded-up handkerchief in one hand and a can in the other. As we watched, he poured some of the contents of the can on the handkerchief, then began sniffing the handkerchief. Dropping the can, he suddenly threw both arms in the air and shouted, "I'm in heaven and it is beautiful." He launched into an elaborate description of heaven, the beautiful colors he was seeing, the purple mountains, the clean rushing steams, and the green meadows. Suddenly he stopped and climbed to the top of the sofa and, standing there weaving back and forth with arms in the air, said, "I can fly like a bird." Then he jumped to the floor, losing his balance and rolling to the corner of the room. About that time we got a good strong whiff of ether. Roger was on an ether jag. Where had he gotten it? After sobering up, he told us he had brought a can of the stuff home from the experimental lab at the biology department. He wanted to conduct an experiment on himself to determine the effects of ether on the human being. It was easy to see that ether had a profound effect. It had completely changed Roger's personality from a quiet, serious person to one who was totally uninhibited, one who was hallucinating. (Later on, Roger became the dean of the School of Medicine and vice president of the University of Tennessee.)

It seemed that a good part of my ROTC training consisted of learning the art of modern warfare, communications, tactics, map reading, and all the other things a good soldier should know.

Out on the floor of the huge armory, we were put through the paces by Sergeant Purchla, an old army veteran. We had close order drills, with the sergeant barking out the orders and counting the cadence, "One, two, three, four, to the rear march; column right; column left; about-face; attention; at ease; parade rest," and all the other commands in the manual.

All of our equipment was left over from World War I. There were 155mm howitzers, 75mm guns, and five-ton Holt Caterpillar tractors. Each company was divided into squads of eight men each. Each squad was assigned a gun or a howitzer. We were drilled in the art of setting a weapon in place and firing it. I noted early that the number one man in the gun squad had the easiest job and he also got to sit on the little seat to the right of the gun breech, so I worked myself into that position. All I had to do was open and close the breech block by moving a handle and set the range by turning a crank. The rest of the squad had to move around, getting the shell and shoving it into the breech, swabbing the tube after the gun was fired, picking up the trail and moving it around to position the gun. Learning to handle the tractor was more interesting. The tractor was maneuvered by the movement of what looked like oversized handlebars mounted on a post directly in front of the seat and by the manipulation of foot pedals. These clumsy monsters moved at slow speed even when the throttle was wide open. The tractor was simple to steer so I had no problem—push on the right pedal and push the handlebar right for a right turn and do the same with the left handlebar and pedal to turn left. What nearly flunked me, though, were the arm signals. Communicating verbally was impossible because of the roar of these tractors, so the army had devised an elaborate system of arm signals. There were signals to start, signals to stop, signals to speed up, signals to slow down, signals for right by squad and left by squad, column left and column right, and on and on. We were given detailed instructions on the use of arm signals by a regular army captain and then ordered to mount our mechanical charger. The captain led us out to the drill field to practice our maneuvers. Suddenly, he gave the signal "Column right." I already had forgotten what this indicated, so as the rest of the column was going along to the right, I took off alone in the opposite direction. The captain waved his arms, his face bright red with anger. Everyone stopped and he came running over and gave me a lecture on the rudiments of tractor driving, ordered me off the thing, and sent me back to the armory for more instructions. After two or three more tests, I finally mastered the signals.

I had chewed tobacco since I was about fifteen years old, and when I went to college, I didn't quit. Chewing tobacco had a soothing effect on my nerves and being in the army sure made me nervous. During inspection one day, the commanding officer stopped immediately in front of me and, looking me straight in the eye, asked, "What do you have in your mouth?" "A chew of tobacco, Sir," I answered. "That will be ten demerits," he said and walked on. I decided right then that this was really a sissy outfit—wouldn't even let a man enjoy a good chew.

One day the captain said, "You are to be in charge of the wire-laying crew." I had never been in charge of anything since I had been at Purdue. Now I was to have a position of authority. Our mission was to lay one line of communication to the observation post from the portable switchboard and another line to the gun position. All of that was to take place in the countryside west of the campus. We were assembled on the drill field, given a briefing and a set of maps, and sent on our way. Our tractor had a reel of rubber-insulated, heavy copper wire in tow. Each man in the crew had a specific job to perform, and I was the boss. Going down a gravel road, we came to a creek that we crossed over a concrete bridge. I ordered the crew to halt and took out my map. Yes, this was the spot marked on the map as the location of the switchboard.

We unloaded the portable switchboard from the tractor, and the men carried it down under the bridge and started to connect it to the line that had been reeled out. Two men were to be left to man the switchboard. Everyone began to sniff. Something smelled awful. About that time one of the men spotted the body of a badly decomposed dog lying in the creek. The two switchboard men began to protest loudly. "You can't expect us to sit next to this dead dog," groaned one of them. "I do expect that," I replied, with a ring of authority in my voice. "This is war, and the switchboard has to be at this location, dog or no dog."

I took the rest of the crew and proceeded to lay the line on to the observation post and gun enplacement. After the problem in communication was completed, we were ordered to take down the switchboard and rewind all the cable back on the reel. The instructions were to run the tractor at low speed with two men walking behind the reel, letting the cable run through their hands to feel for breaks. After a few minutes, I decided we were going to be late getting back to the drill field for dismissal, so I ordered a speedup. The driver put the tractor in high gear, and the men behind let go of the cable. We all piled aboard the tractor and went merrily down the road. The reel was spinning like a top, and the cable was running back on without a hitch. I had forgotten one detail. When the last hundred feet or so of cable hit the reel, it was like a king-size backlash on a fishing reel. The writhing cable came flying through the air like a big snake entwining the entire tractor. Cable was woven in and out through the treads, around the radiator and engine. What a mess. I carefully surveyed the situation and quickly made a command decision.

"Men, get out your wire cutters." Each man had a set of tools fastened to his belt, and each kit contained a pair of wire cutters. The men eagerly got to the job of slicing up the cable that failed to get back on the reel. Soon I had an armload of expensive rubber-covered copper cable. No piece was more than two feet in length. The emergency delayed our return to the drill field. We were the last to arrive. The captain was fuming, pacing up and down in front of the rest of our company. With all the dignity I could muster, I climbed down from the tractor, marched up to the captain, presented him my armload of cuttings, stepped back, gave him a snappy salute, an about-face and stepped into line with the rest. I thought he was going to have a stroke. I was never put in charge of anything again during my two years in ROTC.

Purdue was more difficult than I had imagined. I don't recall that I ever got homesick, but coming back to school after Christmas was one of the hardest things I ever had to do. As the days went by before the approaching exams, I felt like a condemned man waiting for the day of execution. I received my examination schedule and saw to my horror that chemistry was the first on my list of final exams. Until then, I knew I had an average below passing. I tried to study, but the more I studied, the less I knew. I just couldn't remember all those formulas. Finally came the night before the exam. I sat at my study table in my lonely room. The room was dark except for the light from my study lamp, glaring down on my opened chemistry book. Jim was already asleep. He didn't have to worry. He didn't have to take chemistry.

I crawled into bed and lay there for awhile, staring into the dark. Little symbols were running around my head—H_2SO_4, HC_1, $AgHO_4$. They kept running into each other and getting all mixed up. It's a miracle they didn't finally get together to form some exotic explosive mixture that would have blown my brain to pieces. Finally, I dropped off to sleep.

The next morning I just wanted to "get it over with." As I walked out the door, the cold chill hit me. The gray sky was spitting out a cold rain mixed with sleet. It was as if even the elements had only contempt for this upstart who thought he could leave that small country town and come to a prestigious university and make his mark. When I opened the test book, I could barely believe my eyes. We were to answer any ten out of twelve questions and had three hours to complete the examination. Of the twelve questions, I actually knew the answer to ten. It didn't take me long to complete the examination. I turned in my exam book and walked out of the room, almost dancing. Going down the steps to the sidewalk I looked up at the sky. It was still a cold, gray, damp day, but for me the sun was shining. My final grade for the semester was a "B." After the ordeal of the chemistry exam, the rest of the tests were a breeze, even math.

Starting the second semester, I had gained confidence in myself and the subjects I was taking were more interesting. My math grades through differential and integral calculus were all A's. The beating I had taken at the hands of Dr. Hazard really taught me something. His methods were certainly unorthodox, but they were most effective. I no longer hated him.

Spring football practice was going to start soon. My fractured hand had healed, and the coach told me he was expecting me at spring practice. I kept in condition during the winter by working out in the gym. I ran around the indoor track and even tried some wrestling. By opening day of spring practice, I had put on some weight and was ready to go. A week or so after the competition of spring training the list of freshmen numeral winners was posted. My name was on the list. I was presented with a black, heavy wool sweater with the gold numeral "35" affixed to the front. I was a bona fide member of the class of '35 freshman football team. I constantly wore my sweater as I went about the campus. I was so proud.

I didn't think I was big enough or talented enough to play varsity football, and I knew that football would take a lot of time I needed for study if I were going to be a success in engineering, so I decided to concentrate on my education, leaving football to the experts. I had had a lot of fun and proven to myself I could succeed in the sport even though I wasn't particularly talented.

G. A. Young was a man I'll never forget. I first met him when he greeted the incoming class of mechanical engineering students. He stood at the front of the auditorium, a short, stocky man in a rumpled suit, the head of the School of Mechanical Engineering. "I want you to know I think of you all as my boys," he said. "My name is G. A. Young, and I don't want you to call me professor, doctor, or mister. I want you to call me 'GA.' The door of my office is always open. You don't need an appointment to see me. If you have a problem, no matter how small or insignificant, you'll know where to find me. Come in and we'll talk things over and find a solution." With that introduction, he started to tell us about our school. He informed us that these meetings would continue throughout the year, and since it was considered a noncredit course, attendance wasn't required. No one in the class would have missed one of these sessions for anything. GA had many stories to tell us about the university—things that had happened since the university was founded—the traditions and the customs that had developed over the years. His eyes would light up, and his voice would ring with emotion and enthusiasm. He loved the school and his job.

GA was highly respected in the field of engineering, and his reputation as an expert in the field of tank car rail transportation was without par. He frequently told us about his trips as an expert consultant. He would chuckle and boast: "They paid me five hundred dollars a day, and actually I spent only two or three hours of the day doing what I was being paid to do. The rest of the day I played golf." I suspect he was prouder of his golf score than he was of his achievements as an engineer.

Years later as an intern at Methodist Hospital, I noticed a familiar name on a list of new admissions: GA Young. Could it be? I went up to the floor and got the chart. The information on the admission sheet on the front of the chart confirmed it. It was my GA. I walked through the door, and there in bed was GA, much older than when I had last seen him. He looked tired, but there was the old twinkle in his eyes and the grin across his face when he saw me standing there in my white intern uniform, stethoscope hanging around my neck. "Boy," he exclaimed as he held out his arms, "what in the world are you doing here? I thought I had made an engineer out of you." After all those years, he recognized me. He didn't remember my name, but he knew I was one of his boys.

Bill Miller was a professor in the School of Mechanical Engineering. He was a big man with an ample waistline. All of his students loved him because he treated us as equals, never putting us down. He was very intelligent and knew how to teach. I had him for an air-conditioning course, and I also had him for the steam laboratory.

Bill and I had something in common—we both chewed tobacco. I would sit in class with a chew in, and Bill would be up front also with a chew in, lecturing on some aspect of air-conditioning, drawing diagrams on the board. Suddenly he would stop and walk to the rear of the room, raise the window, and unload a thick stream of tobacco juice. I would be right behind waiting my turn. After Bill had turned from the window, I would unload, close the window, and return to my seat. That act was repeated several times during the course of the hour.

One day we were running an efficiency test on a steam engine in the lab. Two platform scales had been set up with a tank on each one. One tank held the feed water for the engine, and the other contained the condensate that was collected from the exhaust. The weights of the contents of each tank were used in computing the efficiency. Bill and I were chewing tobacco as usual. He sidled over to where I was working and said, "Mitch, you spit in that barrel and I'll spit in the other so we won't foul up our computation. I figure that way things will balance out."

At Christmas time we kept alive one of the many traditions. Each member of Bill's class brought a package or plug of chewing tobacco to the last class before Christmas. At some time during the period when his back was turned, the signal was given, and Bill was pelted with chewing tobacco. He would whirl around looking surprised, but it was well known that he always came to class the last day before Christmas with an empty bushel basket to carry his loot home.

8

From Engineering to Medicine

I CONTINUED TO WORK on the farm during summer vacation. We had completed thrashing on the Kimes's place, and all that remained was a huge stack of straw. Dad wanted the straw stack baled and engaged a man to do the job. He had a standard stationary baler with a gasoline engine mounted on top to power the machinery. Of course, it was pulled between locations by a team of horses. He had a distance of several miles to come from his home to our place. It was a hot day, and Dad decided I should take a team and meet him a few miles down the road so that our fresh team could replace his team. I knew he was coming out west on the National Road so I went south through Spiketown. At Spiketown one road angled off to the east and the road I was on went on south to the National Road, where there was a filling station; I knew I could get a cold bottle of pop and a candy bar there. I tied the team to the fence, got my pop and candy bar, and sat down under a shade tree.

Suddenly I thought about the road that angled off at Spiketown. That was the road I should have followed because further to the east it joined the National Road. I jumped back on the team and started at a gallop back up toward Spiketown. When I got there, there was no sign of the baler, but the tracks of the baler wheels in the dust told me I had missed the meet. I galloped on back toward the farm and finally caught sight of the baler. When I pulled up, we were in sight of the farm. I told the man I was sorry I had missed him and offered to replace his team with mine, but he said there was no need; his team wasn't tired so I started on up the road. About that time I saw a cloud of dust up ahead, and my worst fears were realized. It was Dad in his Model A. He skidded to a stop, his face red as a beet, cigar clamped between his teeth, and wearing his ever-present straw sailor hat. "Why didn't you change teams?" he growled. I meekly told him what had happened. With both hands, he lifted his hat, jammed it back down on his head and exploded, "Damn," and roared on down the road.

He always brought out a warm lunch that Mom had prepared for me but that day I wondered if I would eat. Nevertheless, about noon he showed up and handed me the basket, without saying a word. That night when I came in, Mom asked what had happened. "What do you mean?" I asked. "Well," she said, "I knew something had happened because your dad came home before noon and kept stomping around the house and through the kitchen muttering to himself." By the next day Dad and I were back on good terms, and nothing was ever said again. That was Dad's way. He was quick to explode, but just as quick to forgive and forget.

Even with the hard work, the farm was a rewarding experience. The outdoors was stimulating. The clean, fresh air I remember most: in the summer, the smell of new-mown hay and the sweet smell of wild honeysuckle, with the bees gathering nectar to make their honey; the smell of growing corn on a warm, humid night; the cool, crisp air in the fall, with the pungent odor of burning leaves; the cold air in the winter that stung the nostrils; the white blanket of snow, untouched by grime and dirt or disturbed by footprints; the firm, clear ice on the creeks, broken only where the water bubbled over a riffle of rocks; the awakening in the spring with the first flowers popping up in the woods; the croak of frogs; the songs of returning birds and the smell of the good earth as the plow first dipped its point down to bring up the soil that had rested through the winter. To me these were the good things about the country that city folks had no opportunity to enjoy.

We hauled the hay from the Kimes's place and put it in the hayloft of our barn. Almost every time I passed the Murphy farm, I would come upon little George sitting out front in the middle of the road in his wagon with his dog hitched to the front. He was like a statue. I would yell at him to move out of the way, but he would just sit there, staring up at me as if to say, "I am here and you will have to figure some way of getting around." Eventually, I would wrap the lines around the standards on the wagon, crawl down from atop the load, and lead the dog, wagon, and George to the side of the road so I could pass.

On down the road was the Pleasant Grove School, a one-room schoolhouse. A swarm of bees had taken up housekeeping under the eaves, and as I came along with a load of hay one day, they came out to greet me. I was afraid they would attack the horses and start a runaway if I relaxed my hold on the reins. I gripped the lines tightly with both hands and held on. I was getting by the dangerous spot when one bee sat down on my nose. I couldn't let go to knock it loose.

All I could do was sit there looking cross-eyed at the thing. Finally, he sank his stinger in and took off.

I was unloading a load of hay at the barn one day when the hayfork became fouled up. We had what was called a harpoon fork. It was a long steel rod, with two sharply pointed metal pieces hinged to one end. The sharp metal pieces were in a position parallel to the main shaft until they were stuck in the hay. A pull on the trip rope would then bring the two points out at right angles to the shaft. The big rope attached to the shaft ran up to a pulley on the carrier that ran along a track stretching the length of the haymow. The rope ran through a pulley at the other end of the haymow and down through a pulley at ground level, then on out to where it was attached to a team. After the hayfork was anchored in the hay on the wagon, a signal was given, and the driver would start the team up. This pulled the hay up to the carrier, where it was locked in place and carried along the track and dumped into the mow. The hot job was working in the mow throwing the hay around.

One day I was in a hurry, and the load of hay got jammed in the carrier. I dumped the hay back down on the wagon, but the carrier was still jammed. A ladder was fastened to the side of the barn, so I started up the ladder as fast as I could climb. I didn't look up to see where the carrier was, and before I knew it, I received a blow on the top of my head. I had hit the sharp harpoon with my head. The blood poured out and down over my face and into my eyes. I held on to the ladder, cussed a little, got the carrier untangled, went back down the ladder and over to the horse tank. I dunked my head into the cold water, and finally the bleeding was checked. I went back to work. As Dad said, "Hard work builds character," so I built a bit more character that day.

PURDUE WAS ALWAYS EXCITING, but as I came along through my junior and senior years, it became more interesting. Having gotten the basics out of the way, I was introduced to the technical aspects of mechanical engineering—thermodynamics, heating and ventilation, machine design, and certain aspects of electrical and civil engineering. My major was aeronautical engineering, and most of my senior year was spent learning the basics of aerial navigation and the design of airplanes. One project was to produce an original design of an airplane, including the engine.

I was soon invited to join the Purdue Glider Club. We flew from a field that was given to the university by its great benefactor, David Ross. The club owned one glider. It was called a primary glider and it was just that. It looked somewhat like the Wright Brothers' plane without an engine, except it was a high-winged monoplane. There was no fuselage. The wing was supported by a center post. A long wooden piece extended back to support the tail assembly. There were no wheels, just a wooden skid that supported the entire assembly. A small wooden seat was fastened above the skid in front of the vertical post. The pilot sat on the seat with a safety belt around his waist, holding the control stick with his hand, his feet on the rudder bar. Out in front, on the end of the skid, was a big clasp with a trip wire running back to the pilot. After limited instructions from the more experienced pilots, the novice was strapped into the seat, the tow wire hooked into the clasp on the end of the skid. Then it was time to take off.

A tow car was the means of propulsion. It was stripped down to nothing but the running gear. There were oversized tires on the wheels to give better traction. A thousand-foot wire cable was hooked to the rear of the car, and the other end was fastened to the hook on the glider. One man stood at each wingtip, balancing the glider as the tow car stretched the cable tight. At the signal from the pilot, the car started forward into the wind. The men at the wingtips ran alongside until the wing picked up enough draft to stay level. At about forty miles an hour, the glider lifted off and started to climb. The tow car kept moving on until the glider was high up into the air. Then the pilot pulled the release, dropping the cable. Depending on the amount of updraft, the plane might soar a minute or two or much longer. Finally, the pilot banked and turned and came back to the field, landing on the skid. It was like riding a big kite. We really never thought about the danger involved, sitting unprotected on a small board out in the open with no parachute.

One day I was all set to take off, my ever-present cigar between my teeth. Everything went well. The tow car started off smoothly, the glider picked up speed, and the liftoff was good. Suddenly, when the glider was about forty feet in the air, the main support wire to the wing snapped. The whole thing came down in one big pile. The others came running to get me out. They dug down and there I was, my mashed cigar still in my mouth. I crawled out and didn't even have a scratch, but right then I made a decision. I was going to learn to fly something that had an engine.

The land given to the university by David Ross was an excellent site for an airport, but there were no funds for development. However, exercising good old Yankee ingenuity, the university was able to get the job done. One day I sat in the office of Dr. G. Stanley Meikle, the director of Research Relations for the university, and listened to the amazing account of how the feat was accomplished. Dr. Meikle had made it a top priority item, but we were in the depths of the Great Depression. The university was hard put to get enough funds to keep itself in operation. Faculty salaries were pitifully inadequate, and there was no money available for new equipment or capital improvements.

One day Dr. Meikle went to see President Elliott, and they discussed the airport project. Finally Dr. Elliott said, "Stanley, we simply have no money for such a project, but I can let you have a thousand dollars from the President's Fund to use in any way to try to get things started." Dr. Meikle first thought of talking to Mr. Shambaugh, who owned a small airport south of Lafayette, about buying his hangars and moving them to the Purdue site, but he quickly abandoned that idea. The hangars were old sheet metal buildings and, even if they could be moved without breaking them up, they would not be satisfactory. Finally, he decided to gamble. He took the money and made a trip to Washington. He lobbied the Congress and made such a favorable impression that Congress agreed to put up fifty thousand dollars in funds if the state of Indiana would match the grant. He then made a trip to Indianapolis, where he again used his powers of persuasion on the legislature. The legislature voted to match the federal funds, and the ball was rolling. An eighty-thousand-dollar brick hangar, complete with repair shops, offices, and control tower, was built. (The building is still in use today.)

He next persuaded the federal government to move the weather station from Wolcott to Purdue. The airport was in business. Captain Aretz, who was a seasoned pilot and instructor, was employed to supervise the airport activities. He had been a flight instructor in World War I and looked the part. He was a tall, slender man with a weathered face and a well-groomed mustache. He always wore riding breeches and boots. He immediately started giving flying lessons, using a Waco F plane that he owned.

Although I continued as a member of the Purdue Glider Club, I still wanted to learn to fly a plane with an engine so I checked with Captain Aretz. I found that lessons cost twelve dollars per hour. I did not have that kind of money, but with careful saving, I finally had enough money for my first hour of instruction. What a thrill it was climbing into the rear cockpit of the Waco F the first time! I had never flown in an airplane before. "Cap" had given me some basic instructions beforehand and told me he would fly me around and would talk to me from the front cockpit as we flew. We communicated by a primitive speaking tube arrangement. The only instruments were an altimeter, a gauge that measured the revolutions per minute of the engine, a simple compass, an oil gauge, and a gasoline gauge. The throttle was mounted on the left side of the cockpit and could be moved back and forth on a quadrant. Forward movement opened the throttle and movement to the rear closed the throttle. The engine switch was mounted on the instrument panel in front. There were dual controls—rudder bar and stick—in the front and rear cockpits. I got settled in, my seat belt fastened, flying helmet with chin strap fastened, goggles down over my eyes, both feet on the rudder bar, and both hands on the stick, which stuck up between my legs. After the mechanic turned the propeller over, I switched on the ignition. Then, grabbing the tip of the propeller with both hands, the mechanic gave a kick with one leg and a mighty pull. The engine coughed and came to life. Cap looked at the wind sock, taxied out to the end of the field, and turned into the wind. He sat briefly to let the engine warm, then pushed the throttle full forward. Slowly we picked up speed, bumping across the uneven terrain.

The stick was pushed gently forward, the tail came up, and suddenly the bumping stopped. We were airborne. Gradually we climbed until we were almost a thousand feet up; then we made a sweeping left turn and continued to climb. It was a different world aloft—banking first to the left, then to the right, climbing and descending. The roar of the engine seemed to become less noticeable. The wind in my face was exhilarating. Cap kept talking to me through the speaking tube, telling me what he was doing and why. I could feel the movement of the rudder bar and stick as he maneuvered about. Finally, he let me try my hand. My movements were clumsy—too far forward or backward on the stick (which later placed me in a dive or approached a stall, but I was in no danger because Cap corrected my movement by his hand on the stick). My use of the rudder was just as clumsy, but I soon realized these controls were sensitive and only a touch was needed to change direction.

Gradually I began to get the hang of things. My coordination improved, and my turns became smoother. The hour flew by and it was time to land. Cap made his approach and went into the final glide. Gently we came down and he reduced the power. Finally he cut the throttle clear back, and it felt as if the bottom dropped out. At that point he pulled clear back on the stick, and the wheels touched the ground with scarcely a bump. As we rolled to a stop, Cap turned around with a grin on his face, "How did you like it?" he asked. The grin on my face was my answer.

My glider experience was a help in learning to fly an airplane since the basic controls were the same, but the addition of power from the engine provided more flexibility. I wasn't at the mercy of the wind currents in powered flight. It took me several months to get in my flight instruction. Each time I managed to get some cash, I put in some time. Cap was very patient. He didn't push me but gradually gave me more leeway.

I practiced takeoffs and landings until it seemed I could do them in my sleep. One day we went out for some more instruction. I was soon doing all the flying, and Cap was going along for the ride. I had all the confidence in the world. I took off, flew around for awhile, when Cap suddenly said, "Let's go in." I made my approach and came in for a smooth landing. Without a word, Cap unbuckled his safety belt, flipped up his goggles, and climbed out. "She's all yours, take her up," he said and nonchalantly strode off. There I sat all alone in the cockpit. Where was all that confidence I had? My mouth got dry, and it felt like someone had shoved a wad of cotton in it. I said to myself, "George, it's now or never," so I revved up the motor and turned into the wind. Everything that I had been taught came clearly to mind. I pushed the throttle forward. I picked up speed and gently pushed the stick forward, keeping the rudder bar steady. As I became airborne, I gradually brought the stick back little by little. I was flying all by myself. What a great feeling! After circling around, I came in for a landing—the moment of truth. Gradually I brought the plane down when I felt the bottom drop out. I cut the engine and brought the stick back, but I had jerked the stick instead of gradually bringing it back and I bounced and was airborne again. Back I came to the ground, bouncing the second time, but this time I eased off and the wheels touched and stayed. Well, at least I got the thing down without wrecking it. Cap greeted me with a grin, "You didn't fly too badly, only a two-bounce landing."

I continued to fly as often as I could scrape a few dollars together to pay for my flying time. My proficiency improved, and before long I was making good takeoffs and smooth, three-point landings. I found flying to be very relaxing. It is impossible to describe the feeling of soaring into the air, climbing higher and higher, leveling off and then banking first to the left, then to the right. "Free as a bird" is the best description I can give. There is no one to interrupt your thoughts. The freedom of flight high in the sky is most exhilarating.

One of my friends owned a Fleet airplane. Occasionally, he let me fly it. It was a beautiful open-cockpit plane with clean lines. It was stressed for stunting, and every time I took it up, I would climb to an altitude of six or seven thousand feet and throw it into a spin. What a thrill pulling up into a stall, then pushing the stick forward as the spin began—first slowly, then faster, until it seemed as if the plane were spinning like a top. Then it was time to give a kick on the rudder bar and to pull back the stick, slowly climbing to a higher altitude and leveling off.

I liked to chew tobacco while flying, but there was one problem. I found that spitting out into the slipstream was not the thing to do. I tried it once and got it back in my face and all over my goggles. I devised a way I could chew and fly at the same time without splattering myself or the plane. I placed a large wad of mechanics waste in the bottom of the cockpit and used it as a spittoon. When I got through flying, I removed the waste and tidied up any spots caused by near misses.

There were a number of students who were flying, and we decided to organize a flying club. Three of us got together and formed the Purdue Flying Club. We wrote a constitution and bylaws and presented our petition to the university. The club was approved and given official status as a university organization. (It is my understanding that the Purdue Flying Club still exists.)

Amelia Earhart, the world-famous aviatrix, came to Purdue in 1934 as a counselor on careers for women and remained on the staff until her death in 1937. On occasion she lectured on various topics in the field of aviation, and I had the privilege of attending those lectures. At a dinner party in the house of the Purdue president, she once discussed her ambition to fly around the world. Two other dinner guests that night guaranteed a total of fifty thousand dollars toward the purchase of a suitable plane for the proposed flight, with the object of collecting essential scientific data. A Lockheed Electra was purchased and outfitted as a flying laboratory. In fact, the plane was named the *Flying Laboratory*. She had as her navigator Captain Fred Noonan of the U.S. Army. The flight around the world at the equator began in Miami, Florida, on June 1, 1937. She reached Lue, New Guinea, on June 19. Ahead lay the most perilous leg of the journey, 2,570 miles over the ocean. Trouble developed and her plane went down somewhere near Howland Island. Despite a widespread search, there never was a trace of the lost plane and its occupants. The mystery has never been solved, but it had been conjectured that there might have been some involvement by unfriendly forces. That was but a few years before the attack on Pearl Harbor.

Arriving back on campus Sunday, April 14, 1935, after a weekend at home, I found everyone excited. A prominent visitor had suddenly descended on Purdue. The famous aviator Wiley Post had made an emergency landing at the Purdue airport.

Post was one of the famous, if not the most famous, aviators of that day. He had made a solo trip around the world in his plane, the *Winnie Mae,* and had set a number of speed records. On that occasion he was attempting to set a new transcontinental speed record, flying from west to east. His plane had a speed of 170 miles per hour at the usual altitudes, but Post felt the speed could be greatly increased by flying in the stratosphere. The air, of course, offered much less resistance at that altitude. A supercharger was required. (His speed could be increased to 260 miles per hour by flying in the stratosphere.) At that altitude, he knew he needed a special suit in order to survive the low pressure to which his body would be subjected. That was long before pressurized cabins. He devised a pressurized suit that was a crude version of the suits astronauts later would wear. The suit, topped by a helmet resembling a diver's helmet, made him look like a man from another planet.

The retractable landing gear had not yet been developed, so Wiley devised another gimmick to cut down on wind resistance. He had the underbelly of the plane reinforced and a heavy landing skid built in. Then he altered the fixed landing gear so that it could be jettisoned after takeoff. Of course, when he landed, he did a belly landing and was immobilized until the landing gear could be forwarded to him and reattached to the plane.

His plane had developed supercharger trouble, and Post had to make a forced landing. Since the Purdue airport was closest, he flew there, making a perfect landing on the skid without damaging the plane. The greatest difficulty he had was getting out of the suit. The inexperienced students who had never seen anything so strange finally got his suit off after loosening about forty wing nuts. There was nothing he could do until his landing gear arrived, so he remained the guest of the university for several days. He was most enthusiastic about our aviation facilities.

The day following his arrival, I arrived back at the fraternity house after morning classes and was given a message to call the university. I wondered what I had done to warrant such a call. I was asked to report to the Union Building to attend a luncheon honoring Wiley Post. I was overwhelmed. I couldn't believe my ears. I expected to be one of several hundred guests and thought that the function would take place in the grand ballroom; but when I arrived at the Union, I was directed to one of the small private dining rooms. Entering the room, I saw some of my classmates who were members of the flying club, and there stood our hero, Wiley Post, a rather short, stocky man with a burr haircut and mustache with a black patch over one eye. (He had lost an eye some time in the past.) The group attending the luncheon totaled about a dozen, and here I was one of the group. It was a leisurely luncheon, and Post was common as we were. He was friendly and a great conversationalist. After the plates were cleared, we sat back and listened to him tell of his experiences. That was one of the highlights of my life, being privileged to sit across the table from such a famous person, asking questions and hearing firsthand the account of his exploits. He was not boastful at all but rather "down to earth" in his manner.

He told us about his trip around the world and about the places he had visited. One experience he related was having to make an unscheduled landing in Russia. He brought the *Winnie Mae* down in a field somewhere out on the steppes near a peasant's house. When he finally stopped, the people rushed out wide-eyed to greet him. The first thing he did when he climbed out of the plane was to ask for a drink of water. They couldn't understand English, and he couldn't speak Russian. Finally, he gestured as if he were drinking from a glass. They smiled and shook their heads and went back to the house and brought him a tall glass filled with a clear liquid. He was quite thirsty, so he turned the glass bottoms up; then he realized as he sputtered that it wasn't water. It was the national drink of Russia, vodka.

When the landing gear arrived, we bade our distinguished visitor good-by. On August 15, we were deeply saddened to learn the great man had been killed. He and his close friend and fellow Oklahoman, the renowned Will Rogers, were on a flight in Alaska when their plane crashed. They were killed instantly.

Shortly after the unscheduled visit of Wiley Post to the campus, Professor George W. Haskins, head of the Department of Aeronautical Engineering, received an invitation to the charter meeting of the National Collegiate Flying Club, to be held in Washington, D.C. The letter also invited student representatives. Professor Haskins read the letter to our class, and we immediately started planning on how we could get to Washington. Permission was obtained from the university to be away from classes for the period of time required. Finally, eight or ten of us made the trip at our own expense.

We took turns driving and reached Washington late that night. We had the name of the hotel but had no idea how to get there. Something we hadn't counted on was the irregular layout of the streets. I was driving up a street that I later learned was Connecticut Avenue and actually passed the same building three or four times. I could swear I had never made a turn.

We found the hotel and fell into bed, exhausted. The next morning the meeting began. We were amazed to see the size of the crowd. There were representatives from practically every college and university in the United States. I got acquainted with the group from the University of Maryland, and they asked me to stay with them during the conference. I was glad to accept their invitation because it meant I would not have to pay for a hotel. One of our hosts was the Secretary of the Treasury, William G. McAdoo, who also was an aviation enthusiast and had played a leading role in organizing the conference. McAdoo had made elaborate arrangements to entertain us while in Washington. We were taken from our meeting place in the Carlton Hotel by motorcade to inspect Bolling Field, Washington headquarters of the Army Air Corps, and then on to Anacostia Naval Air Base. I had never seen anything like it before in my life. We rode in the chauffeured touring cars normally reserved for the top Washington brass, and we were escorted by motorcycle police. Down through the heart of Washington we rode, through red traffic lights with sirens screaming and red lights flashing. What an experience for a country boy!

We were also escorted to the Department of Commerce, where we saw the first Link Trainer. It looked like a midget airplane mounted on a pedestal. It was used to train pilots in blind flying, relying only on instruments. We were given a chance to try our hand. I stepped into the cockpit, and a hood was closed over the top of the cockpit. I was in complete darkness. The controls, rudder bar, and stick were the same as on a standard airplane. When all was ready, I started up the machine.

The Link Trainer responded beautifully. It climbed, dived, turned, and banked. It was a terrific sensation sitting there in the dark, trying to read instruments, wondering whether I was flying upside down or right side up, and wondering when I was going to crash. After that experience, I had much more respect for those pilots who must fly through all kinds of weather and rely entirely on instruments.

The big social event was a dinner dance the night before we left for home. One of my friends from Maryland arranged a date for me with one of the coeds. She was most attractive, decked out in a formal gown. All I had to wear was the suit I had worn since leaving Purdue. By that time, it was badly wrinkled and no doubt had a stain or two. We arrived at the Shoreham, one of the finest hotels in Washington. There was a reception first, then a sumptuous meal followed by entertainment and dancing in the adjoining famed Blue Room. By the time the entertainment started, I thought I was doing quite well with my date. Several couples were standing just inside the Blue Room watching the entertainment. My date was just in front of me. She turned and smiled, and I smiled back. Shortly, she turned and smiled again, and I thought, "Boy, I'm really doing great." Then she said, "Would you mind moving your foot. You are standing on my dress." What a letdown.

The final session was held the next day, and I returned to College Park to pick up my suitcase and bid farewell to my new friends. On my way back into Washington to pick up my passengers, I was stopped by a motorcycle policeman. He stated I was going forty miles per hour in a thirty-mile zone. I didn't argue, but I told him that I was on my way to pick up my friends, that we were all students at Purdue University and had been in Washington for a very important meeting, and that we had to be back at school by noon the following day. I didn't impress him. He asked for my driver's license and I told him I didn't have one. In fact, Illinois issued no driver's licenses. Then he wanted to see the certificate of title for the car. I told him in Illinois it was not required to carry that with you. Then he said, "How do I know this isn't a stolen car? I guess I'll have to take you in and lock you up until we can check this out."

I was really sweating then and was trying to figure a quick way out. Suddenly I remembered that Sam Prevo from Marshall was in medical school at George Washington University and his father had sold the car to my father. I told the cop I could get verification by calling Sam, but that wasn't good enough for him. Then I played my ace. "I will call Secretary McAdoo and he will vouch for me." I said, "The Secretary was the one who arranged the meeting, and I'm sure he will straighten this out." "Well," said the policeman, "you are free to go, but watch your speed." Still sweating, I started on down the street, driving twenty-eight miles an hour. I picked up my passengers and we drove all night, arriving back at Purdue on schedule.

From our standpoint, the meeting was a success because some members of our delegation were elected officers of the national organization. It was also agreed to hold the club's first national air meet at Purdue's new airport the summer of 1935. The Purdue Flying Club was an immediate success, with quite a contingent of enthusiastic members. One of our first projects to raise money was a moonlight dance at the airport. We received permission to use the new hangar. We moved all the planes out and parked them on the apron. We scrubbed and waxed the floor, set up tables and chairs around the floor, and installed appropriate lighting. We asked the dean of women and her escort to be the official chaperones and she accepted. We hired a band, sold tickets, and prayed that it would be a beautiful, clear, moonlit night. It was a beautiful night, the crowd turned out, the music was good, and the dean had a wonderful time. Our first club project was a success.

Our club took the leadership in making all arrangements for the National Air Meet that summer. The university cooperated all the way. We were amazed at the number of entries from all over the country. There were contests in bomb dropping (attempting to hit a bull's-eye drawn on the ground from an altitude of several hundred feet, using a sack of flour as a bomb), dead stick landing (attempting to touch down on a line drawn on the ground after cutting the engine), ribbon cutting (ascending to an altitude of three or four thousand feet, throwing a roll of toilet paper over the side and coming back to cut the ribbon streaming down [The time was clocked from the instant the roll went over the side until the wing had cut the ribbon in two.]). Ribbon cutting was tricky; the best way to do it was to make a split S—moving the plane down at full throttle and coming back up and over in a steep bank. There were other events, and the entire meet lasted two days.

Our visitors were very impressed by our airport, which at the time was the only university-owned airport in the country.

The following year, the meet was held at the Wayne County Airport in Michigan (later the site of Ford's Willow Run Plant and now the Detroit International Airport) under the auspices of the University of Michigan. Even though I had graduated from Purdue, I was still in the graduate school and continued as a member of the flying club, so I flew in that meet. I drove to Detroit, rented a plane there, and flew on to Wayne County. They had made a rule that all contestants had to wear a parachute so I rented one. I was cramped. My head was up against the top of the cabin, and I had to reach down to hold the stick. I competed in the ribbon cutting but did not win a trophy.

I DIDN'T DO MUCH socializing until my senior year at Purdue, and even then I rarely joined the social scene. Studying kept me busy and, besides, I didn't have the money.

Two events that stand out in my mind were the junior prom and the "Riveter's Rassel." I didn't attend the junior prom until I was a senior. That was a formal affair, and I didn't have a tux. I decided to splurge and bought a double-breasted one with satin lapels. As was the custom, I bought a corsage for my date and a carnation for me. When I started to put the carnation on, I found no buttonhole in the lapel. I figured that the tailor had made a mistake, but I resolved the problem. I went to the kitchen, got an ice pick, and poked a hole through the lapel and ran the stem of the flower through. Later at the dance, I found that everyone else had just pinned the flower to the lapel. Every time I wore that suit afterwards and saw that hole, I would chuckle at how dumb I was.

The "Riveter's Rassle" was more my kind of affair. No dressing up. Instead, the worse you looked, the better. I started getting ready about three weeks before the dance by letting my beard grow. There was to be a contest for the heaviest beard, and by the night of the dance I thought I was in the running. I found an old pair of pants that had been white at one time but were a dull gray now from dirt and stains, and I tore some holes in an old T-shirt. I put the outfit on with a rope over my shoulder to hold up my pants. I wore a dirty cap and an old pair of shoes that were full of holes. Before I left the house, I rolled in the coal pile, cleaned the flues in the boiler and rubbed the soot on my exposed skin, rubbed some garlic in my armpits, ate some garlic, and put in a chew of tobacco. I picked up my date, who was wearing an old formal that was full of holes. She had a large artificial rose in her hair, holes in her stockings, and run-over shoes. Also, she had poured a bottle of cheap perfume all over her dress. We were a smart-looking couple. I didn't win the beard contest, but my picture appeared in the paper.

Occasionally, about once a year, we had a dance at the fraternity. We had some members who were very talented in rigging up gimmicks. The bathroom on the second floor was reserved for the girls. One ingenious soul rigged up the toilet seats so that when they were in the down position, contact was made with a switch activating a record player that played the "Star Spangled Banner." That almost caused a riot.

EACH SENIOR was required to write a thesis. I picked the subject "Letters of Application for a Job." I hoped that the exercise would give me a head start in the job market. The depression was still on, and jobs were very tight. I devised varying approaches. Letters were sent to several hundred corporate headquarters. The majors—General Motors, Ford, and so on—were well covered, and the smaller companies were not ignored. The responses received from all the companies could be summed up in one statement—no jobs available.

I realized that after four years of study and hard work I was going to receive a B.S. degree in mechanical engineering but have no job. The Army Air Corps was actively recruiting aviation cadets. That sounded great. I loved flying, and with the training offered, I could obtain a commission as a second lieutenant and be flying the latest model airplanes.

I was given the application form, but there was one catch. I wasn't twenty-one yet so I had to have my parents' signatures. I called home and did a hard sell on Mom and Dad. Dad finally said he would sign the papers so I went home for the weekend. Reaching in my suitcase for the envelope with the forms, I found they were missing. In my excitement to get home, I had left them in my desk.

I told him I would send the forms to him as soon as I got back to school. The next day he called me. He had been thinking it over and had changed his mind. He didn't want me in the Air Corps. I was disappointed but knew I couldn't argue. Once he made his mind up, that was final. He had never been enthusiastic about my flying. Knocked out of going into the Air Corps, I was really up against it. What was I going to do after I graduated? No job and no prospects of getting a job.

Then I began to think how Dad had pressured me to study medicine, which still had no appeal for me. More years of school—and I never liked school. Leaving engineering, which I really loved, was taking a gamble because there was no assurance I would be accepted in medical school. For the first time in my life, I was faced with making a decision that would determine my future. Until now, everything had involved no real complications. Now the straight-line course I had charted had run into a roadblock, and I was going to have to change directions.

I decided to try medicine. Dad had no idea what I was considering, and when I told him, he almost fainted. He was about the happiest I had ever seen him, and, of course, Mom was pleased too.

Dad took me down to Bloomington to meet the dean of the Indiana University School of Medicine, and I can say I was most unimpressed. The dean sat behind his desk at the far end of a large room. Next to him was the desk of his secretary. Along one wall was a row of chairs occupied by anxious young men. As the person next to the dean finished his conversation, he got up and left the room. Everyone then moved down one chair toward the dean. I thought, "This is a hell of a way to run a railroad."

The dean was chewing out almost every student. There was no privacy, and I felt sorry for these victims. Finally, it was our turn. Dad informed the dean that he was an Indiana graduate and that I was interested in entering medical school. The dean learned that I was a Purdue man. His manner became rather insulting. I felt the same way about him and his school. There was a fierce rivalry between the two universities. He told me I would have to come to Bloomington the next fall and enroll as a freshman in premed. I asked him how many years I would have to spend before entering medical school. He said, "Two, three, or maybe four, and even then you won't be assured of acceptance."

I challenged him. "I've been in Purdue four years, and I'm graduating with a bachelor of science degree. I've taken many of the courses that I would be taking here, so what would I be taking during the additional years here?" I asked. "Oh, I would expect you to take a number of courses in philosophy," he answered. I could see I wasn't making any headway, so I asked him for a list of courses that I would need.

Grudgingly, he gave me the list. I saw that every course listed was available at Purdue. Then I said the wrong thing. "These courses are all given at Purdue, so I'll go back there and enroll next year to finish up my requirements for medical school." I thought he was going to explode, but instead he gave me permission to send in an application later.

9

George Washington University School of Medicine

AFTER GRADUATION from Purdue in the spring of 1935, I went back to take my premed courses in graduate school. I originally had planned to cover the required subjects over a two-year period, but I did not like school that well. I decided to do it in one. I was enrolled with freshman students in biology, with senior students in embryology and bacteriology, and with sophomores and juniors in anatomy. In essence, I covered the complete biology curriculum in one year. I was taking a six-hour course in organic chemistry and courses in quantitative and qualitative analysis. Only one section in each of these latter courses was available and they met at the same time, so I got permission from the head of the department to take them together. I alternated attending lectures in each course. In addition to a few other courses, I carried a total of about twenty-five hours per semester.

In the fall of 1935, I formally applied at the Indiana University School of Medicine. I heard nothing until after Christmas, when I received a letter noting that I hadn't taken the MCAT examination. I had never heard of such an exam. The dean hadn't mentioned it, nor had the letter that accompanied the application form. I was furious. "What kind of place is that down there?" I asked myself. I went roaring over to the campus to find out about the exam. I was directed to a certain professor, and when he heard my story, he was outraged. It seems that the exam I was to take was a proficiency exam on medical and scientific subjects. It had been given at Purdue a few weeks before. The Purdue professor said, "Those dirty so-and-sos. I'll give you a special exam." I took the exam and apparently made a good grade.

A while later, I wondered what was going on in Bloomington, so I wrote. I received a letter telling me that they didn't have my application on file. Apparently, they had conveniently lost it. At that time my Dad and I paid a visit to an old retired professor of the School of Medicine. Dad had had that professor, and they had remained good friends. The professor said that it was painful for him to say, but he felt there was some hanky-panky on occasion. Sometimes applications mysteriously disappeared. He said he was having lunch with the dean in a few days, and he would discuss the situation with him.

About two weeks later, I received a letter from Bloomington. They had found my application. By that time I'd had about all of Indiana University I wanted, but the final blow came about the first of March on a Saturday morning. I went to the post office to get the mail. There was a letter from the dean of the medical school. I opened it right there. I was not accepted. It seems the six-hour course I had taken each semester in organic chemistry was considered to be too elementary to meet their standards. I knew then that the dean had no intention of accepting me at the time Dad and I met him the year before. I was furious. I stomped back to the fraternity house, plotting what I was going to do. When I got there, I had my mind made up. I had brought my mother's car back when I was home the previous weekend. One of my fraternity brothers was in the living room as I came in. "What are you doing, Mac?" I asked. "Nothing," he answered. "You want to go to Bloomington?" I asked. "Sure," he replied, and so we took off.

Along the way, I told him the whole story. I pulled in next to the building that housed the dean's office. Nothing looked different from the year before. He was sitting at his desk, and as before, the chairs were lined up along the wall with the students playing musical chairs. I didn't enter into the game. I walked straight up to his desk.

He looked up over his glasses and frowned. Before he could speak, I said: "Sir, my name is Mitchell. I'm sure you don't remember me, but I was here a year ago last fall with my father, Dr. R. A. Mitchell. I talked to you about entering medical school. You gave me a list of subjects I should take. I have taken those subjects, have completed all of the other requirements, and this morning I received your letter telling me I'm not good enough to go to your school. Now I didn't come to beg or plead with you to reconsider. I came here for one reason only—to tell you that you can take your school and stick it." Before he could answer, I was on my way out.

What was I going to do? I had spent four years getting my engineering degree, had spent a year in the graduate school getting my premed, had applied to only one medical school and had been turned down, and it was March of 1936. I had expected to enter medical school that fall. I got back in the car, told Mac what had happened, and said, "We're going back to Marshall."

When I walked in the back door at home, Mother was in the kitchen. When she saw me, she exclaimed, "What in the world are you doing here?" "I want to talk to Dad," I said, not answering her question. She called Dad, and home he came from the office. When I told him what had taken place, he became very upset, not at me, but at the dean. "What are your plans now?" he asked. I had been thinking all the way from Bloomington about what I was going to do next and I had a plan. "Well, Dad, I've done it your way, and it didn't work, so now I'm going to do it my way," I said. "Sam Prevo is a junior at George Washington University School of Medicine, and I'm going to write him to see if it would be possible to get into school there this year." Dad told me I had his approval and to go to it, so Mac and I took off for Purdue.

Sam Prevo was a local boy, a big guy with a baby face who was liked by everyone. He was happy-go-lucky but had a good mind. During his summers home from medical school, he spent considerable time around Dad's office. That night I wrote a letter telling Sam about all that had happened. I outlined all the courses I had taken or was taking then and the grades I was making and asked him if he could help me get into school.

Within a week I had a reply in which Sam told me he had talked to the faculty members of the admissions committee and that I was accepted, providing I maintained my grades. I was to send one hundred dollars to hold my place in the class. I didn't realize until later what a tremendous job he had done. A junior medical student had convinced the faculty committee that a young man whom they'd never seen or heard of, who had not submitted an application or transcript of grades, was a suitable candidate for admission to the medical school. I was more astounded when I discovered after arriving in Washington that there had been four hundred applications that year and only ninety-five had been accepted. Sam had a wonderful personality and was well liked and trusted by the faculty. No other person could have achieved what he had.

That summer I again worked on the farm and sometimes helped Dad around the office or went with him on house calls. When September came, I was ready to start on my great adventure. I went by train from Terre Haute to Washington. My cousin Frank was also starting dental school at Indiana University in Indianapolis. Our folks saw us off at the station and Frank rode the seventy miles or so with me to Indianapolis. By the time we arrived there, I almost had him talked into going on to Washington with me.

I had a great trip, eating dinner in the diner and getting a good night's sleep in a berth in the Pullman. When I arrived in the Union Station at Washington the next morning, I looked out the window and saw Sam standing on the platform. I was tickled to see him because I had been wondering where I was going to go when I got there and where I would stay. After getting my luggage, we took a cab to the fraternity house at 1271 New Hampshire Avenue NW, the site of Alpha

Kappa Kappa medical fraternity. Sam was a member, and he assumed that I would also be a member. He didn't ask me whether I had other plans. It was a week before school started. Sam took me around and introduced me, got me a room, and before I realized it, I was settled. I was in a large room that ran across the front of the house on the second floor. My two roommates were sophomores, both of Irish descent—James Patrick Murphy O'Grady from West Virginia and Bob McMahon from Pennsylvania.

The house was typical of the older houses in Washington. It was a three-story brick with steps leading up to a stoop at the front of the house. Other steps went down from the front walk to the lower level, which housed the kitchen and dining room. The main floor had a hallway opening off to a very large living room with two or three small bedrooms to the rear. The two top floors had bedrooms only. The house was owned by Tim Chillemi, an Italian who at one time had been a bootlegger. Tim rented out the whole house to the fraternity and took care of the cooking and housekeeping. He was a character in his own right, as I learned later.

During my first week in Washington there was no school, but I had to get registered, pay my fees, and get my schedule. It seemed as if the boys in the fraternity did nothing but party. I thought, "If this is going to go on all year, I'm going to have to find another place to live." They were all good people, though, and were doing everything they could to help me adjust and get started off right in school. The first day at school was devoted to meeting with professors and getting assignments.

I was accustomed to a spacious college campus with grass, shrubs, flowers, trees, and beautiful buildings. What I found at 1335 H Street in downtown Washington was a dismal-looking, five-story building, grimy with what seemed to be a hundred years of accumulated dirt, located next to a similar structure, which I was told was the university hospital. Inside, a long, cold, dark corridor extended back past the dean's office to a wooden stairway. Although there was an old, creaky elevator, freshmen and sophomores were required to use the stairs. As I neared the stairway, I noticed there was a strong odor of formaldehyde. Later on, I discovered that the vat containing cadavers was just to the left of the stairway.

As I climbed the creaky stairs to the fifth floor, I was reminded of a climb to the gallows: I had been warned that the faculty spared no one. We assembled in the histology laboratory: there were ninety-five of us, ninety-two men and three women, but there was no member of the faculty present. Suddenly, the door opened and in strode a tall, distinguished-looking gentleman in a long, white lab coat. His hair was snow white, and he had a face that looked as if it had been chiseled out of New England granite.

"Good morning, Ladies and Gentlemen," Dr. Jenkins said, without any show of emotion. He then instructed us as to the rules under which we would operate during the next year. I had the feeling that if any one of us deviated from these rules one iota we would be drawn and quartered. Then he got down to serious business. He held up a copy of *Gray's Anatomy,* for all to see, and then very slowly he said, "No man who has ever lived in the past, no man who will live in the future, nor any man living today knows everything between the covers of this book, but, Ladies and Gentlemen, by the end of this year I expect each of you to know everything in this book. Your assignment for tomorrow is to familiarize yourself with the first fifty pages of osteology. Good day, Ladies and Gentlemen." With that, he turned and slowly strode out of the room. We were all stunned. Looking around, I didn't see a smile on any face, and then we began to talk. What kind of a place was this? What were they trying to do to us? The other professors appeared a bit more human, but we all knew there was to be no monkey business.

I had been through what I thought was a pretty rough time as a student at Purdue for five years, but that was elementary compared to what I was beginning now.

Dr. Jenkins made such a strong impression on me that I went straight back to my room and started studying osteology. I had never heard of *Gray's Anatomy,* and as I started to read, it seemed to make no sense. In fact, many of the words were derivations of Greek or Latin, and I was constantly referring to my medical dictionary, trying to understand what I was reading. I studied all afternoon, all evening, and most of the night, getting only an hour or two of sleep. Red-eyed and dead tired, I went to class the next day, wondering if it was worth it.

We worked in pairs at the white iron tables of the dissecting laboratories. Each pair was assigned a cadaver, a brown, leathery-looking body reeking of formaldehyde. Gradually, we became accustomed to the odor. Everyday, Monday through Friday, from 1:00 to 5:00 P.M., we worked in the anatomy lab; we were also there from 8:00 A.M. to noon on Saturday. It wasn't long before we settled into a routine of dissecting out and identifying muscles, nerves, and blood vessels. Dr. Jenkins and his assistants were constantly roaming about, stopping to give a quick quiz here and there. "What is that muscle? What is the origin and insertion? Show me the obturator muscle. What is its function?" So on and on, day after day, we labored and learned. Frequently, we had surprise written quizzes plus the regular written exams, and then there was the semester final exam. Dr. Jenkins was considered the czar of the freshman class, and it was his intention that all of his students were going to learn anatomy well. His methods were harsh, but I soon realized that I was learning anatomy and that if he had eased off any I most likely would have done poorly.

Of course, anatomy wasn't the only course. There was histology, with lectures and laboratory and countless hours of peering through a microscope and, of course, quizzes and written examinations.

Early on I found I had a problem at the fraternity house. My two Irish roommates were very congenial and easy to get along with, but they liked to play poker. They didn't have to study as hard as I did, so they spent considerable time enjoying their lighter pursuits. They usually stopped on their way home from school Saturday noon to pick up a wee bit of refreshments; then when they arrived at the fraternity house, they started a poker game in our room. Several others would join them, and the game went on all afternoon, all evening, all night until Sunday morning. They took time out for Mass, then resumed the game until early Monday morning. Trying to study in that atmosphere and trying to sleep with all of that going on in the room was impossible. Finally after about three weekends, I told them the game had to stop or I was leaving the fraternity. They were surprised. It had never entered their minds that they were disturbing me. They both apologized and moved their game to another room in the house.

I settled into a routine, getting up early every morning, walking the mile or so to school, leaving school late in the evening, walking back to the house on New Hampshire, and then to the books till late at night. There were times when I would have given anything if I could just take off to go to a movie, but I knew I just couldn't spare the time. Occasionally, we had dancing in the living room on Saturday nights. A console radio furnished the music—the "Lucky Strike Hit Parade" was the most popular show. Sometimes it was Bennie Goodman, Tommy Dorsey, Shep Fields, Eddie Duchin, or another of the big bands of the day.

Finally, Christmas vacation was not far away, but first we had final exams. My last exam was on Saturday morning, the day vacation started—anatomy with Dr. Jenkins—the toughest of all. After finishing the exam, I knew I had done well and felt as if a weight had been lifted from my back.

We had completed the dissection of the head and neck, and it was the rule that after all the tissue had been removed, the bones had to be cleaned up and turned in at the end of the year. The best way to clean the bones, we were told, was to boil them in a solution of lye water. My partner and I sawed the skull in half, front to rear, and each took a half skull home with us to clean over the vacation. Fragments of tissue still clung to the bone. I wrapped my half in a soiled lab coat and left school. I felt so good that I decided to go to a movie downtown at the Capital Theatre before going back to the house to pick up my suitcase and catching a train that evening. Down the street I went with my head rolled up in the coat under my arm. I got my ticket, went into the theater, and found a seat about halfway down in the middle section. I soon noticed the people around me begin one by one to leave their seats and move to another part of the theater. Soon I was all alone. I was puzzled. Then it suddenly dawned on me that there was a strong odor of formaldehyde emanating from the head. I was so used to the odor that I no longer even noticed it. I packed the head in my suitcase with all my clothes and headed for Union Station to board the train for the journey home. I wonder what would have happened if my suitcase had fallen open.

I can't say I was ever homesick, but I sure was happy to see my folks, with nothing to do for two weeks but relax, eat all of the good home cooking, and bask in the love shown by Mom and Dad. It all ended too soon. Before long I was back on the train, headed back to school. While at home, I had boiled the head in the lye solution in a bucket set over an electric hot plate in the basement. It didn't smell the best, but the odor didn't stay around long. I now had a nice snow-white half skull.

The second semester Jim O'Grady and I moved to a different room in the rear of the house. Although smaller, it was quite adequate. Sometime after I returned, I received the one and only letter I ever received from Dad. Mom told me he would ask her, "Alma, have you written the boy lately?" He wanted me to have frequent letters with all the news but wanted her to do all the writing, so I was surprised when I received a letter in his distinctive handwriting. I wondered why in the world he was writing. I wasn't long in getting an answer to my question. The whole letter was devoted to telling me about two patients he had treated, both of whom had died. They were two young boys whom he had delivered and watched grow up and who were in their early teens. Donald, who had lived next door to us since birth, had received an injury to his knee that became infected. The knee had become quite red and swollen, and he had developed a high fever. There was no question about the diagnosis. He had a cellulitis with a blood stream infection of dreaded streptococcus. That was long before the day of antibiotics. The treatment consisted of hot packs, aspirin, and prayer. Dad knew what the ultimate outcome would be, but he couldn't accept it. He vividly described to me his sitting by the bedside of the delirious boy with that terrible feeling of helplessness while watching him die.

The second case was that of bulbar poliomyelitis. As the family doctor, he had been close to the boy. The diagnosis too was clear to him, but again there was no treatment—polio vaccine had yet to be developed, and the iron lung was yet to be invented. Again he described his feelings as he sat by the bedside—the boy's breathing became ever more difficult. As he became weaker and weaker, he continued pleading with Dad to help him breathe. Finally it was all over, and Dad was filled with a feeling of frustration and grief.

After reading his letter, I understood why he had written to me. He needed someone close to him who had some understanding of medicine to share his sorrow and frustration, someone who could understand what he was going through as a skilled and dedicated doctor who had been defeated by the Grim Reaper. At that time, his sharing his thoughts with me and my feeling the same frustrations, it seemed as though we were the closest we had ever been.

My friend Sam Prevo, who was now a senior, had a job that furnished room and board at the Millard Prep School for West Point. That was a private school for students who had been selected to attend West Point but who had yet to take the entrance exams. The curriculum was designed to give the student intense courses of study in all the subjects covered in the entrance examinations. The students were housed in a large mansion and led the life of a West Point plebe, and the rules were very strict. Sam was one of the proctors. He was responsible for seeing that his group of students studied the long hours required and also for enforcing the strict rules of discipline. The entire course covered a period of six months, so Sam's duties ended about March 1. The prep school was located not far from our fraternity house, and Sam dropped by occasionally to visit.

About 9:00 P.M., as Jim and I were studying, in walked Sam with a suitcase. He went over to the couch and stretched out. "This is too short for me to sleep on," he said. "What are you talking about?" we asked. "Oh, I'm moving in with you tonight. The school is closed and I don't have any place to stay." We knew he was serious. Sam never did any advance planning. We finally dismantled the twin beds and moved the mattresses to the floor. Sam and I slept on the floor, and Jim slept on the couch. The next day we moved the couch out and set up another bed so that there was no more sleeping on the floor. Except for the crowding, it wasn't too bad because Sam was always out at night (he never studied) and Jim and I could study in peace.

Springtime in Washington was delightful. Taking a walk around the Tidal Basin and viewing all the Japanese cherry trees that had just burst into bloom was one of the prettiest sights I had ever experienced. The only problem was that the balmy days gave me spring fever and it was more difficult to concentrate on the books. Finally came exams and my first year of medical school was ended. I was amazed at how well I had done. My grades were well above average. I was eager to return to Marshall.

ON THE ADVICE of Bill Coldren, I got a job at the local ice company managed by Everett Smitley. At 6:00 A.M. I went to work. In those days, mechanical refrigerators were scarce. Most people still used an icebox for refrigeration. Iceboxes came in assorted sizes and shapes. Some held 100 pounds, while others could hold no more than 25 pounds. Some opened on the side, some from the top, while a few were quite large with a shoulder-high ice compartment. John Edwards and I were given a 1-1/2-ton truck with side boards and end gate. Our route covered the business district and south part of town. After backing up to the loading platform, we went into the cold room and, using our hooks, slid 300-pound blocks of ice out and onto the truck and tucked a large canvas tarpaulin cover over the load. I learned right off there was a trick in using the hooks and moving the ice. John had been working there for some time so he taught me the tricks of the trade. The large blocks were scored so that it was easy to cut them into 25-, 50-, 75- or 100-pound chunks by chipping along the scored line with an ice pick. To carry the larger chunks, I learned to slide the ice to the back of the truck; then standing on the ground, I placed the hooks firmly into the ice. With my back to the truck, I would reach over my shoulder and grab the handle of the hook and walk off with the ice on my back. To keep from getting soaked, I wore a heavy rubber back pad with each arm hooked through a canvas loop and a canvas strap across my chest. Wearing the thing on a hot summer day was very uncomfortable. It took us all morning and usually half the afternoon to make our rounds.

The ice customers put a card in the window indicating they wanted ice and a number at the top of the card to indicate the amount. If the customer was away, we went into the kitchen, put the ice in the box, and picked up the money or ice ticket. In those days no one worried about leaving a house unlocked. After finishing our route, we returned to the plant and worked the platform. A lot of people came to the plant to get their own ice because they could save some money.

Everett, the boss, didn't worry too much about truck maintenance. The trucks were old, and it seemed something was always in need of repair, so if they were going to be kept running, it was up to us as amateur mechanics to get the job done.

I also covered a fifty-mile country route three afternoons a week. Going south out of Marshall on Route 1, I stopped at every house displaying a card in the window. At Snyder, I serviced the grocery store, then on down to Walnut Prairie, where I took care of the general store. My route then took me east almost to the Wabash River, then north to Darwin. Frakes Store in Darwin had a huge refrigerator with a big compartment across the top that held 300 pounds of ice. There was a trick in getting the ice into that compartment. After getting 100 pounds on my back and holding the handle of the hooks over my left shoulder with my right hand, I walked up and stood alongside the front of the box. Having swung the doors of the compartment open, I gave a huge hunch with my left shoulder and at the same time twisted my right wrist, thus pitching the large hunk of ice into the box. This worked well except on one occasion. Just as I gave the hunch and twisted my wrist, the hooks slipped. Instead of jumping out of the way, I tried to catch the hundred pounds of ice in my arms. The whole thing came down on my right big toe. I sat down on a nearby box and proceeded to say a few choice words while holding my foot. When I got back to town, I stopped at home. Mom wanted to know what had happened, and when I took off my shoe and sock, the toe was swollen and fiery red. It looked like a red balloon and was pulsating like a neon sign. I expected to get a lot of sympathy from Mom, but instead she doubled up laughing. I didn't get an X-ray, but I know I must have fractured the toe because I couldn't wear a shoe for two weeks. I worked wearing a house slipper on that foot.

In spite of all the work I did on that truck, I couldn't keep the brakes in working order; in disgust, I disconnected the brake rods and twisted them around the posts on the side of the truck bed. I soon learned how to stop without brakes by shifting down from high to low gear and finally into reverse. I continued making my country trip with one or two tons of ice on board and no brakes. I never had an accident, but I came close on one occasion.

After leaving Darwin one day and heading back to Route 1, I almost met my end. I still had about 500 pounds of ice aboard and was in a hurry to get back to Marshall. Not far from Route 1 the road went down a hill, over a single-lane bridge, and then on up another hill. As I started down the hill toward the bridge at a good clip, I saw a car approaching on the far side of the bridge. Because I had no brakes, there was nothing I could do. There was no time to shift down, so I held on tight and hoped the other car would stop. He did. I sailed over the bridge and past the car, whose driver was sitting wide-eyed with the color drained from his face.

Carrying ice was hard work, but I liked it. We worked from 6:00 A.M. until the work was done, which was usually midnight. After the platform was closed down at 9:00 P.M., we usually had to take two trucks to Paris, sixteen miles north, to the plant where the ice was manufactured to replenish our inventory. I worked a seven-day week with every other Sunday afternoon off. My pay was the grand sum of twelve dollars per week.

John and I had a great time working together. We both liked to talk, we seemed to have plenty to talk about, and there was always a lot of kidding. We both smoked cigars, and I chewed tobacco. Everett said one time that with our gift of gab, he could send us to West Union with a box of cigars, and that before we left, we would own the town.

THE DAYS FLEW BY, and it was time to get back to school. It was good to see my friends. We had been unable to come to an agreement with Chillemi so we had no fraternity house. Arrangements had been made for our entire group to live in a boardinghouse where the tenants were government employees, both men and women. We eventually found a better arrangement, a house owned by an elderly widow. We had the whole house to ourselves, and a woman was hired to do the cooking. Although we were too far away from school to walk, the streetcar line was nearby and ran directly down to within a half block of the school. O'Grady and I were roommates again. O'Grady hadn't changed his ways. He was still the happy Irishman.

Two seniors, Jamison and O'Connor, had a room on the third floor. Jamison was from Pennsylvania, and O'Connor was from Brooklyn. Jamison was of medium height and was rather quiet. O'Connor was a tall, typically cocky Irishman. The year before, O'Connor had tried to intimidate me because I was a lowly freshman and he was a junior. I thought this was kid stuff and didn't let it bother me. He liked to come up to me, stick out his chest, grab a cigar from my pocket, light up and swagger off, blowing smoke. While I was home for Christmas, I bought a trick cigar, which would explode shortly after it was lit. The first night I was back at school, I went to dinner with the trick cigar conspicuously sticking out of my breast pocket. Sure enough, as soon as dinner was over, O'Connor walked over and grabbed the cigar. I hurried upstairs and waited to hear from below. It wasn't long until I heard a loud explosion followed by a string of expletives. That was the last time I gave up a cigar to O'Connor.

Jamison and O'Connor were quite a pair. Nearly every Saturday night they went out on the town for an evening of fun. They had worked out a system whereby they took turns bringing each other home. One stayed relatively sober in order to bring his inebriated partner home safe.

Late one Saturday night I came home, unlocked the door, and started down the dark hall past the living room. As I turned left into the hall leading past the dining room, I saw a faint glow of light coming from the room. I was puzzled, but when I looked through the doorway I began to chuckle. There stretched out on his back on the dining table was O'Connor, his arms folded across his chest with a large white lily lying across his hands. The light was coming from two candles—one at his head and one at his feet.

I chuckled all the way up to my room. I knew exactly what had happened. It had been Jamison's turn to get O'Connor home, and after getting him this far, he had passed out. It was then that Jamison decided, "To heck with it, I'm not going to carry him all the way to the third floor. I'll leave him here, and what better way to leave him, but on the table laid out like a corpse." About 6:00 A.M., we were awakened by the screaming of our cook, who had just discovered O'Connor's "corpse."

Sophomore classes were more interesting. Maybe I had matured some and was more relaxed, having gained confidence from Dr. Jenkins's tough anatomy course. Incidentally, some of those who had been there the year before had not been so successful and were no longer with us.

Bacteriology was taught by Dr. Parr. He was called "Guinea Pig" behind his back. A round little man with a black mustache and large, horn-rimmed glasses, he really looked like one of his laboratory animals. (Maybe he had been around them for so many years that he had taken on a resemblance.) Dr. Parr had been born and raised in nearby Edgar County, back in Illinois. It was a small world. He introduced us to the secret world of the microbe: streptococci, staphylococci, bacilli, pneumococci, aerobes, and anaerobes. The "bad guys" and the "good guys"—we learned how they spread and how they reproduced. In the course we learned how to stick a vein. We practiced on our partners, and our partners practiced on us. It was a bloody scene at first, but it wasn't long until we became quite skillful. The blood saved from spilling on the floor was used in producing blood agar, which certain species of bacteria grew on in profusion. Long hours were spent looking through the microscope, learning to identify the different types of bacteria.

Dr. Vincent Di Vigneaud, professor of biochemistry, was world renowned in his field, having been awarded the Nobel Prize in Chemistry. Chemistry was not my favorite subject, but I managed to get through the course. There were two experiments we performed that stand out in my memory.

We were required to go on a three-day diet of all protein, all fat, or all carbohydrates. I chose the all-carbohydrate diet because I liked sweets, and I thought I could live on candy bars for three days. When I received my instructions, I found it wasn't going to be that easy. Chocolate was not included—only pure sugar candy without any flavoring—potatoes without butter, salt, or pepper. Every food item I thought I could eat and enjoy contained other than pure carbohydrates, so I was stuck with sugar, unflavored sugar candy, and dry, unseasoned potatoes for three days. Also, I had to collect every drop of urine I passed so everywhere I went I carried a gallon jug. I encountered many raised eyebrows and grins as I traveled to and from school on the trolley car. One of my fellow students had the misfortune of dropping his jug on the tile floor of the corner drugstore, thus fouling up his experiment and having the embarrassment of watching his urine slowly spread over the floor, to the amusement of the people in the store. At the end of three days, I had to conduct a complete chemical analysis to determine the effect of a strict diet of carbohydrates on the urine.

The other experiment I remember well was the fractional gastric analysis. I had to swallow a gastric tube and periodically, using a syringe, aspirate the stomach contents and analyze the specimen. Since I don't have much of a gag reflex, I had no trouble pushing down the tube, but a number of my classmates were unable to get the tube down. In that situation, we had to hold the guy and someone else pushed the tube down. The tube didn't bother me at all, and during the three-hour period, I walked around with the tube hanging out one side of my mouth and a cigar hanging out the other side.

Pathology was very interesting. We spent considerable time in the laboratory studying microscopic slides of the pathology found in different diseases. It was here that we were introduced to the postmortem examination of the human body. These weren't embalmed and pickled cadavers, but bodies that only a few hours before had been living beings. I thus learned early that I must completely dissociate myself from personal squeamishness if I were to cope.

Dr. Roger Choisser was professor of pathology. He was a quiet man who knew the subject well and who was skilled in imparting his knowledge to others. He was an excellent teacher. He had spent many years as a medical officer in the Navy.

When I was home for Christmas that year, Uncle Earl Mitchell asked about my courses. When I mentioned Dr. Choisser's name, his face lit up and he walked over to a picture on the wall. "Is this Dr. Choisser?" he asked, pointing to a man standing in the group. "Yes, that's him," I answered. Then I saw that this was a picture of a class in the Navy Medical School during World War I. Standing close by Dr. Choisser in the picture was Uncle Earl. Dad then joined in the conversation, and he and Uncle Earl started discussing the Choisser family. They had been raised on adjoining farms near Harrisburg and had played together as children. Uncle Earl informed me that I had mispronounced Dr. Choisser's name. He said that when he'd been on the farm his name was pronounced "Sozier."

Dr. Albritton was professor of physiology. He was rather old-maidish. We conducted various experiments on live animals, mainly rabbits and dogs. The animals were kept in cages on the top floor of the medical school, and it was a strict rule that the windows were to be kept closed at all times. The reason was that the *Washington Times Herald* newspaper was next door. "Cissy" Patterson, the owner and publisher of the newspaper, was a rabid antivivisectionist and was in the forefront of a crusade to abolish animal experimentation. The windows were kept closed so that no sound of barking dogs could drift over to the newspaper offices to remind Miss Patterson that we in the medical school were engaged in doing what she violently opposed. All experiments were conducted without causing any pain to the animals. They were completely anesthetized before any procedure was started; if a particular animal was going to be harmed, it was destroyed while anesthetized after the experiment was completed.

Dr. Roth was professor of pharmacology. We were introduced to the art of compounding prescriptions, and we probed the mysteries of the action of specific drugs on diseases. We learned to write prescriptions using the Latin words and symbols that have been a part of medicine since ancient times.

As with any group of students, we had our share of pranksters. One of the members of my class usually brought his lunch to school in a brown bag and placed it up on the high window ledge in the student lounge. One day he came in at noon, took down the sack, and pulled out a beef sandwich. He took a big bite and immediately began to sputter and spit. Someone had replaced the beef in the sandwich with a large slice from a cadaver.

Down around the corner from the fraternity house was a small delicatessen and magazine stand run by Mr. and Mrs. Dobbins. We dropped by usually around 9:00 P.M. to pick up some delicious sandwiches to munch on while studying. During my freshman year, when we had been dissecting the head of our cadaver, I left the anatomy lab late in the day and put one of the ears that had been removed in my pocket. That night when on the way to the delicatessen to get my sandwich I stuck my hand in my pocket and found the ear. That gave me an idea. I walked in, ordered my sandwich, then said to Mrs. Dobbins, "I have a surprise for you. Close your eyes and hold out your hand." When she opened her eyes, she let out a bloodcurdling scream, threw the ear into the air, and ran me out the door.

10

On the Medical Service

WHILE I WAS IN MEDICAL SCHOOL, I visited several different churches. Although I was a Methodist, I occasionally attended the Baptist or the Presbyterian church. Foundry Methodist had a large congregation and was quite impressive. I wondered why it was called "Foundry" and found someone who knew the story behind the name. During the War of 1812, when the British were marching on Washington, a wealthy man who owned a large foundry saw that the factory was directly in the path of the oncoming army. According to the story, he prayed that the Lord would spare his business from destruction and pledged that he would purchase land and build a fine church if his prayers were answered. Miraculously, the British troops bypassed the foundry. True to his word, the church was built and given to the Methodists—hence the name, Foundry Methodist Church.

I attended the New York Avenue Presbyterian Church most of the time because of the minister, Peter Marshall, one of the finest speakers I had ever heard. He was a handsome man of athletic build with a fine head of sandy hair. He had a booming voice with a thick Scottish brogue. Although his sermons were seldom over ten to fifteen minutes in length, he could pack more into those few minutes than most ministers could say in thirty minutes. The church itself was historic and well preserved. The pews were of the type seen back in revolutionary days. The Lincoln family attended that church, although the president did not actually belong. A plaque affixed to the end of a pew marked his place. His son Robert Lincoln gave the chimes and the clock in the tower of the church in memory of his father. Just across the street was the medical school, and we kept track of time by listening for the old church clock to strike.

Peter Marshall was also the chaplain of the United States Senate. After his death, Mrs. Marshall wrote a number of books about him, including collections of his prayers and other writings. Her most famous book was *A Man Called Peter,* later made into a movie.

DURING THE SUMMER of my sophomore year, I went back to my job delivering ice. The first day back I had to stop off on my way home for lunch at a house I had missed that morning because the card wasn't in the window. Everett, the boss, was with me in the truck. I was to drop him off at his house for lunch and pick him up on the way back. I stopped in front of the customer's house, grabbed the twenty-five pounds of ice, and ran up the walk toward the back porch. I knew from the year before where the icebox was located—into the kitchen from the porch, across the kitchen, through a door onto a side porch, where the box sat in the corner just outside the door. There was no one in the kitchen so I went across to the door. I opened the door and had the ice up in the air ready to drop into the box, but since last year there had been some remodeling. There was no porch. It was now a bathroom, and sitting on the toilet just inside the door where the icebox used to be was the big fat lady of the house holding a roll of toilet paper. I almost dropped the ice in her lap. "Where in the hell is your icebox?" I sputtered and backed out. When I got back to the truck, Everett knew something had happened. When I told him, he almost fell out of the truck laughing.

When I got home, I had to tell Mom and Dad what had happened. But Dad was not amused. "Son, I'm afraid you're in trouble," he said. "The husband of that woman called me this afternoon and he was furious, and you're going to have to make peace with him." He let me splutter through supper, and finally he started laughing. That was Dad's idea of a joke.

AFTER WORKING ALL SUMMER, I returned to Washington to begin my junior year. It was hard to believe that I was starting on the final half. I had successfully completed my basic sciences, and now I was going to get into the real studies—medicine, surgery, obstetrics, gynecology, pediatrics, psychiatry, and all the rest. I would be carrying a real doctor's bag with stethoscope, blood pressure gauge, and all the other instruments needed to examine patients. I also would be wearing a white coat and going into the hospital to see patients. We all felt important, swaggering along with black bags in hand and stethoscopes hanging around our necks.

It didn't take long, though, for the instructor to take the wind out of my sails. I was assigned a patient to interview in the OB/GYN clinic one day. She was an attractive young lady wearing a big overcoat. In my most professional manner I asked every question on the checklist. The only positive finding was that she hadn't menstruated for six months. I left the space for tentative diagnosis blank. The patient was then sent to an examining room to be examined by a staff physician. I was summoned to the examining room, and a staff physician (a female) started giving me a chewing out in front of the patient. "I notice you apparently don't have any idea what could be the problem with this patient," she said. "That is right," I answered. "She had no complaint except she hadn't menstruated for six months." Then very sarcastically the female doctor asked, "Didn't it occur to you she just might be pregnant?" I quickly looked at the patient and sure enough, her belly was bulging as if she had swallowed a good size watermelon. As the patient was leaving, I stopped her and asked why she let me make a fool of myself. "Why didn't you tell me you were pregnant?" "I didn't know I was pregnant," she said. "Well, didn't your husband notice and didn't he suggest that there was a possibility you might be going to have a baby?" She blushed and answered, "Oh my, no. We never talk about things like that."

I was attracted to surgery and could hardly wait for the opportunity to do some cutting. One day a big man came to the clinic with the complaint of a large lump in the palm of his hand. He was examined by the resident with several of us watching. The patient stated he had been hit in the hand by buckshot quite some time before. The lump had gotten larger, quite hard and painful, and limited the use of his hand. He wanted the buckshot removed. I got the jump on my classmates and asked the resident if I could operate. With his permission, I asked the nurse to get the instruments. The patient was sitting up in an examining chair with his hand stretched out, palm up, on an arm board. The nurse scrubbed the hand and prepped it for surgery. Then I injected Novocain. I scrubbed my hands and slipped on the sterile gloves. I was ready for my first operation. I grabbed the hand and took the scalpel in my hand. The lump was about the size of a marble and I knew it was going to be duck soup. Just make an incision down till I hit the lead shot, spread the tissue apart with a hemostat, work around the shot, loosening it up, and then simply lift it out. I planned a couple of sutures to close the wound and then would apply a dressing.

I made the incision properly and began to work my way down to the shot. I kept going deeper and deeper and still no shot. My classmates were hanging over my shoulder watching. They began to give advice. Maybe I was in the wrong place. I began to dig—first to one side, then to the other. I began to sweat. Glancing at the patient, I saw he was sweating, too, and had begun to turn a sickly gray color. I quickly had one of the boys flip the chair back so that the patient was lying horizontally. The color began to return to his face. After about fifteen minutes, I was ready to throw in the towel. Then the hospital radiologist wandered in. "What are you doing?" he asked. I thought that was a silly question. Any damned fool could see I was cutting on a man's hand. I told him I was taking out a buckshot. "Hmm, that's interesting. I'll bet you a steak dinner you'll have to get me to help you by using the fluoroscope before you find it," he said in a patronizing way as he strolled out. I wanted to slit his throat. I was determined not to give up, but after another fifteen minutes with no luck, I threw down my scalpel and walked across to the X-ray department. "I give up," I told the radiologist. "I know when I'm licked." We put the patient on the X-ray table, and even with the fluoroscope where we could visualize the shot, it took us fifteen minutes to remove it. That was a most humbling experience, but later I realized I had learned a valuable lesson. Never underestimate a given situation and never take anything for granted.

We spent considerable time in the lecture halls taking notes as we listened to top professors in all the specialties. Most of these men were busy in their practices but still gave enormous amounts of time to teaching. Their services were donated. It was a matter of their passing on knowledge to us, continuing the precedents set when they were students, learning from the specialists of their day.

We were impressed by the various professors who came into the parking area next to the medical school. Most of them had chauffeured limousines. One was a flamboyant urologist with a waxed handlebar mustache. He was always impeccably dressed. He had a lavender limousine, and his chauffeur wore a lavender uniform that matched the car.

We not only attended clinics and made rounds with staff members at the University Hospital but also traveled about Washington to other hospitals, including Children's, Garfield, Columbian Eye, Emergency, and Gallinger.

At Children's Hospital, we were introduced to the use of steam for treatment of respiratory infections such as croup and laryngotracheobronchitis in children. Children suffering from such conditions were wheeled in their beds into a large room similar to a walk-in refrigerator, with a slatted floor to provide drainage for the condensed steam. The door was closed and valves were opened, permitting steam to flow into the room from a number of pipes around the walls. It was amazing to see the soothing effect of the warm vapor on the respiratory system of these little patients. Instead of raspy breathing and harsh coughing, the patients almost immediately started normal breathing. Today the wheeling of a bed into a room full of steam vapor has given way to the small warm or cool mist vaporizer on the bedside table.

Gallinger (D.C. General today) was the so-called city hospital, composed of many hundreds of beds occupied by "charity patients."

It was our primary teaching hospital. We called it "the cesspool" because of the constant stench of unemptied bedpans. Almost every disease found in the books could be seen there. It was sobering to take histories and do physical exams on these patients. I quickly began to see the tremendous scope of the practice of medicine—all of the things that could go wrong with the human body and the great responsibility of a doctor.

Not many of us had automobiles so getting about the city created a transportation problem. Those with cars loaded the rest of us in so that we managed to get by. I usually rode with Mary McLaughlin, one of three women in the class. Good-natured and of Irish stock, she had been orphaned early in life. Her older brother, a physician, had assumed the responsibility of seeing her through school. She had a Chevrolet coupe with a rumble seat. I always got the rumble seat, rain or shine. Riding with Mary was taking your life into your hands. She was forever running red lights or making illegal turns, and she did these things with the innocent air of a child. It seems as if I spent most of every ride with my hands over my eyes. We decided that Mary, with a St. Christopher medal dangling above the windshield, was not only blessed by the luck of the Irish but had an angel perched on each shoulder. We never had an accident.

I HAD BEEN ELECTED president of the fraternity in my junior year. (I think I got the job because no one else wanted it.) I was rather pleased at first but soon learned that there could be headaches. Any problem that arose was the responsibility of the president. Tim Chillemi, once again our landlord, was an aficionado of the game of poker. Occasionally, the brothers in the fraternity took part in a friendly game with Tim. One Friday night before dinner one of the brothers tipped me off that Tim was running a professional game with outside patrons. I immediately collared Tim, and he admitted that he had been running a game, but "Docta Mitch, this is just a friendly game and I make a little money serving sandwiches." "Nevertheless, Tim, this has to stop—no more games," I said. "The next thing you know we'll be raided, and even though the boys in the fraternity are innocent, we'll be in trouble with the school and probably be thrown out." "Please, Docta Mitch, just one more time. Tomorrow night. It has already been arranged, and then no more," pleaded Tim. "All right, Tim, tomorrow night but no more." Me and my soft heart. Why couldn't I say no and stop the whole thing?

The next night it was cold and foggy with a light drizzle. Occasionally, we brought dates to the house on Saturday night and had a dance in the living room, dancing to the radio music of the big bands. About 10:00 P.M. one of the boys came in the living room, his eyes as big as saucers. "I've got to see you right away," he said, so we slipped out into the hallway. "What's the problem?" "We're being raided," he answered. He and his date had gone downstairs to the kitchen to fix a sandwich, and while they were sitting in the kitchen, a man ran through and out the back door. Right behind him came a policeman with his gun out. Sam Prevo was in the living room with his date (the dean's private secretary), so I got him out in the hall. About that time, a detective came charging up the back stairs with his gun drawn. "What are you doing here, Doc?" he asked when he saw Sam. "What are you doing here, Blackie?" Sam shot back. "We're raiding the place," answered Blackie. "Well, there is nobody up here involved. These are all medical students, and they know nothing about anything downstairs, so stay down there and, furthermore, we want no publicity about this," Sam replied. "Okay, Doc, that's the way it'll be," and with that Blackie disappeared down the steps. Sam had many friends in the police department, including Blackie, so we were fortunate that he was there that night.

We were still worried, though, because the editor of the *Times Herald* didn't have any love for the medical school and we could just see the headlines—"George Washington Medical School Fraternity Raided." The only recourse the school would have would be expulsion of the fraternity group.

We all stood at the front windows and watched as the police brought out the poker players. They filled one paddy wagon, and a second pulled up. The last one brought out to the wagon was Tim, a big cop on each side. About midnight, I got a call from Tim—"Docta Mitch, I'm sprung. I'll be home in time to cook breakfast." I was furious about the whole thing. I gave Tim a chewing that I'm sure he didn't forget. The poker sessions were ended. The detective kept his word, and nothing was leaked to the press. Tim wasn't so dumb. He had selected his poker clients with care. Those picked up in the raid that night were all prominent people, including an attorney, a judge, and a physician. They were all released, but Tim had to pay a small fine for running a restaurant without a license.

I managed to get through the rest of my junior year without any major problems except at midyear exams. I made a condition in preventive medicine, which was a minor course taught by Dr. R. R. Spencer. Dr. Spencer had done research on Rocky Mountain Spotted Fever and was involved in the development of a vaccine for the disease. He volunteered to submit to the bite of an infected tick and was given the vaccine that he had helped develop.

Pappy Willard and I drove out to the Spencer home one night to take the makeup exam. Neither one of us had studied, and it suddenly dawned on us that if we flunked the test we would be expelled automatically. The policy at George Washington was two conditions in four years—any more would mean expulsion. One flunk was cause for expulsion. Dr. Spencer greeted us with a friendly smile, and after we were seated, he said, "I've decided to give you the same test over again, but instead of writing the test, I will ask ten questions and you take turns answering them." The test took only about fifteen minutes, and we each made a grade somewhere between 90 and 100. Dr. Spencer shook hands, and we went running out to the car. We were not going to get the boot.

PAPPY WAS GETTING MARRIED as soon as school was out in June, but he had a problem. He had the job as night physician at the District of Columbia jail, and he had to take over as soon as school was out and was allowed no time off for the next year except for school. Since I was going to be in Washington most of the summer doing obstetrics, I volunteered to take Pappy's job for two weeks while he was on his honeymoon.

I reported to the jail to start my tour of duty about 4:00 P.M. The huge brick and stone structure had been built before the Civil War and housed Confederate prisoners during the war. I rang the bell; a small peephole was opened and a guard peered out. I gave him my name. He unlocked the door, and I walked into a vestibule that was surrounded on three sides by steel bars. The guard unlocked the gate, and I went inside. I was introduced to the other guards and was shown my quarters (a former prison cell) on an upper floor. An opening had been cut through to an adjoining cell that was my closet and dressing room. I was introduced to a trusty, who was to take care of my room and my clothes, including shining my shoes.

The jail had a huge central gallery, with the cellblocks extending out like spokes in a wheel. Each block was four stories high. In an alcove of the dining hall was located the facility's electric chair. According to the guard, the chair was kept covered by a white sheet until the morning of an execution. Then, the tables were pushed back, the chair was brought out and hooked up to the cables, and the prisoner was brought in and executed at 10:00 A.M. "I'm sure not many show up for lunch on the day of an execution," I said. "Hell, it doesn't bother the others. The b——ds eat twice as much," he answered.

I held sick call every evening in the dispensary. Monday night was the big night. All the prisoners who had been held in the precinct lockups over the weekend were taken to court on Monday and, after sentencing, were brought to the jail. Most were severe alcoholics, and a more bedraggled, pitiful group I have never seen. Their clothing was torn and ragged; some had no shoes and their feet were bloody. They were beginning to have the "shakes" from alcohol withdrawal. I found they were drinking everything from cheap wine to rubbing alcohol.

My assistant was a prisoner who was a pharmacist. I was curious as to why he was in jail. When I asked him, he just grinned and told me he had the bad habit of writing bad checks.

The first night I was there I went to bed in my "private cell," and the next morning when I awoke the sun was streaming through the barred window. My first thought was "What have I done to land in jail?"

I had to check the "hole" every day. The hole was actually a small room below the main level. In the middle was a cage of steel bars. A prisoner who had been convicted of murder was in solitary while I was there. He had been put there for an undetermined period of time for throwing food at a guard. Except for when we were there, the hole was in total darkness. The prisoner was stripped to the skin. Around his middle was a wide leather belt that was locked so it couldn't be removed. Extending out from the belt were two chains, one on each side, with a wide leather cuff at the end of each chain. His wrists were locked in the cuffs. He had a pallet on the concrete floor for a bed, and a bucket in the corner served as a toilet. He was given two slices of bread and all the water he wanted for each of three meals, with the fourth meal being a complete meal. He had to be seen by a doctor each day; hence, the reason for my visit. He was weighed daily and his weight recorded on the chart on the wall.

Those prisoners who had trusty status occupied a dormitory at the front of the jail near the dispensary. They were not locked in cells and had more privileges. "Lights out" was extended to a much later hour at night. They also were allowed packages from home, including cakes. It seemed as though someone had a birthday almost every day so there were plenty of cakes. Of course, they had to have ice cream to go with the cake, so they'd give me the money and ask me to get the ice cream from a nearby drugstore. In return for that favor, I was invited to the party. The dormitory was organized almost like a club. There was room for only so many in the dorm, yet there were more trusties than there were beds. When a trusty was released, creating a vacancy, the remaining members of the club balloted on the men who were on the waiting list.

The jail was an eerie place late at night. On occasion, when I had to go down to the rotunda after lights out, I could hear the snores of the men in the cellblock. When someone having a nightmare screamed out, the sound echoed off the walls and ceiling. Open gas jets furnished the only light, and the gentle breeze that seemed to waft continuously through the building caused the flame of the gas jets to flicker, casting grotesque shadows on the wall.

THE SUMMER WAS extremely hot and sultry as only the summers can be in Washington, and the day I reported to Gallinger Hospital seemed to be hotter, if possible, than it had been so far that summer. I had finished my stay at the jail, and it was only a short move over to the nearby hospital for the obstetrical rotation. The resident physician explained that I was to be on continuous duty for the next month. I was to leave the hospital only when I could be spared to get something to eat. The hospital did not provide meals. The only place to eat was a restaurant about a block away, and it was really a "greasy spoon." The nursing supervisor kept a close watch to see that no one took any food from the kitchen, not even a glass of milk.

There were four medical students on the service, two from George Washington and two from Georgetown. We were all assigned to one sleeping room. It was an ordinary-sized hospital room with four hospital beds lined up side by side, with no space between them. If you were in the bed farthest from the door you had to climb or roll across all the other beds. There was no air-conditioning, and there was only one window. To make matters worse, a new wing to the hospital was under construction; even if you had the chance to get some sleep during the day, which hardly ever happened, the riveters outside the window kept you awake.

We rotated new patients among the four of us. We were required to do a complete history and physical on our assigned patients: take them through delivery and follow them through postdelivery until they were discharged. We assumed total responsibility for each patient. Many hadn't seen a doctor until they arrived at the hospital in labor. It seemed that a full moon or a bad thunderstorm always stimulated labor. On those occasions, the elevator ran continuously up to the floor, the door opening and coughing out a new patient, and back down to get another. Since many of the women had received little, if any, prenatal care, they frequently had complications, the most common being hypertension, a forerunner of eclampsia. Of course, most of them were overweight and had abnormal urines and marked swelling of their legs. One of the dangers was that the patients could develop eclampsia, convulse, and die.

After I had made the delivery, I was required to sit by the table with my hand on the patient's belly, squeezing the uterus down tight to prevent bleeding. We were required to do the procedure for an hour after delivery before taking the patient back to the room. It seemed as if I saw every sunrise over the Potomac, sitting there half asleep with my hand squeezing the uterus, trying to keep from falling off the stool. If the patient had an elevated blood pressure and there was any danger she might have a postpartum convulsion, we were required to sit at the patient's bedside on a hard, straight chair, the room darkened, for at least three hours. There could be not the slightest noise—not even the rustle of a paper—for fear the patient might convulse. Only when the blood pressure approached normal levels could we leave the room. Sometimes it was impossible to get the history and physical completed before the patient delivered because most of them were not first-time mothers and when they hit the hospital they were ready. One of the boys from Georgetown had been there several days when he delivered his first baby. Every patient he had been assigned had delivered just as he stepped out for a minute to go to the bathroom or some other reason. Finally, he had a patient whom he seemed to be getting along with quite well. He was sitting at the bedside, taking a history while the patient was on a bedpan quietly answering all his questions. Suddenly she interrupted him, saying, "Pardon me, Doctor, but I've just had the baby." He jumped up, jerked back the sheet. Sure enough, there was the baby in the bedpan. He reached in the bedpan and extracted the screaming infant. Holding it high by its feet, he took the bedpan in his other hand and marched out of the room with a proud look on his face and announced, "My first delivery, and from a bedpan."

I just couldn't take the food at the "greasy spoon," but I had an ace in the hole. When I could get away about meal time, I'd take off for the nearby jail and ring the bell at the front door. The guard looking out the peephole would recognize me and open the door. "Come on in, Doc, and let's eat." I don't know how I would have survived for that month if it hadn't been for the good meals at the jail.

The student nurses felt sorry for us and smuggled in food at night. Sometimes they would bring us a homemade cake or even fry pancakes in the diet kitchen. On these occasions we would station "lookouts" down the corridors to keep watch for the night supervisor. If the nurses had been caught, they would have been disciplined severely.

One of my classmates, Buck Weaver, was always hungry. One night he sneaked into the kitchen and rustled around for something to eat. The only thing he could find was a quart bottle of milk in the refrigerator. He had just drained the last drop from the bottle when a student nurse walked in. "Where did you get that milk?" she asked. "Up there," he said, pointing to the top shelf of the refrigerator. She burst out laughing. "What's so funny?" asked Buck. "You just drank a quart of breast milk we pumped from one of the patients," she answered, doubling over in laughter.

One of the first things we checked on our patients were the lab reports. We were particularly interested in whether there was any venereal infection present. One night I had a patient ready to deliver. As I stood ready to perform the delivery, she had a hard contraction and the bag of water bulged out in my face like a big bubble. Suddenly the bag burst, and I was soaked from my waist down. I was terrified.

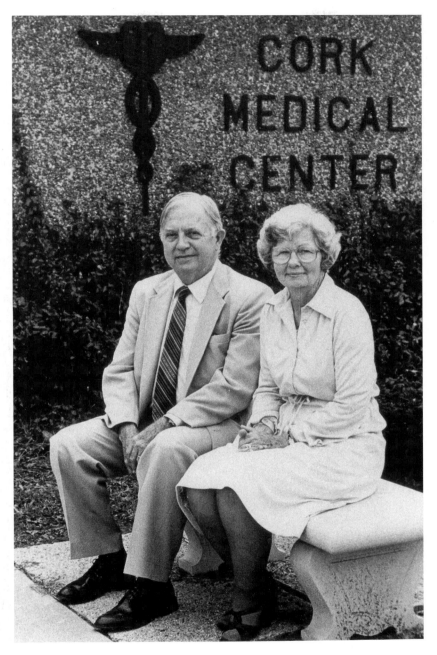

George and Millie Mitchell outside Cork Medical Center, Marshall,
Illinois, 1980

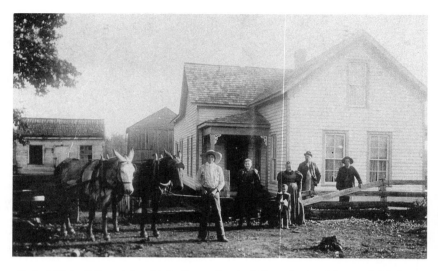

R. A. Mitchell (in white shirt), the author's father, during his youthful days as a southern Illinois log hauler near Harrisburg

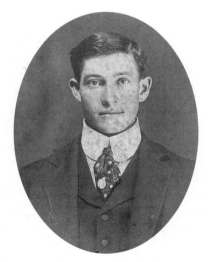

R. A. Mitchell, ca. 1904

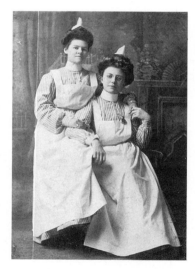

Alma Trice (*right*), the author's mother, 1904

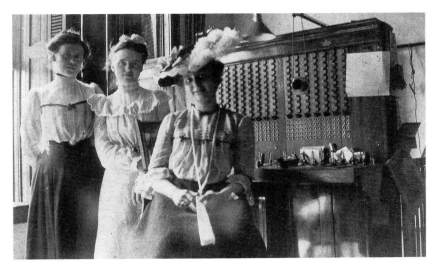

The Marshall, Illinois, telephone switchboard and operators, 1900
(*courtesy Drew Casteel*)

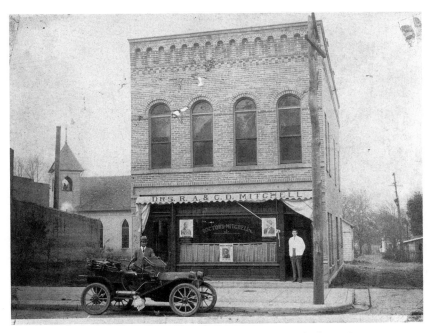

The Mitchell Building on the Courthouse Square, Marshall, 1910.
Dr. R. A. Mitchell stands at curb; Dr. C. D. Mitchell stands in the doorway.

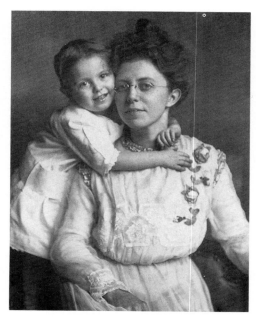

The author and his mother, 1917

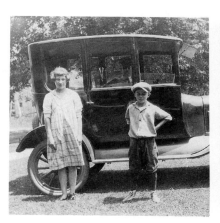

Sylvia Short and the author in front
of a Model T, ca. 1922

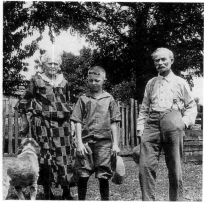

The author and his maternal
grandparents, Sarah and David
Trice, at the Heltonville, Indiana,
farm, ca. 1924

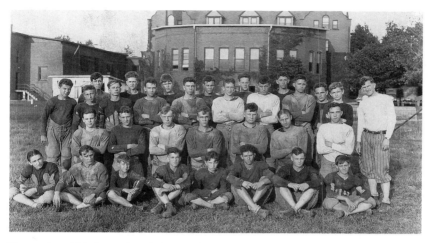

The author (*third row, fourth from right*) and fellow members of the Marshall High School football squad, 1930

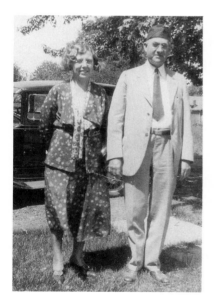

The author's parents, 1931

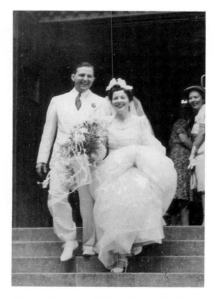

The author and his wife on their wedding day, June 21, 1941, McKee Chapel, Indianapolis

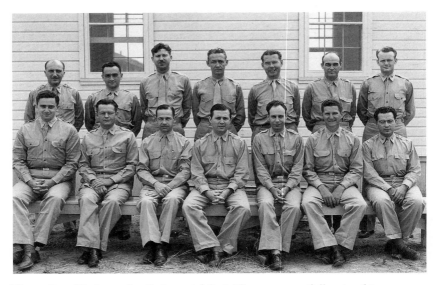

The author (*first row, fourth from right*) at Albuquerque, following his commission in the Medical Corps of the Army Air Corps, ca. 1941

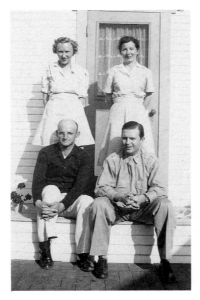

The Mitchells (*right*) with Lois and Kennie Long, 1942

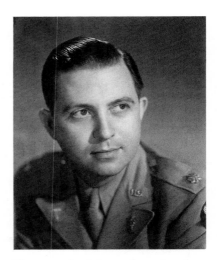

Photograph of the author taken by George Cukor's *Winged Victory* film crew, ca. 1943

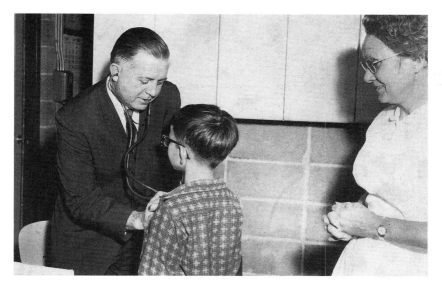

The author conducting a school examination, ca. 1950; nurse Clara Norton
assisted Dr. George for more than forty years.

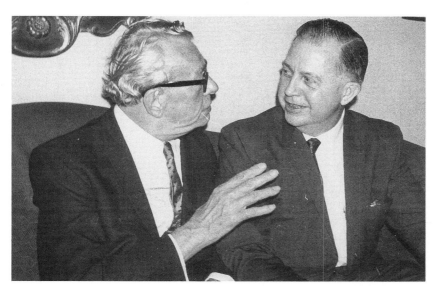

The author with Senator Everett Dirksen (*left*), 1968

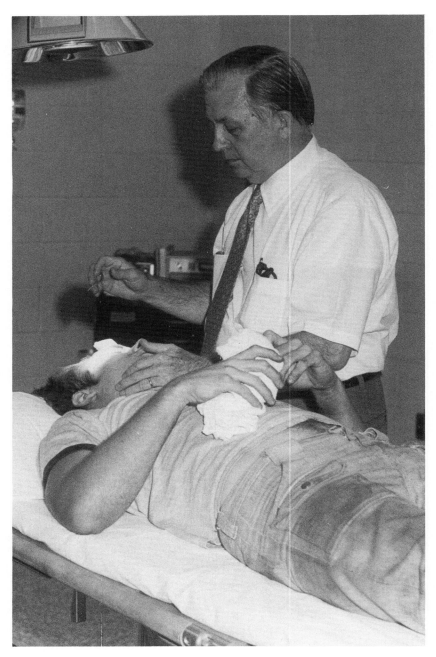

The author with a patient at Cork Medical Center, Marshall, Illinois

The patient had a venereal infection. I thought, "What a helluva way to get a venereal infection!" I quickly delivered the baby and ran down the hall to the showers. I stood under the shower for almost a half hour scrubbing and scrubbing with soap until I was almost raw and the bar of soap was down to a sliver.

There were too many patients for so few nurses. As most of the babies were breast fed, the infants had to be taken from the nursery out to the mothers for feeding every three hours. The poor nurses were on the run all the time, and it was impossible to get the job done carrying one baby at a time. Consequently, they carried two or three at once cradled in their arms like a load of stove wood. They went from bed to bed dealing them off the top. One day there was quite an uproar. A mother started screaming, "You gave me the wrong baby! You gave me the wrong baby!"

The month at Gallinger was one of the hardest months I experienced, but I learned a lot. I don't know how many babies I delivered, but when my time was up, I left with a feeling of confidence. My partner on "outdoor OB," as we called it, was Jim Winn. Jim was what I called a refined person. He was a member of a wealthy family from the East, whereas I was a Midwestern farm boy. There was a lot about life he hadn't been exposed to, but I liked him very much.

For "outdoor OB," we were provided a small apartment, actually a bedroom and bath, in a building not far from the university hospital. We were expected to stay in the room and await calls from the hospital switchboard directing us to the scene of a home delivery. When a call was received, we rushed to the hospital and picked up the delivery bag. We were required to furnish our own transportation, but I was in luck because Jim had a Packard club coupe, a luxury car.

The bag, which was actually an oversized suitcase, was crammed with sterile towels, drapes, instruments, pans, and the medications we needed. We had little, if any, information concerning the patient we were to deliver. We were on our own except for the phone number of an obstetrician we could call if we felt we were getting in over our heads.

Our first call came in the middle of the night. We raced to the hospital, dressed up in our freshly starched white uniforms, picked up the bag, and tore down the street toward the great unknown. We had a map of Washington, but looking for an address in the middle of the night was almost like looking for a needle in the haystack. Finally, after stopping several times and looking at house numbers with a flashlight, we found the place. The husband was out in front anxiously awaiting our arrival. We jumped out of the car and went briskly up the walk, with me carrying the big suitcase. At each delivery one of us was the doctor and the other was the nurse. We had flipped a coin before we started and I lost. I was the nurse so I carried the bag.

We were led into the house and down a hallway to the room where the patient was in bed. We made every effort to appear calm and in complete control, just as if we had been delivering babies for years. Jim examined the patient, listened to the fetal heart, palpated the abdomen, and checked the blood pressure, duly noting his findings in a notebook. The labor pains were getting closer, and it was evident delivery was near. I turned the patient around crossways in the bed and placed two straight chairs about three feet apart at the side of the bed and placed one of her feet on each of the chairs with her buttocks at the edge of the bed. I then prepped the patient by scrubbing her belly and buttocks with green soap. In the meantime, Jim had laid the instruments out on a sterile towel on a nearby table. Jim scrubbed up at the kitchen sink, and I helped him into his sterile gown and gloves. He then sat down in a chair in front of the patient. The contractions became stronger, but there was no sign of the head coming down. I could see a look of concern showing in Jim's eyes above his mask, but neither one of us said anything. Finally, we could see the bag of waters beginning to show through the opening. With each contraction the opening expanded more, until suddenly the waters broke with a gush. Then things began to really move. With a towel in one hand, Jim had exerted a little pressure below the opening and placed his other hand over the head to control the speed of delivery. He gently extended the head and brought it out; then the arms, torso, and legs emerged with the next contraction. Jim laid the squalling baby up on the mother's abdomen and clamped and tied the cord. He had done a fine job. Then he waited for the placenta to appear.

We had been taught never to exert any pressure on the abdomen to expel the placenta, just to wait until the placenta separated and popped out of the vaginal opening. Jim sat and waited, but no placenta showed. Jim began to sweat, and the father began to look at us as if he wondered whether we were qualified or not. Finally, Jim got up and motioned me to a corner of the room for a consultation. We had not run into that sort of thing in our days at Gallinger. Jim suggested I go for help. I excused myself and went out to the car. I drove down the street to a filling station that was closed but had a phone booth outside. I called the doctor who was our backup. It was evident that he was displeased about being awakened in the middle of the night by an inexperienced medical student. After he had listened to my description of the predicament, he said very sarcastically, "Did you think to look inside the vagina?" I hurried back, and Jim and I had another whispered consultation. He returned to the patient, sat down in the chair, and quickly took a peek inside the vaginal opening. There, all nice and cozy, lay the complete placenta. Jim lifted it out and popped it into the pan, like a pro, looking up with a broad smile on his face. He then did the usual massage job on the uterus through the abdominal wall. In the meantime, I cleaned up the baby and put the required silver nitrate in the eyes. Then I diapered and gowned the little thing and placed it in bed with the mother. My nurse's work wasn't done yet because I had to bathe the patient, put clean sheets on the bed, clean up the mess, and pack the suitcase with the dirty drapes and instruments.

We left a happy father and mother with their new baby and wearily went to the car. Dawn was breaking as we went back to the hospital to leave the bag to be restocked. Tumbling into bed, we felt pretty good. We had just successfully completed our first delivery on our own.

The first thing we did upon returning from a delivery was to go directly to the bathroom. We both stood in the dry bathtub and stripped down, leaving our clothes in the tub and inspecting each other closely for bedbugs.

One hot, humid morning we were summoned to a flat, where we found a large woman in hard labor. The room was very small, and it was crowded. It contained a large double bed over by the one window, a table, two or three chairs, and a four-burner kerosene cookstove going full blast. On top of the stove was a huge kettle of boiling water that emitted a cloud of steam. The heat was unbearable. We moved the patient into the usual position with her feet on two chairs. Again Jim was the doctor, and I was the nurse. After the patient was prepped, Jim dressed in sterile gown and gloves, crawled over the bed, and got into position with his back to the window. There was no room for him to move. The pains were close together and hard, and with each pain the patient let out a scream. To add to the problem, with each contraction a gush of blood shot out of the vaginal opening, but there was no sign that the head had come down. It was obvious things weren't going well. I stepped out into the hall to compose myself, and the old granny followed me out and started talking. "Doctor, I don't know why she didn't go to the hospital. She always has such a hard time, and this is the first time she ever tried to have a baby at home." Any confidence I had had suddenly vanished. I hurried back into the room to tell Jim I was calling for help, and there sat Jim wide-eyed, looking at the bag of waters bulging out in his face. With each contraction it got bigger, and Jim leaned back a little further until he was almost leaning out the open window. Suddenly the thing burst, showering Jim with a mixture of blood and amniotic fluid, soaking him to the skin. The baby shot out, landing in his lap. With that, the bleeding stopped. Jim picked the slippery baby from his lap and laid it across the woman's abdomen. It lay there, squalling. Jim finished the job, and I proceeded with my nursing chores, cleaning and dressing the baby, bathing the patient, and putting clean sheets on the bed. Granny and the mother were both grinning from ear to ear.

The following day we went back to check on the mother and baby and found the mother had a fever and was chilling. Our diagnosis was postpartum pyelitis (kidney infection). That was before the advent of sulfa drugs or any of the other antibiotics. The standard treatment was baking soda dissolved in water. We left the directions with granny and instructed her to give the patient several glasses of water each day.

The following day we checked back and found the mother had a normal temperature and was feeling great. When we came into the room, I noticed a plate full of sliced onions on the table next to the bed. When we told granny that the temperature was normal and that the infection was under control, she didn't act surprised. "Oh, I knew she would be all right today," she grinned, "It was the onions. They always get rid of the fever."

One dark night we were looking for an address in a particularly squalid section of Washington. After what seemed like hours, we finally located the right house. We went in the dark hallway and climbed the creaking stairs to the second floor, entering a room lit by a single kerosene lamp. After our eyes adjusted to the dim light, we could see a woman lying quietly in a bed over in one corner of the room. The floor was bare, and there was no other furniture. The patient was alone. No granny was in attendance. We walked to the side of the bed and looked at the patient. She obviously wasn't having any labor pains so we thought we had been called out on a false alarm. She looked up and said, "Docta, you are a little late. I already had the baby." We looked around on the bed, but there was no baby.

"Where is the baby?" Jim asked. "Well, I always squats down in the corner to have my babies," she answered in a soft voice. In the far corner of the dimly lighted room I could see a large pile of crumpled newspapers. I walked over and started gently moving the papers with my foot. Then I heard a cry. I flipped on my flashlight, and down on my knees, I started pulling paper out of the pile. Then I saw the baby on the floor kicking its feet, the cord still attached to the placenta. Jim picked the baby up, and I picked up the placenta and we gently carried the baby and placenta over to the bed and laid them down. The cord was tied and cut. Again I had the job of cleaning up the mess and bathing the patient. On the way back to the apartment we marveled at the way nature takes care of things without the assistance of a doctor.

The next night we went back to check on the mother and baby. In the dim light of the kerosene lamp, we could see that everything in the room was spotless and the baby, dressed in a lace gown, was lying in a crib with clean white sheets. Over the crib was mosquito netting to protect the baby from the mosquitoes and flies that were buzzing about. We discovered there was no inside plumbing in the house except for a cold water tap. It was hard to believe that here in the shadow of the Capitol there was such a concentration of poverty.

Others who had been through home deliveries had plenty of stories to tell. My fraternity brother, O'Grady, the Irishman, was out alone on a delivery one night. When he arrived the patient was alone. He examined her, and it appeared it was going to be awhile before she delivered. He sat and watched her for quite some time. The longer he sat, the sleepier he got. He kept eyeing the bed she was in. Finally he couldn't resist the temptation. "Move over," he said as he pulled back the sheet. "When you are ready to have the baby, wake me up," he mumbled, dropping off to sleep.

Bill Bailey came running into the room one day all out of breath. He had just gotten out of bed and had been to the bathroom. "What in the world are these things?" he yelled as he stood scratching. Bill was on second call and had delivered the baby the night before. I took a good look and laughed, "Billy, you've got bedbugs." He was horrified—a gentleman from a fine Virginia family infested with bedbugs!

After delivering babies all summer long I was ready for a rest. I had only a couple of weeks before I started my senior year so I hurried home for a short visit.

11

Internship at Methodist Hospital

DAD WAS NOT in good health, although he would not admit it. He was very sensitive and never discussed his health problems. On one occasion he had slipped out of town and entered the University Hospital in Indianapolis for a checkup. When he was admitted, he gave his name as Roscoe Addison—not Roscoe Addison Mitchell—and gave his occupation as a farmer. Mom and I frequently had discussed his health after we learned that he had hypertension. Mom put him on a diet to lose weight, giving him lots of salads and nonfattening foods. He never complained, but when at the table he only picked at his food. We soon found out that after leaving to return to the office he stopped at the local restaurant to eat a big meal of his favorite high-calorie foods. When Mom discovered what he was doing, she abandoned the diet and returned to preparing the food he enjoyed. We decided that rather than make him miserable it was best to let him enjoy life, even though we felt he was soon going to be in trouble.

I spent all my time with him at the office and on house calls, trying to take the load off him. I drove the car and carried his bag. We both enjoyed the companionship we had those few weeks.

One morning in September we started out to make his round of house calls. The day was hot and humid, he seemed to be more tired than usual, and his face was flushed. I knew his blood pressure must be high. About midmorning we made a call on an elderly woman living on North Seventh Street. Dad slowly got out of the car and shuffled up the walk. I walked by his side carrying the bag. The patient was on the second floor, and he was breathing heavily when we got to the top of the stairs. As he was finishing the examination, he received a phone call about a farmer five miles away who was injured and needed help. We found the man lying under a tree with a dislocated right elbow. Dad gave him a hypodermic and instructed the family to bring him to the office.

The family brought the man in and laid him on the examining table. Dad's brother Earl, who was associated with Dad in practice, started the anesthetic of drip ether. When the patient was anesthetized, Dad took hold of the wrist and told me to take hold of the arm just above the elbow and pull. He started pulling in the opposite direction and reduced the dislocation. Suddenly he stopped, lay the arm across the man's chest and, without saying a word, started walking toward the door. He staggered, striking the door casing. I sent the nurse out to see if he was all right. She screamed for me to come quickly. I ran into the waiting room to see him slumped in the chair, his feet straight out in front of him. He was unconscious, breathing heavily, with his mouth pulled to one side. My uncle was unable to leave the anesthetized patient so, leaving the nurse to watch Dad, I ran next door to Dr. Weir's office. Unfortunately, he had gone to lunch. I called his house, and he came immediately.

There was no question: Dad had suffered a cerebral hemorrhage. We decided to take him home. I called the ambulance but told them not to bring him home until I had told Mom what had happened. When I walked in the back door, Mom was putting lunch on the table. "Where's your Dad?" she asked. "Mom, you know what we have talked about so many times? Well, it's happened. Dad had a stroke." When she heard that, she grabbed her head with both hands, pulled her hair straight up and let out one scream. Then it was over. She quietly said, "You bring him home, and I'll have the bed ready."

Later that day we moved him to the hospital in nearby Paris. His condition was critical for several days. He remained unconscious, and it appeared he was going to die. He began to improve and regained consciousness, but he was completely paralyzed on the right side and unable to utter a word. The hemorrhage had destroyed the motor and speech areas of the left side of the brain. Mom never left the hospital except to come home to launder his gowns and get a few hours' sleep. She was content to sit by his bed.

I had decided not to return to school that year. I felt Mom needed me. The crops were going to have to be harvested, and the livestock needed to be cared for. We had a tenant who would look after things, but I knew that Dad, if he were able, would be out checking on things every day. Since he was not able, Mom would have to take his place. After he regained consciousness, he seemed to know what I was planning to do. He had started to communicate by scribbling on papers with his left hand. Although it was hard to decipher, I got the message, "Go back to school."

I called Katie Breen, the dean's secretary, and told her about Dad. She told me not to worry and that she would take care of my registration and to stay home until I was satisfied he was out of immediate danger. As a result, I was about three weeks late getting back to school.

It was all I could do to leave those two I loved so much—Dad lying helplessly in bed and Mom sitting loyally by his side. I had a sad ride back to Washington. My classmates were all concerned and did everything they could to help me get back into the routine. I received a daily bulletin from the hospital. Sometimes it was encouraging, and then there were the bad days. Dad progressed to where he was out in a wheelchair and Mom could push him down the corridors to see other patients. The hospital was a familiar place to Dad. He had been on the staff for years.

Mom soon developed a routine. She stayed with Dad from early morning until 10:00 or 11:00 P.M. Then she drove the sixteen miles home by herself, laundered his gowns, and went to bed. She was up by 4:00 A.M., ironing his gowns. She drove out to check the farm operation, then on to the hospital where she gave Dad a report on the farm. I don't know how she was able to hold up to the grueling schedule. She seemed to have some inner strength that kept her going.

It was hard to attend classes and to concentrate. This was my all-important senior year. I managed somehow to begin applying for internships. I applied at Methodist Hospital in Indianapolis and at Barnes and City hospitals in St. Louis. With tongue in cheek, I decided to apply at the Indiana University Medical Center—the school that had refused me three years before.

One night I got a call from Mom, "Your Dad is worse. Will you come home?" I caught the first plane out of Washington and was home in a few hours. A friend met me at the Indianapolis airport and drove me directly to the hospital. After a few hours, Dad rallied and began to improve. I stayed for several days.

Before returning to school, I drove to Indianapolis to check on the internship at Methodist Hospital. My first appointment was with Dr. Ottinger, who had been Dad's classmate at Indiana and who served on the intern committee. He was very sorry to hear about Dad. He told me that the intern class selections had not been completed but assured me that I would be accepted. On my way out, I passed the office of Dr. Gatch. Seeing the name on the door aroused a devil in my soul. Dr. Gatch, I knew, was the dean of the Indiana University School of Medicine at Indianapolis. I opened the door and walked across the waiting room to the receptionist's desk. I explained to her that I had applied for an internship at the Medical Center, and I wanted to discuss it with Dr. Gatch. She informed me that Dr. Gatch wasn't in but his partner, Dr. Owen, who was on the committee, would see me. I was shown into his office. When I told him what I had on my mind, he said he could call Dr. Thompson, who was also a member of the committee, so that I could talk to him too. After Dr. Thompson arrived, I told them that I just happened to be in town and thought I would inquire about the application I had made for the internship. Dr. Owen told me that the committee had not met yet to go over the applications so they had nothing to tell me. "Well, Gentlemen," I said, "I know you are busy and I don't want to take up your time, but I am quite interested in the Medical Center. I have already been accepted at Methodist, but if you could guarantee that I would be accepted at the Medical Center, I possibly would not accept the Methodist offer." They looked at each other for a few seconds, and then Dr. Owen said, "We wish we could give you that guarantee, but I believe you will understand that would be very difficult since we have not examined any of the applications as yet."

With a big smile I shook hands and said, "Well, Gentlemen, thank you for your time. I just thought I would talk to you first before I accepted the Methodist offer. Really what I meant was I just thought I'd give you a chance." I left two very puzzled men standing there in the room as I walked out the door. I laughed all the way down the hall. I had gotten at least a small bit of revenge, I thought, for the way I had been treated three years before. Later I received a telegram from the Medical Center offering me an internship. I already had accepted the offer from Methodist so I had the extreme satisfaction of turning them down.

It was near mid-November when I received the dreaded call. "Hurry home. Your dad is dying." It was at night, and there were no planes leaving Washington at that hour. I spent a sleepless night and caught the first plane out in the morning. When I arrived at the hospital, Dad was unconscious and barely breathing. Mom, pale and haggard, was sitting by the bed holding his hand. She was not a large woman, but she looked so tiny sitting there. I joined the vigil. We didn't leave the room. Once he seemed to get stronger, and I spoke to him. He gripped my hand, and I felt he knew I was with him. Nearly twenty-four hours after I arrived, his breathing became more and more shallow and finally stopped. I tried to give him artificial respiration, but the heart had stopped. He was gone. The long struggle was over.

The life of a great man had come to an end at the age of sixty. He never wanted fame or fortune, only to serve the people he loved. The outpouring of sympathy following his death was indicative of the degree of love my father's patients had for him. I have his picture in my private office, and to this day, occasionally his old patients will come in just to stand looking at the picture to recall how he cared for them.

Returning to school after we had put Dad to rest in the little cemetery at Lewisville, Indiana, I was saddened by the thought that I no longer had a dad, a dad who was so proud that he had a son following in his footsteps and before long could be working alongside him in the practice of medicine—the dream he would never see come to pass. I also wondered about my mother. How was she going to cope with all the responsibilities that Dad had assumed before? And what about the business affairs? I could not be there to help. I soon found I need not worry. Mom was strong-willed and intelligent; she had many friends she could call on for advice. She conducted the sale that disposed of the livestock, and she converted the farming operation to a strictly grain farm. She disposed of the property in Florida, which had been a losing proposition; she bought out my uncle's interest in the office building, collected the amounts due on Dad's practice, and, in a sense, consolidated his assets into a manageable operation. It was amazing to see how she, a person with no apparent business experience, so quickly learned. She kept her finger on every aspect of the business. When I came home at Christmas, she brought me up-to-date on what she had done and I could find no fault. That was a great relief to me.

The last year of school went by swiftly, and my courses were most interesting. It was hard to realize that I would be graduating soon. The closer I came to final exams, the more excited I became. I didn't fear examinations as I had when I was a freshman. Four years of a demanding curriculum had given me confidence in my abilities. I breezed through the final exams; when the grades were posted, I was pleased that I had made high marks in every course.

There was a waiting period of nearly two weeks between the end of finals and graduation day. For the first time in four years I could completely relax. No more school. No more books. No more worrying about exams. It was hard to realize that I was through, but then I suddenly thought about a policy of the medical school. Every senior had to be evaluated by a faculty committee. They not only looked at grades but also probed into the background of each student. Was he of good moral and ethical character? That committee had the power to declare a student ineligible to receive a diploma, even though academic requirements had been mastered, if he did not measure up morally and ethically. I was confident I would measure up, but still there was that nagging question—would they think so? I didn't have long to await the answer. The list was posted on the bulletin board. The entire class would receive their diplomas. Finally, I could relax completely.

Sam Prevo proposed we go fishing off Solomons Island in the Chesapeake Bay. As we drove along in the early morning mist through the scrub pines, I saw in the east above the treetops the superstructures of a fleet of ships rising up like so many ghosts. Sam told me these were ships from World War I that had been "mothballed." I wondered, if they could speak, what they could tell us about the great sea battles they had been through—the sinking of both enemy and allied ships, the submarine attacks, and the eventual victory in the "war to end all wars."

We arrived at a small pier jutting out into the bay. A fishing boat was tied up at the end of the pier, and we arranged a charter with the owner of the boat. We climbed aboard, and Sam settled himself in the stern. After he was comfortably seated, he pulled out a bottle of bourbon and carefully positioned it between his feet. The captain started the engine and shoved off. As we pulled out into the bay, he handed out our fishing lines and shrimp for bait. I was ready for some serious fishing. I jiggled my line up and down, eagerly awaiting the strike of a big fish. I glanced over at Sam and saw his line hanging limply over the side. Sam had uncorked his bottle and was enjoying a swig. After a long wait, I got a strike. It was a good one. The fish took the bait, and I set the hook. Then the battle began. After several minutes, I landed a large sea bass, the largest I had ever caught. I was so excited I could hardly get the hook out. Sam was still sitting comfortably in the stern—fishing line hanging loosely over the side, enjoying another drink. I looked over the side and saw the baited hook hanging out of the water. I decided Sam hadn't come to fish. We brought my prize fish back to the fraternity house, and Chillemi stuffed and baked it for dinner that night. It was delicious.

A few days before the big day, Mom arrived in town. She was as excited as I was, and it was so good to see her. I had arranged for a room for her in a nearby guest house. Sam most graciously had offered me the use of his car while she was in town. We had a great time sightseeing around Washington and the surrounding countryside. One day we took the ferry from Annapolis across Chesapeake Bay to the eastern shore. Her father, Grandpa Trice, had come to Indiana from the area, and Mom knew he had a sister, whom she had never seen, still living there. After making several inquiries, we located the farm where she was living with her daughter and son-in-law. She was quite old but was still mentally alert. We had a good visit with her, talking about family and things of the past. As we drove back to the ferry, I noticed how bright Mom's eyes sparkled. She had gotten to do something she had never dreamed she would have the opportunity to do. I believe that was the high point of her trip.

The baccalaureate service for the graduating class was held in the magnificent Washington Cathedral, located on the heights in northwest Washington overlooking the city. It was built in the manner of the great cathedrals of Europe, with a spire reaching high into the heavens. Skilled craftsmen had slowly constructed it stone by stone. The services were held in the main nave with its high vaulted ceiling. The mighty organ boomed out and seemed to engulf us completely with the sounds of its beautiful music. The service was most impressive and left us with a feeling of complete awe.

A few nights later came the climax. We paraded solemnly into Constitution Hall in our caps and gowns, the hood with the gold bars indicating the degree of Doctor of Medicine draped around our shoulders. I have no memory of who spoke or what was said. The only memory I have is of looking up at Mom sitting there with a grin on her face and tears in her eyes as I received my diploma. If only Dad could have been there.

It was time to leave Washington. I had managed to get all the things together that I had lived with for the past four years. I got my trunk and suitcases packed and was ready for the baggage truck to arrive to take my trunk to the station. After the trunk had been picked up, I was to take a cab and pick up Mom on the way to the station. As train time came nearer and nearer and the baggage truck had not arrived, I began to panic. Finally, I ran out to the street and hailed a cab. I told the driver my predicament and he agreed to take us, trunk and all, to the station. I loaded my suitcases in and he tied the trunk on the back of the cab, and we took off. Mom was ready. I rushed her out to the cab, pushed her in with her suitcase, and off we went. I told the cab driver we had only a few minutes to make the train. He raced down through Washington rush hour traffic, dodging cars right and left. We stopped at the entrance to the Union Station and I hailed two redcaps. I instructed one to take Mom and her suitcase to the train. The other redcap I took with me in the cab. The cab driver drove down into the lower level and unloaded the trunk at the baggage room. I paid the driver, tipping him well, and quickly checked the trunk. Then I grabbed some suitcases, the redcap grabbed the others, and we raced through the station, dodging people right and left. I saw an unhappy conductor grimly standing by the door with a look of disgust on his face. He had to hold the mighty train for several minutes waiting for me. Mom was standing there with a firm look on her face. She had told him he was not leaving without her son. Tossing the redcaps a tip, I pushed Mom on board and the train started. We lunged into our compartment and dumped our luggage. Mom plopped into the seat; I can still see her, sprawled out with her hat cocked over the side of her head and her hair looking as if it had never been combed and brushed. We were in Baltimore before we had caught our breath and stowed our luggage. "Son, is this the way you always catch a train?" she spluttered as she tried to catch her breath. "That's right, Mom—I wanted you to do it the way I have all these years."

I had time to relax and enjoy Mom's home cooking for a couple of weeks before I reported to Methodist Hospital to begin my internship. I enjoyed seeing my friends, going out to the farm, and talking things over with Mom. She was in good health and seemed to be enjoying life, but she still couldn't forget Dad. She frequently talked about him and would remind me that "this is what your dad would say" or "this is what your dad would do."

MY INTERNSHIP BEGAN July 1. I was told to report the day before. When I arrived at the hospital, suitcase in hand, I was amazed by its size. I checked in and was given my room assignment. The intern quarters were located on the fifth floor of the south wing of the hospital. The room was large, and I found that I had two roommates, Lowell Jackson and Robert Sloan. I was a total stranger to the entire group of interns so I spent the rest of the day getting acquainted.

Many of the fledgling doctors were graduates of Indiana University School of Medicine. The rest of us came from schools around the country. We were to receive room, board, and laundry plus ten dollars per month for our labors.

I found that my first assignment was on the surgical service and that Dr. Goethe Link was the surgeon with whom I would be working. I was to report to him in surgery early the next morning. I got up early, put on my new white uniform and white shoes, ate breakfast, and went down to surgery. I had been told by some of the Indiana boys that Dr. Link was one of the most prominent surgeons in the Midwest. Dr. Link was a short man who was partially bald with a rim of snow-white hair. He looked at me through his rimless glasses as he shook my hand. His eyes seemed to be probing my very soul. He took me into the dressing room, showed me a locker, and threw me a scrub suit. I changed clothes and walked into the scrub room, where I found him standing in front of a scrub sink with the water running. He took a mask with a wire threaded through the upper border, placed it over my nose and mouth just beneath my eyes, pinched the wire down across the bridge of my nose and tied the strings over the top of my cap-covered head and the other strings around my neck. The wire pinched over my nose made it difficult to breathe, and I went around all morning talking through my nose. I couldn't understand why he did that until I saw that he also was wearing his mask with the wire formed over the bridge of his nose. The wire kept the mask close to his face so that his breath didn't escape upward to fog his glasses. I, however, did not wear glasses.

Another thing I couldn't understand was why he was starting to scrub at 7:30 A.M. for 8:00 A.M. surgery. The standard scrub was ten minutes in length. I soon discovered what it was all about. He threw me a sterile brush, and I started scrubbing, using green soap that was very irritating to my skin. We scrubbed about ten minutes, and I was following his every move. Suddenly he threw down his brush, picked up an unsterile towel, squirted some green soap on the towel and proceeded to wash the inside of his mouth. That procedure I passed up. He then started his scrub over again. We scrubbed right up to 8:00 A.M. By that time my hands and arms were red and raw. The final act was the immersing of our hands and arms into a pan of alcohol. I thought I was on fire! Holding my hands high with alcohol dripping off my elbows, I followed Dr. Link down the hall into the operating room. The patient was asleep on the table, prepped and draped. The nurses all seemed to be standing at attention as we entered the room. Dr. Link formally introduced me to all. The operation was the removal of a gall bladder. I had never before assisted in a major operation. I know I must have been clumsy, but Dr. Link never lost his temper. He quietly explained what we were doing and instructed me in the proper procedure. I was amazed at how quickly I learned. There was no question that I was working with a master of the craft. As soon as we finished a case, we scrubbed and operated again. It seemed as though that went on forever. I have forgotten how many cases we did that day, but by the time we had finished, I thought there was no skin left on my arms.

After surgery, I went as instructed to a desk in the lobby of the hospital and picked up a list of new admissions to my service. I was required to do a complete history and physical on these patients that afternoon before they went to surgery the next morning. I hardly had time to get anything to eat. Finally, finishing up late that night, I fell into bed completely exhausted. I wondered if it was really worth it.

I enjoyed surgery and before long, with the help of Dr. Link, had sharpened my skills to the point that we were working smoothly as a team. His main interest was thyroid surgery, and he had probably performed more thyroidectomies than any other surgeon in the state. He used silk sutures and ties throughout in his thyroid cases long before that was being done by anyone else. In tying the vessels he used fine suture material and insisted on cutting the suture "on the knot." That was no easy task, but I got so I could do it without any problem. When I finished his service, he paid me the highest compliment. He told me he would like to keep me permanently as his assistant.

When I came home and told Mom that I was working with Dr. Link, she was surprised and pleased. It seems that Dr. Link had been one of her instructors when she was in nurse's training, and he also had been a member of the medical school faculty when Dad was a student. Now he was training me. I learned that he was quite wealthy and had varied interests outside of medicine. He had a large observatory on his estate and was quite an astronomer. Later he gave that observatory to Indiana University. During the time I was at Methodist, he took a three-month vacation and spent it at the University of Arizona, taking some special courses in advanced mathematics.

It was amusing making rounds with him. He never used a stethoscope. Although his patients had been thoroughly worked up before surgery, he insisted on checking them himself. His greatest fear was having a patient die during surgery. He would walk into the patient's room, throw the sheet back, and put his ear to the patient's bare chest. It was particularly amusing to see him trot into the room of a female patient with ample breasts, throw the sheet back, and root around with his ear between the breasts until he could hear the heart.

One night while on duty awaiting calls, I was sitting by the desk of the night supervisor of surgery. It was after midnight, and I saw Dr. Link come down the hall. He turned and went back and finally returned, pacing up and down. I asked the nurse if he had an emergency scheduled, although I knew he never did any emergency surgery at night. "Don't you know what is going on?" she whispered. "No, what?" I answered. "He's just like all new fathers," she said, "his wife is in labor." He was past sixty. She then told me his first wife had died and he had remarried. The second wife had been a student nurse not long before, and I later learned she was in the class ahead of the woman I later married. At home, the Link baby was placed in a nursery as sterile as an operating room. Rumor had it that any toy that fell to the floor was never given to the baby again.

Forty years later I picked up an Indianapolis paper, and there was an article on Dr. Link concerning an award presented to him by the Indiana State Medical Association. He had passed the century mark.

It didn't take long to slip into the routine as an intern. The hours were long and the work was hard, but it was interesting. There was no forty-hour week. We started out in the morning and worked all day long until all the work was done. We got every other weekend off, from Saturday noon until Monday morning. Each of us had a partner, and we took turns taking call at night. In addition, we had to take a turn at six weeks of continuous night duty during the year. One intern served the south wing, including the emergency room, while the other took the north wing. The two interns were kept busy all night long, starting intravenous fluids and checking on patients.

I had been there about two weeks and was on surgical call. I was sitting near the surgery supervisor's desk when the phone rang. A young nurse I had never seen before answered the phone. I overheard her conversation. When she said there was no one by that name there and hung up, I became suspicious and asked whom the call was for. "Someone by the name of Mitchell," she said. I was furious. "Don't you know who I am?" I yelled. "I'm Dr. Mitchell." It turned out the call was from a former girlfriend in Washington. I later discovered the nurse was Mildred Miller, assistant supervisor of surgery. When we had arrived to start our internship, a group picture had been taken, and it was placed in the Indianapolis paper along with a story. Soon it seemed every nurse who was single had a copy of the picture. They checked out all the interns as to their marital status. It seems the nurses had picked me out of the bunch to become the boyfriend of Miss Miller. She was away on vacation when we arrived, and when she returned, they informed her they had selected her future husband—me—and on our first meeting I blew it. She told them the day after the telephone incident that she wouldn't have anything to do with me even if I were the last man on earth. I stayed out of her way.

Several weeks later, I was assisting a plastic surgeon in a complicated, tedious piece of facial surgery. The surgeon was sitting on a stool, but I was standing bent over holding retractors for a long time. My legs ached and my back was about to break. Miss Miller came into the room and stood watching. She went out and came back in with a stool and slipped it behind me. She saved my life. After surgery I apologized for my rudeness over the telephone incident. I thanked her for getting the stool and told her I would like to take her out. I was amazed when she accepted. One date followed another. We became good friends. She was a quiet, unassuming person with a great deal of intelligence. She worked hard and was dedicated to the profession of nursing, which she loved. I discovered she was a neurosurgical nurse and scrubbed on all the neurosurgical cases of Dr. Hahn. She had a tremendous amount of responsibility but handled it very efficiently. It wasn't long before I knew that this was the woman I wanted to marry.

Surgery was a busy place. There were eighteen operating rooms, and the schedule each day filled a large blackboard that covered an entire wall. One day I was scheduled to assist an orthopedic surgeon in doing an open reduction of a fractured femur. The surgeon used lots of gadgets and designed most of the instruments and equipment he used. The leg was elevated up above the table, and I was standing on a footstool holding retractors. The patient was draped with sterile sheets. The surgeon asked me to get an instrument from the back table. Someone had placed a kick basin on rollers behind me, and as I stepped back off the stool, my foot went into the pan, the basin scooted back, and I fell forward across the patient, almost knocking the contraption holding the leg off the table. The whole field was contaminated. All the drapes were removed and the leg repositioned. I scrubbed again and new drapes were put in place. I received quite a scolding from the surgeon.

Dr. Gatch, the dean of Indiana University School of Medicine, did a lot of surgery. He was scared to death of the new gas anesthetics. He was sure there would be an explosion so he used the old-fashioned drip ether. Although a fine surgeon, Dr. Gatch had the reputation of being absentminded. The boys from Indiana University had many stories about him. One day he entered the room of a patient with a private duty nurse. He wanted to discuss the patient with the nurse. They stepped into the bathroom and closed the door, and Dr. Gatch sat down on the stool. After the discussion had ended, he stood up, flushed the stool, and walked out.

It was rumored that Dr. Gatch went to the Terre Haute Union Hospital to operate one day in a chauffeured limousine. As he entered the hospital, he told the chauffeur that he would be there about two hours. The chauffeur waited and waited. After about three hours, he went inside and inquired if Dr. Gatch was about to finish with surgery. "Oh, Dr. Gatch left about an hour ago," he was told. He drove back to Indianapolis and found Dr. Gatch behind his desk. "Where have you been?" demanded Dr. Gatch. "Well, Doctor, if you remember, I took you to Terre Haute this morning and waited several hours for you to finish your surgery. Finally, they told me you were finished and had gone so I came back here." "Oh, my goodness," said Dr. Gatch, "I forgot that. When I finished, I came back on the interurban."

Frequently, surgeons from Indianapolis went out to smaller hospitals around the state. Dr. Gabe asked me to go with him to assist on a hysterectomy at a small town several miles away. The surgical resident said that it was quite an honor to be asked. Dr. Gabe was a colorful man. He did everything with a flourish and prided himself on being able to do an operation in record time. I was told to arrive at his house for breakfast at 6:00 A.M. The resident informed me that promptness was expected. The next morning my finger was on the doorbell exactly on time. After breakfast he showed me around. In the basement was a movie theater complete with projection booth. In the living room was a large grand piano. He sat down and played a composition or two before we left, and he played beautifully. He told me that his two hobbies were music and photography and that he practiced the piano three hours a day. We got into his big Cadillac and, even though it was a warm day, he slipped on his pearl-colored suede driving gloves. The patient was prepared and anesthetized, and we started the operation. The anesthetic was drip ether being administered by the local doctor, who was a general practitioner. I noticed the blood was getting dark, which indicated the patient wasn't getting enough oxygen. I also could hardly see any respiratory movement of the chest. I looked over the shield at the head of the table. The doctor was pouring ether in the saturated mask and the patient's face was black. We stopped everything, started oxygen, and finally the patient pinked up and resumed normal breathing.

Because interns and residents are subjected to a great amount of stress, they sometimes need to find ways of letting off steam. We indulged in pranks and other things that might appear to be silly. For example, we once discovered that the terrace on the roof of the hospital was a great place from which to fly kites in the spring. Everyone got busy making kites in all sizes and shapes. All were covered by green cloth from scrub suits and gowns swiped from surgery. Before long, a myriad of kites could be seen flying high up above the hospital. Competition was keen to see which kite could go the highest. All went well until one day when the wind was extra strong and gusty. Suddenly, one of the large kites was caught by a strong downdraft and, despite the operator's wild maneuvering, plummeted to the streetcar trolley wire over Illinois Street, some two blocks away. The motorman had to make an emergency stop and wasn't able to proceed until a line crew came out, turned off the power, and removed the kite. The next day an official notice from the superintendent of the hospital appeared on the bulletin board: "Kite flying is prohibited from the roof of the hospital."

One night some of the boys were sitting around the supervisor's desk in surgery waiting for calls. Things were slow, and they were looking for something to liven things up. Someone suggested a surgery cart race. Two carts were taken down to the south end of the corridor; one man lay belly down on each cart, and another man pushed. At the signal, they started running full speed, pushing the carts toward the other end of the corridor. Unfortunately, things didn't go as planned. At the other end stood a large glass case filled with Dr. Hahn's neurosurgical instruments. One man lost control of his cart and couldn't stop. Cart and rider crashed into the case, breaking all the glass, and scattering all of the delicate instruments over the floor. My future wife, Millie, was upset because she was responsible for the care of all those instruments.

Another night an insurance agent had a big party in the Riley Hotel across the street. All interns and residents were invited. R. B. Moore asked if I was going since it was my night off. Since I had no interest in going to the party, I told RB I would work for him.

About midnight we had an emergency surgery. While the anesthetist and I were waiting for the surgeon and patient, we saw the double doors open at the far end of the corridor. There stood two of our colleagues with RB draped between them. He had passed out, and they had brought him back to the hospital. They took him up to bed, and we went on with our surgery.

The anesthetist and I were laughing about RB and his predicament while we were operating. We decided what he needed was a cast on his arm. After surgery we went back to orthopedics and gathered up several rolls of plaster of paris. When we got upstairs, we found the boys had gotten RB in bed, but they couldn't keep him there. He kept rolling from one side of the bed to the other. We had no side rails to put up so we moved the mattress onto the floor. At least he wouldn't fall out of bed. We rolled up the sleeve of his pajama top and applied a heavy cast from his shoulder to his wrist. The heavy cast acted like a counterweight, and each time he rolled over, the weight of the cast flipped him over quickly.

At breakfast next morning, RB appeared. He was wearing a frown, walking drooped to one side from the weight of the cast, and nursing a nasty hangover. He wanted to know why he was wearing a cast. We told him he broke his arm at the party the night before. Suddenly I got an idea. Jackson's father had just given him a new car. Now Jackson and RB were always at each other's throat. "Don't you know what happened, RB?" I asked. "No, what happened?" he answered. "You took the keys to Jackson's car out of his pocket and took off with the car, wrecked it, and broke your arm." "Oh, my God!" was the answer. At that point Jackson got in the act. RB asked him if that was true. "Don't speak to me, you SOB," said Jackson and stalked out.

I had another idea. RB had been wanting his father to buy him a car but hadn't been able to convince him yet. His father was a teetotaler, and if he thought RB had had a drink, he would never get the car. I went out into the hall and called the hospital operator, asking her to page Dr. Moore and tell him his father was in the lobby to see him. When RB answered the page, I thought he was going to faint. After he came back from the phone, he realized that he had been hoaxed. "I don't have a broken arm. Please, someone, take this cast off," he pleaded. "We can't because it was put on by an orthopedist and he will have to take it off," we told him and walked out leaving poor RB to sweat. Finally, someone removed the cast, and he arrived a half hour late for surgery with one of the toughest surgeons on the staff, who gave him a royal "chewing."

Since our income of ten dollars a month didn't take us far, we were pleased when we received the news that we could go on the professional donors' list. There were no blood banks then. Patients needing a blood transfusion had to be supplied by volunteers from among family members or friends. In the event none of them were suitable or, in an emergency, blood came from professionals who were always available. The fee was fifty dollars a pint, which to us was big money. We all immediately went on the list—everyone gave blood as often as possible. The limit was supposed to be one transfusion every three months, but we all tried to shorten the waiting period. One of the interns seemed to be selling blood every month or two. He had repeated bouts of tonsillitis and was advised to have a tonsillectomy. After surgery he began to hemorrhage, so much in fact that he required several transfusions. After he recovered, the intern got the cold shoulder for quite awhile from the boys who had to give him blood. Needless to say, he didn't sell any more blood.

One day a notice issued by the hospital superintendent appeared on the bulletin board. We were informed that the fee for a pint of blood was being reduced to thirty-five dollars. We blew up. We had been told from the beginning that the hospital had no responsibility for collecting the fees for donors. That was strictly a deal between the donor and the patient or family. If the fee was paid to the donor, the money was left at the cashier's office, but that was the only way the hospital was involved.

We held a meeting of all interns and residents to decide what counteraction we could take. While we were at it, we decided to air some other grievances we had. Among them was the quality of food, the poor conditions of the showers, and the repairs needed on the pool table.

The possibility of calling a strike was brought up and abandoned. The patients weren't to blame, and they would be the ones to suffer—we all were dedicated to abiding by the Hippocratic oath. Finally, we came up with an idea that would strike at the Achilles heel of the hospital administration and yet would not endanger any patients. We would refuse to start any IVs or blood transfusions. In those days all IVs and transfusions had to be administered by a physician. All staff physicians ordered a large number of IVs, and if we refused to start them, the physician would have to leave the office or get up in the middle of the night to go to the hospital to do the job. This we knew would cause an uproar among the staff physicians. We drew up the ultimatum, and a committee from our group delivered it to the superintendent, who himself was a patient in the hospital at the time. We didn't have to wait long for a response. A new notice suddenly appeared on the bulletin board, rescinding the previous notice. A committee of staff physicians came to our quarters to inspect and to hear our complaints. Immediately, the showers were fixed, the pool table was repaired, and the food got better.

MISS MILLER AND I continued to get better acquainted. The more I saw of her, the more I thought of her. Visiting her on my nights off call became a regular thing. I was completely happy with her, something that had never happened to me before. Christmas was approaching, and I began looking for a suitable present. One day as I was window shopping, an electric roaster caught my eye. That was the perfect gift. Now I could find out if she could cook, so I made the purchase. I had the roaster wrapped in Christmas paper, and on Christmas Eve carried it to her apartment. When she unwrapped the gift, I looked closely to get her reaction. She seemed pleased, but I wondered if it weren't the last thing in the world she wanted for Christmas. She must have gotten the hint because not long afterwards she invited me to her apartment for dinner.

The apartment was quite tiny—a kitchenette and a living room with a sofa that made into a bed. When I arrived, she was preparing a feast. She knew I loved chocolate pie and had already baked the crust and placed it on top of the refrigerator to await the chocolate filling. Suddenly, the window blind nearby flew up with a bang that shattered the pie crust. I thought she was going to cry, but then I began laughing and told her that because it shattered so easily, I knew that the crust wasn't tough. She was preparing the salad dressing, and when she took the wrapper off the Roquefort cheese, she got a strong whiff. "They sold me cheese that is spoiled," she said. I took a close look at the cheese and saw it was covered with mold that emitted an odor that was somewhere between dirty feet and spoiled milk. "Don't worry—I'll take it back to the store and exchange it while you're finishing here." I took the cheese back to the nearby store and exchanged it. When I got back, we unwrapped it, and it smelled just like the other. Then we realized that neither of us knew any better. That was the true odor of good Roquefort.

Jackson, my roommate, and I were off call on alternate nights, and after I had dated Miss Miller several months, I found out that he was going out with her on the nights I was working. I was furious. I stormed into her apartment and began to tell her what I thought of her. "You're two-faced, and I could never trust you. If this the way you play the game, you can go straight to hell." Then I stormed out.

Things between us became quite cool. I ignored Miss Miller when I saw her in surgery and never spoke. Her friends became very concerned; with their help a reconciliation took place. Jackson never saw her again on a date, and finally on Valentine's Day of 1941, I gave her a diamond, a jewel purchased with money I had earned as a blood donor.

Miss Miller, who was now just Millie to me, and I decided we must make plans to be married. I had taken her home with me several times, and Mom was completely charmed by her. We decided to be married in Indianapolis, to Mom's pleasure because she and Dad had been married in Indianapolis. She had been a Hoosier neurosurgical nurse, and Dad had just started in practice. Our plans made the occasion seem as if history were repeating itself.

Because of recurrent throat infections, Millie was advised to have a tonsillectomy. After the operation, she was given time off to recuperate and went to be with her aunt and uncle in Dana. I didn't want her to make the trip alone, so I took the day off and we went by train to Dana. This was my first meeting with Aunt Nellie and Uncle Ward. They gave me a cordial greeting and fed me supper before Uncle Ward took me to catch the bus back to Indianapolis. Gradually, I was meeting Millie's family. I went to Monon with her to meet her father, mother, sister, and the rest of the family. Millie's youngest sister I met when she visited Indianapolis. I don't know what kind of impression I made, but I liked all of them.

Millie wanted to be married in McKee Chapel, a Presbyterian church. She was Baptist and I was Methodist, so we decided on neutral ground. She planned every detail, selected her attendants, and I selected mine. We went to talk to the minister, and he asked a lot of questions. I guess we gave the right answers because he said he would be delighted to perform the ceremony. The best part was his refusal to accept a fee because his family had suffered considerable illness and had been so well treated that he would never accept a fee for a doctor-nurse wedding. The date was set: June 21.

12

The Gathering Storms of War

I BECAME QUITE INTERESTED in orthopedics and assisted on every case I could. Dr. Garceau, who was professor of orthopedics at the Indiana University School of Medicine, was my favorite orthopod. We worked well together, and he was an excellent teacher. I thought that I wanted to become an orthopod, and he encouraged me to apply for a residency at the Indiana Medical Center. That wish was not to be fulfilled, however.

Adolf Hitler had invaded the Low Countries and France, and England had become involved. Our government had instituted the draft. We all had to register, and I knew that as soon as I finished my internship I would be drafted. It was then I thought of my friend Bailey, back at George Washington University, who had tried to talk me into enrolling in ROTC. I remember telling him I would rather sleep that extra hour than go out and play soldier. I also remembered his reply: "You'll be sorry when we get into war, and I'll be an officer giving you orders." I should have listened to Bailey, but there still should be a way I could beat being drafted. I was telling my troubles to one of the staff doctors who happened to be a reserve officer, and he advised me to volunteer and ask for a commission in the Medical Corps. The same doctor gave me my physical, and I received notice that I was accepted and would be assigned as a first lieutenant in the Army Air Corps. I wanted to stay out of the infantry if I could. I had to take another physical given by a regular army medical officer before receiving my commission and official orders. I was directed to report to Colonel Weaver in the federal building downtown. Colonel Weaver was the Chief Medical Officer of the Fifth Corps.

When I walked into Colonel Weaver's office, I was given a warm greeting because he was the father of my classmate Buck Weaver. We spent almost an hour visiting, and finally he decided we had better get on with the examination. I was sitting in a chair about four or five feet in front of his desk. "You know the most important part of the physical is the eye test," he said. "I don't happen to have an eye chart, so I guess we will have to use something else." He scrounged around in his desk and came up with a blotter with an advertisement printed on the back in big letters. He held it up and asked if I could see it. "Yes, I can see it," I answered. "Good, you've passed your physical and will soon receive your commission and your orders," he grinned. I was assured I wouldn't be called to active duty until I had finished my internship on July 1.

I received notification that I was commissioned as a first lieutenant in the Medical Corps, and my orders assigned me to the Albuquerque Air Base. The effective date of active duty was July 15, 1941, and I was to serve one year. Fortunately, I didn't know what was coming—World War II. That one year stretched to March 1946. I requested to be relieved of my intern duties the middle of June but was refused. The only way I could leave early was to get one of the incoming class of interns to assume my duties. I got the list of interns and wrote letters asking for help and offering to pay them. The rest of the interns in my class thought I was getting a raw deal, so they helped me write the letters. Finally, I got a response from one man who agreed to come in early, but it cost me $100; my pay for the whole year was $120. I decided to take the state board examination before I left Indianapolis. One of the other interns wanted to do the same thing, so we went down to the statehouse to talk to the secretary of the Board of Medical Examiners. We told her that we had graduated from medical school outside the state, and we had heard that unless we were Indiana graduates, we were doomed to fail the examination. We were determined that we wouldn't put down the registration fee of fifty dollars until we knew this wasn't so. She laughed and assured us that no names appeared on the exam books, just a code number.

The exams were given over a three-day period and were to conclude just a day before June 21. With everything that was going on, I had no time to study, and it was with trepidation that I walked into the room for my first exam. I had moved in secrecy from the intern quarters to the Riley Hotel the night before because I had learned the boys were laying for me and were planning a bit of hazing. After those three days of exams, I felt as if I had been through a wringer. I moved from the Riley Hotel to Speedway to stay with my old friend from Purdue, Chet Robbins, and his wife. I had a white Palm Beach suit that I was going to wear for the wedding and had it sent to the cleaners from the hospital. I came back to the hospital during the afternoon of June 20 and slipped upstairs without being seen. Everyone was working. The housemother told me my suit was on the way.

Since I needed a haircut, I decided to go to the barbershop off the lobby while I was waiting for my suit. As I walked in, one of my fellow interns walked out. He grinned and asked how everything was going. I immediately began to have misgivings. I knew I was trapped because there was only one door to the barbershop. When I walked through the door, I was met by a crowd of grinning interns. They had me surrounded—there was no escape. They grabbed me and carried me squirming and twisting down the hall to an elevator. They crowded into the elevator, but the darn thing wouldn't move because it was so overloaded. Some of the boys got off, and the rest carried me, struggling to get loose, up to the surgery floor. Through the surgery department they carried me, with the nurses laughing along the sidelines. Everyone seemed to be in on the joke but me, but I wasn't long in discovering why. Into one of the empty operating rooms we went. They lifted me onto the table and strapped me down so I couldn't move. Now I knew how the patients felt. Next, they stripped down my pants, baring me from my waist to my knees. Then they prepped me. Shaving off all hair, they painted hearts and arrows all over with gentian violet. R. B. Moore was having more fun than anyone, getting even for the arm cast I had helped put on him. They unstrapped me, and I got my clothes back on and headed out of surgery, the laughter of the nurses following me through the door. I raced to where I was staying in Speedway, filled the bathtub with water, and jumped in. I tried to wash off the gentian violet, but even with all the scrubbing, I couldn't remove all of it. It was like being tattooed, and it was several weeks until the last vestiges disappeared. That was the night of the wedding rehearsal and the rehearsal dinner. I was late, but RB and the others were on time.

Millie was worried because I hadn't arrived, and RB would only grin when she asked him if he knew why I was late. I told Millie what had happened, and she said maybe her friends had planned the same fate for her. They had asked that she stay all night with them for old times' sake. I recommended she duck the whole deal. After rehearsal and the rehearsal dinner, we all went to the Wharf Club. Millie had given me her luggage for the honeymoon, and I locked it in the trunk of my car so that her friends couldn't tamper with it. As the evening came to an end, Millie said she just couldn't disappoint her friends so she was going to spend the night with them. After the wedding, I found that she had also received a prep, only they used red Merthiolate instead of gentian violet.

Our wedding day was beautiful. I left Chet's house in Speedway with plenty of time to spare, I thought, but on the way to the church I was stopped by a freight train. After what seemed like an hour, I finally got on my way and arrived at the church just in time. Just as they were ready to start the music, Aunt Nellie's nose began to bleed so there was a delay until the bleeding was under control. Everything from then on went off without incident.

After the wedding, we changed into our traveling clothes and then went out through the usual shower of rice to Chet's car. I left my car in care of Stoney, one of the bridesmaids. Until we had started from the church, Millie had no idea where we were going on our honeymoon. I had told her we were going to fly part of the way, drive part of the way, and go by ship part of the way. I told her we were going to fly first. We arrived at the airport on schedule and were given a royal sendoff, including my mother pointing a toy double-barreled shotgun at me just as we got on the plane.

Millie and I both tried to act very nonchalant as we walked down the aisle to our seats. We didn't want the people to think we were newlyweds, but as I took off my Panama hat, the rice flew in all directions. The part of the honeymoon by air didn't last long. We landed in Dayton about thirty minutes after takeoff. I had made reservations at the Biltmore Hotel. We had our wedding dinner in the Kitty Hawk Room. We ate like royalty. I remember we had filet mignon priced at $1.75 each. The next morning, we went to breakfast, and I picked up a newspaper with the headlines blaring out "Germany Invades Russia." Things were getting worse. About noon Stoney and some of the others showed up with our car. We took them to the airport, and they flew back to Indianapolis.

We continued on with our leisurely honeymoon. I still had not given our itinerary to Millie. We spent that night in Kentucky, then went on the next day to Gatlinburg, and after that to Charlotte, North Carolina. On our way to Raleigh, about noon Millie said she would like to stop to eat. I wasn't hungry; in fact, I didn't feel too well. I told her that I would sit in the car and wait for her. We started on toward Raleigh, and I felt worse and worse. When we stopped in front of our hotel, it was all I could do to get out of the car. We registered, and our bags were taken to our room, which was quite large. I remember a ceiling fan slowly turning—there was no air-conditioning. When I awoke the next morning, I was so weak I could hardly get out of bed. Millie wanted to call a doctor, but I flew into a rage. She said I had been delirious all night, and she was scared. She thought she was going to be a widow before she finished her honeymoon. To this day, I don't know what illness I had. After breakfast, I revived and felt fine.

We arrived in Norfolk after dark and went into the hotel where I had made a reservation. It was strictly third-rate, and after looking at the room, we left and drove south to Virginia Beach. We found a hotel with a vacancy right on the ocean. We were lulled to sleep by the surf breaking on the shore. After a leisurely breakfast on the terrace, we decided to go down to the shore to do some sightseeing. Down the highway, we came to a barricade with a soldier standing by the road with a rifle. When we stopped, he told us the highway from there on was off-limits except to military personnel, and we would have to detour some fifteen or twenty miles. I didn't want to drive the extra miles so decided to pull my newly acquired rank. "I'm a first lieutenant in the army," I informed the guard. "Do you have any identification, Sir?" he asked. I was dressed in my green Palm Beach suit, wearing my Panama hat, and smoking a cigar. "Sure I do," I replied, reaching for my bag behind the seat. I whipped out my orders to active duty. The guard read them. He handed back my orders and suddenly came to attention, saluted, and said, "Proceed, Sir." I was startled by his sudden action. I had never received a salute before. I brought up my hand to return the salute, knocked my hat off my head, and the cigar out of my mouth. It would have been embarrassing enough if I had been alone, but in front of my new wife, it was humiliating. I said nothing but drove away as fast as I could, my face a brilliant hue of red reaching down to my collar. Millie didn't even snicker.

Later, when we started back and came to the barricade at the other end, I said nothing but made a turn and took the long detour. That evening we drove to the waterfront in Norfolk. A large ship was tied up at the wharf. That was the overnight boat to Washington. I told Millie we were ready to start the trip by ship that I had promised her. We were flagged onto the ramp leading into the ship's hold. The car was parked, and we were directed up to the passenger deck and escorted to our stateroom. I really had splurged. I had reserved the largest room and the only one with a double bed. By morning we were coming up the Potomac River. We drove to our room at the Lee House Hotel, and then I took Millie on a tour of the city where I had spent four years as a medical student. We visited the Capitol, the White House, Washington Cathedral, Mount Vernon, Shakespeare Library, Embassy Row, my old fraternity house, and the medical school, where she met my old friend Katie Breen, the dean's secretary.

Katie told me we had just missed Sam Prevo, my Marshall friend who was responsible for my getting into George Washington University. Sam had resigned from the army and was going to be the chief medical officer for an airline. That all sounded very strange. I knew that Sam was stationed at Ft. Bragg, and I didn't see any way, with the war clouds gathering, how once in you could get out. I wasn't to get my answer until years later; Sam was, indeed, released from active duty to go as a civilian doctor with General Chenault who, also as a civilian, was organizing an air force in China that would later become famous as the Flying Tigers. Sam became the chief medical officer of that organization with the rank of colonel. He remained in China until the war was over.

We didn't have much time in Marshall before going to Albuquerque. We did have a chance for Millie to get acquainted with my friends, and they all accepted her warmly. Mom was proud of her new daughter and wanted to show her off to her friends. Millie was great, although in retrospect I'm sure that it was embarrassing to her.

Mom was doing well, but I was concerned about leaving her alone, not knowing when we would return. However, I knew she was tough and capable of running her own business. The day came when we had to leave for the army. We said our good-bys and took off for Scott Field near Belleville, Illinois, not far from St. Louis. I had to stop there to take my final physical exam before proceeding on to Albuquerque.

They told me at the hospital to come back the next day. It seemed there were a number of calcified lymph nodes in my chest X-ray that indicated healed tuberculosis, and a decision would have to be made as to whether it might bar me from the service. We stayed in St. Louis that night, visited the zoo, and attended the summer opera in Forest Park. We returned to Scott Field the next morning, and I got the verdict. I passed my physical and was officially in the army, so it was on to Albuquerque.

We arrived in Albuquerque with our meager belongings and spent the night in a hotel. We were nearly out of funds but weren't too worried. The next morning, while I went to the air base to report for duty, Millie set out to find us a place to live.

I reported to base headquarters, not in uniform, but wearing my trusty green Palm Beach suit, my Panama hat, and smoking a two-for-a-nickel cigar. I had resolved from the beginning that I was not going to take guff from anyone in the military—regardless of rank—because I was a doctor, not a soldier. I was directed through the personnel and finance offices. In personnel, I was told that on Labor Day, all officers and their companions were to spend the day in Santa Fe to attend the fiesta. Later, we were to appear at the Governor's Mansion for a reception. In the evening, we were to attend the Governor's Ball. I was also informed the official uniform of the day was to be blouse and slacks, with a Sam Brown belt and officer's cap.

All I had were two pairs of khaki wash pants, two cotton khaki shirts, an overseas cap, and insignia. I had spent a grand total of $10 or $12 for all of that at Strauss's in Indianapolis. We were not given a uniform allowance, so I was going to have to spend $150, which I didn't have, for a full uniform. After completing all the paperwork, I was escorted to the office of the commanding officer of the base, Colonel Hackett. He was rather short and a little on the obese side. I just walked in, cigar and all, didn't salute or come to attention. I said hello and shook his hand. He offered me a seat, and I sat while he gave me a briefing on military customs and regulations. I drove from base headquarters over to the post hospital. I was told that it was the station hospital, but I had no idea what a station hospital was. Later, I was to learn a station hospital is just above a dispensary in importance. At the hospital, I reported to the sergeant major, a typical old career army man, who took me in to meet the commanding officer of the hospital. I discovered that the commanding officer of the hospital was called the surgeon, even though he might not know one end of a scalpel from the other. That was all confusing. Major Tracey was a very relaxed, quiet man. He was courteous, and we visited for quite some time. He found out about me, and I learned a lot about the military, particularly military medical practice. He asked the sergeant to have all the doctors come into his office to meet me. As I recall, I was the fifteenth doctor on the staff of the hundred-bed hospital.

They were a great group, and I immediately felt at home. We toured the hospital and dispensary, and I was asked where we were going to do our banking. That was the furthest thing from my mind. We didn't have anything to bank. In fact, I was worrying about where we were going to get enough to live on until my first pay two weeks hence. John Minnet, a captain, said, "We all bank at the New Mexico State Bank. It is a new bank, and they have fine people running it. Let us take you down to meet them." I was first introduced to the vice president, a friendly young man. I agreed to do my banking there. Then I asked, "Could you make me a loan? I'm practically broke and need money to live on till payday." "How much do you want?" he asked. Timidly, I answered, "How about twenty-five dollars?" He brought out a note, filled in the blanks, and I signed. We were in business. We weren't going to starve.

When I returned to the hotel, Millie told me she had rented a nice apartment. "How much?" I asked. "Forty dollars a month furnished," she answered, "and we can move in now." We checked out of the hotel, had lunch, and drove to our first home at 1271 East Grand. It was a duplex, and we were on the ground level. It was quite small but adequate—a living room, dining room, bedroom, bath, and kitchen. We had everything except a few kitchen utensils. We went to Woolworth's and came away with a cardboard carton full of merchandise, which I paid for with a ten-dollar bill with change left over. That night when we went to bed, Millie said, "There is one thing we just have to have." "What is that?" I asked. "A bedspread," she answered, "this bed doesn't have one, and I won't live in a house that doesn't have spreads on the beds." I thought that was absurd. Here we were trying to make our money last until payday. We had to eat, and I had to buy gasoline, and she insisted on a bedspread. She wouldn't budge. Right then, I had my first demonstration of her German stubbornness. "Okay, get your bedspread, but we may go hungry." First thing Monday she got the bedspread; when I returned from my first day at the hospital, she took me in the bedroom to show off her pride and joy.

When I reported for duty on Monday, I was placed in charge of the genitourinary ward and also was assigned to sick call. Most of the men in the GU ward were being treated for venereal disease. The average daily census was four to five patients, so I didn't have much to do. Most of the doctors on the staff helped at daily sick call; thus, we had that taken care of in a half hour to three-quarters of an hour. We all went home for lunch, and the day was finished by 3:30 P.M. We took turns as officer of the day. The officer of the day took care of all medical problems after 3:30 P.M. until the next morning and from noon Saturday until Monday morning.

I also had the added duty of taking care of the pregnant wives of the enlisted personnel on the base. All deliveries were performed at St. Joseph's Hospital in Albuquerque. I went to the hospital one morning to make rounds and discovered one of my patients had delivered. She had hemorrhaged badly and had to be transfused. I asked the nurse why I hadn't been called and was told that I had been called repeatedly, but they got only the busy signal. I discovered I was on a two-party line, and the woman on the line spent most of the time gossiping with her friends. I immediately had my phone changed to a private line. Fortunately, one of the other doctors from the base took over when I couldn't be contacted. I was beginning to get bored for lack of something to do, so I asked Major Tracey if I could immunize all the enlisted men. I took a squadron at a time, giving each soldier tetanus, typhoid, and smallpox inoculations. I devised a way to speed up the shots by using a large syringe that held enough vaccine to immunize several men. Instead of changing needles for each man, I sterilized the needle by passing it through the flame from an alcohol burner. Of course, sometimes the needle was so hot that it sizzled when I gave the injection, but no one complained.

My salary was $167 a month plus $40 a month subsistence allowance. At the beginning of the month, we figured we had $7 per day to live on, so we got by on a lot less. Near the end of the month, we had saved enough on our daily budget to have $20 or $25 per day to spend; then we felt we could splurge on a movie. We ate a lot of cheese souffle. We bought an $18.75 War Bond each month and started a savings account. I purchased my uniform at Fred Mackey's Men's Store in anticipation of the big day in Santa Fe and arranged to make monthly payments. That put a strain on the budget, but I had no choice.

On Labor Day, there was a mass exodus of officers and their wives from Albuquerque to the State Capitol at Santa Fe. Millie was nervous because she didn't have any fine clothes, but she did manage to come up with a formal. Santa Fe was decked out with flags and banners for the fiesta. The beautiful old adobe buildings that had stood there through all of the years reminded me of the history of New Mexico. That territory had been settled by Spanish-speaking people, and the architecture of the buildings and the customs bore out the heritage. There were gaily bedecked horses, many with hand-tooled silver saddles. Their riders were dressed in Spanish costumes and wore broad-rimmed sombreros. It was truly a festive occasion. Later in the afternoon after the parade, the wives returned to the hotel where rooms had been reserved so that they could change into their formal gowns. The day was hot, and I was uncomfortable wearing my heavy uniform. We all went to the Governor's Mansion for the reception. The mansion was a beautiful building fronted by a portico supported by round columns. Near the entrance was a large circular table that was used to check our caps. Several state policemen were on duty to handle the checking of the caps. They didn't mark the caps with a stub; instead, they merely took each cap and placed it on the pile. I worried the rest of the afternoon about my cap, which wasn't paid for. Most all of the caps had been purchased at the same store, and the only mark on them was Fred Mackey's Men's Store printed in the lining. How was I going to get the right cap back? On the side porch overlooking the huge walled lawn was a large ice sculpture of an eagle. There was a bountiful supply of food and drink, and I finally quit worrying too much about my cap. As we left, a trooper handed me a cap. I put it on and it fit. That night we attended the Governor's Ball in the Armory. We arrived home late that night, having survived our first military social event.

We had a fine group at the hospital. We worked well together and were good friends. Most of the medical officers were older than I and had been on active duty much longer—Capt. John Minnett, Capt. Sid Seid, Capt. Henry Thomas, and Lt. Bill Schick. Our wives got along well, and we met socially at the officers club or in each others' homes. I was closer to Lieutenant Schick than the others, I believe, because he had been in only two weeks longer than I; his wife was a nurse as was Millie, and we had gotten married about the same time.

I was quite surprised one day to run into Capt. Pat McIntyre, a bomber pilot. Pat and I had been classmates at Purdue and members of the aviation cadet program. Pat went into service and became a full-fledged pilot. I remember we drove to the mesa one night for a steak fry. We spent the evening reminiscing about Purdue. Little did we know what lay in store for us in the months to come. Things were going from bad to worse in Europe. We weren't privy to any military secrets, but we knew it was only a matter of time until we would be embroiled in the biggest and worst war the world had ever seen. We didn't talk much about it, but I'm sure we were all constantly thinking about it. Later, I received word through the grapevine that Pat, who had been in the Philippines, escaped to Australia when the Japanese invaded Luzon. While riding as an observer on a training mission, his plane crashed, and he was killed.

The Nineteenth Bombardment Group and its support unit, the Seventh Materiel, were stationed in Albuquerque. The planes were the best available at the time but were slow and not well armed. Eventually, we began to get some B-17 bombers, which were mammoth four-engined planes armed to the teeth. Deliveries speeded up until all of the old planes had been replaced. In October, orders were received for the Seventh Materiel to move out. Medical personnel had to be assigned to the Seventh, and the rumors flew. Which medical officer would go? One day, it was Sid Seid; the next, it was Bill Schick. Finally, it was official. Sid Seid had been chosen. The dental officer who had been assigned earlier received orders a month before relieving him from active duty. He had served his year. He packed his belongings and shipped them back to his home in Texas, gathered his family together, got into his car, and started to clear the post. When he reached the personnel office to check out, he was handed a telegram from Washington rescinding his orders. He was back in the army.

Major Tracey usually toured the hospital at least once each day accompanied by his faithful dog. The jingling tags on the dog's collar gave advance warning that the major was coming. One day, I heard the familiar jingling and in came the major. "I have a job for you," he told me. "We have received a message that there has been a plane crash, and I want you to go with the base engineering officer to the site of the crash." I was to take an ambulance and a crew of eight men. I also was told to take a medical bag that contained only a fifth of Green River Whiskey. I couldn't see the need for that because we had been informed there were no survivors. I rode with the engineering officer, who was a major, in a chauffeured staff car. As we started, the major told me we had a trip of about 125 miles. He didn't have the exact location but was told to proceed to Vaughn, and then on down the highway toward Roswell. Somewhere we would meet a sheriff's car near a gap in the right-of-way fence. They would then lead us to the scene of the crash. About fifteen miles beyond Vaughn, we came to the gap in the fence, and there was the sheriff's car. They informed us we had another ten miles or so to travel across the mesa to reach the scene. One deputy shook his head and said he had never seen such a gruesome sight. "I was in World War I, and my buddy standing by me in the trench had his head blown off, but this is worse. In fact, it made me vomit," he said. We bounced along behind the squad car and finally arrived at the site. All I could see was sagebrush. There was no sign of an airplane. When I got out of the car, I could see why. The plane had exploded on impact, and there were only small pieces of debris scattered around. An old sheepherder lived in an adobe shack nearby, and he was the one who had reported the crash. During the night, there was a severe thunderstorm. He had heard the sound of a plane overhead, and then the sky was illuminated by a bright light followed by an explosion, another bright flash, and then another loud explosion. The storm was so severe and it was so dark that he could do nothing until daylight. He then went looking for the crash and found it not far from his house. He had no telephone so he had to drive into Vaughn to report the crash to the border patrol. The border patrol drove to the crash site for verification, then radioed the air base at El Paso that, in turn, notified our base.

When we arrived, there were representatives from the FBI, postal department, border patrol, county sheriff's police, and the police department in Roswell. The downed plane was one of the five twin engine planes that had departed from El Paso the night before on a navigational flight. Each plane carried a pilot and four aviation cadets. They had flown to Albuquerque and were on the return flight to El Paso when they ran into a severe storm. They broke formation, and all the other planes made it back safely. It was evident the plane had come in at a steep angle. There was a large crater where the nose and engines had hit, and an indentation about twelve inches deep in the sun-hardened soil marked the impact of the leading edge of the wings. The sagebrush was seared off in a fan-shaped pattern out from the impact point, almost as if it had been burned by a giant blow torch. We started looking for bodies, but all we found were five spots containing bits of human flesh scattered forward of the plane. I made a crude drawing of the crash site and marked the location of the victims. After inspecting the body locations, I split up the ambulance crew and had them go over each spot carefully, beginning in the center and working out, picking up each piece of flesh until we were satisfied every piece had been collected. The pieces of bodies from each spot were put in a sheet and tied up. When we had finished, we had five separate bundles of flesh. After completing our work, we all went to the sheepherder's house to warm up. I was very uncomfortable. It was cold on the mesa, and all I was wearing over my uniform was a flight jacket. It was crowded in the shack, but we got warmed up. That was when the major asked me what was in the bag. I pulled out the whiskey and passed it to the major, and he passed it on to the sheepherder. It was getting dark, so we headed back toward

Albuquerque, our gruesome cargo loaded in the ambulance. We stopped in Vaughn to let the crew rest and get something to eat, arriving back at Albuquerque about midnight. We took the bodies to a local mortuary.

The five bundles had been placed in the preparation room, and we were waiting in the office for the arrival of the mortician. He came in and introduced himself, and as he was leaving to go to the preparation room, I asked him how he was going to embalm the bodies. "Oh, the usual way," he said, "by raising a vein in the arm and leg and injecting the fluid. Why do you ask?" "Oh, I was just curious," I answered. He was back in about a minute, his eyes bugged out. "I've been in this business thirty years and have never seen anything like this," and off he went. He was back in a few minutes with five new washtubs. The remains of each victim were placed in a tub and covered with embalming fluid. Then the remains of each man was placed in a rubber pouch with hardening compound and sealed. My chief concern was establishing positive identification of each victim, so before the embalming took place, I had the provost marshal come over, and we managed to find at least a piece of a finger in each pile of flesh. Fingerprints were made and sent to Washington. We positively identified each man, and the remains were returned to the proper families.

Each medical officer was expected to attend flight surgeons' school at Randolph Field in San Antonio. Assignment to the school was made in accordance with seniority. Bill Schick had two weeks' seniority over me so he was ordered to Randolph Field just ahead of me. We decided that Millie and I would give up our apartment and move into the house he had rented. At San Antonio, he would get an apartment, and when I went to Randolph Field, we would take the apartment there, and Bill and Lois would come back to their house in Albuquerque. Bill's house was much larger than our small apartment.

It was early in November, and the Sandia Mountains just east of Albuquerque had a thick coating of snow covering the uppermost slopes. Major Tracey again walked in my office. "I have another job for you," he said. "What this time?" I asked. He told me that there had been a search on for about a week for a downed plane. A lieutenant and sergeant had taken off to make a local flight. They were to be gone only about an hour or so but never returned. The weather had been good, and no distress calls had been received. An aerial search was conducted for several days, but no trace of the missing plane could be found. Ground search teams had combed the area to no avail. The evening before, a team had gone far up the western slope of the mountain and were starting back down when one of the men spotted the tip of an airplane tail sticking out of the snow. My job was to climb the western slope of the mountain with the engineering officer and ambulance crew and bring out the two bodies.

Early the next morning, we drove across the mesa to the spot at the foot of the mountain that was below the point of impact of the plane near the top of the mountain. The top is about eleven or twelve thousand feet above sea level. We started climbing, the enlisted men carrying two metal litters. It was slow going and, although we were below the snow line, the surface was covered by sharp flint-like rock, and there were large boulders scattered in our path. After a while, breathing became labored because of the decrease in oxygen in the air. Reaching the snow line, our traveling became much more difficult. The snow was nearly up to our knees, and occasionally we stumbled into deep drifts. It was noon when we arrived at the crash scene. The plane had burned on impact. Both bodies were badly charred and frozen. The plane crashed into a box canyon, and looking along the rim, we saw where the plane had clipped the tops of some pine trees and had crashed on the floor of the canyon. It could be determined that the plane had come in from the southwest; on the day of the crash, the wind had been from the southwest. We found out that the pilot was a deer hunter; some surmised that he had been scouting for deer, had become too intent, and had come in too low over the rim. The plane was then pulled down into the canyon by the stiff downdraft pouring over the rim. The bodies were loaded onto the litters and strapped down. There were four strong men to each litter, and we were going down the mountain, but because of the difficulty in breathing, we stopped about every fifty feet or so to give the men a rest. It was night when we arrived back at the base of the mountain. The men were exhausted, and the new pair of heavy flying boots I had checked out the day before were cut to pieces by sharp rocks.

Rumors were flying everywhere. One day, the Nineteenth Bombardment Group was said to be moving out; the next day it was staying. Nobody knew what has happening, but the uneasiness that had started before the Seventh Materiel moved out became more intense. Then I heard that Bill Schick had been ordered back even though he hadn't completed the three months of flight surgeons' school. The rumor was confirmed a few nights later when Bill called from a local hotel. He, his wife, and mother-in-law had just gotten in. When I saw him the next morning, I insisted that he and his wife move back in, and Millie and I would go to a hotel until we could get an apartment. "No, you won't move out," he said, "because I'm not going to be here long." Instead, we compromised: the Schicks moved in with us. It was a little tight, but we had no problems. Bill had been graduated early from the course and ordered back to Albuquerque and assigned as flight surgeon with the Nineteenth. The rumors were confirmed. The Nineteenth was moving out. All Bill knew was that he would be leaving in a matter of days, but he had no idea where he was going. Bill, Lois, Millie, and I went out almost every night doing things we knew Bill enjoyed doing. On Sunday, we went to church on the base, and as we went through the gate, Bill threw a left-handed salute to the sentry. He didn't do it to be cute—Bill was just not meant to be a soldier. He didn't realize he had saluted with his left hand.

The following Wednesday, we were all seated around the table at dinner when the phone rang. I answered, and it was the sergeant at base operations. He wanted to talk to Bill. I knew that was it. Bill finished talking and came back to the table. "We leave in the morning," he said quietly. We finished our meal without any conversation. Millie and I washed the dishes and went to bed, leaving Bill and Lois alone in the living room. The next morning after a quiet breakfast, I loaded Bill's gear into my car. Millie was going to the commissary so she got into the car with me and waited for Bill. After a while, he and Lois came out on the front porch. They stood looking at each other, then after a long kiss and embrace, he hurried out to the car. As we drove slowly down the street, he was looking back and waving to her still standing on the porch. As we went around the corner, he wiped a tear from his eye and said as he showed us a camera he was holding. "I don't know where I'm going, but I'm taking a lot of pictures with this camera Lois gave me."

We drove to the flight line, and I stowed his gear aboard a B-17. There was going to be a delay in takeoff because of weather, so we drove to the hospital and turned the car over to Millie. Bill told her good-by, and she drove away in tears. All the doctors in the hospital, including Major Tracey, went to the mess hall with Bill, where we sat and talked and drank coffee. Bill excused himself and went to a phone and called Lois. They talked a long time. I kidded Bill about the will he had made a few days before. The chaplain had helped him make the will, and I had witnessed his signature. The chaplain told him that to make the will official, he needed to apply a seal, but in the absence of a seal, a postage stamp would do, so Bill stuck on a one-cent stamp. I told Bill that showed what a tightwad he was. The phone rang. It was the operations office—the time had come.

We took a staff car to the plane where I gave Bill a handshake and a big hug. He got aboard, and the plane taxied to the runway. I watched until the plane was out of sight. I drove slowly back to the hospital with an empty feeling in my belly. I had that uncomfortable feeling something was going to happen, but I didn't know what or when.

13

Organizing a Military Hospital

THE FOLLOWING SUNDAY, Millie and I planned to drive to a place in the hills near Santa Fe, where the people in a small mining village had created an elaborate Christmas display complete with live shepherds and animals. We had asked one of the nurses from the hospital to go along. We planned to have lunch in Santa Fe and then to drive on to see the display. It was a nice day with the sun shining and not too cold for early December. After a late breakfast, we were sitting in the living room reading the papers. Lois and her mother had left on Friday to drive back to Chicago, so we were alone.

I turned on the radio, and suddenly the program was interrupted. In a voice filled with excitement, the announcer blurted, "Pearl Harbor is under attack by the Japanese Air Force." We sat in stunned silence for a minute or two. The uneasiness and uncertainty that had been nagging me for months vanished. It finally had happened. We were at war. I checked in at the base. Everything was quiet at the hospital. There was no panic. Since I wasn't needed, and there was nothing I could do, we decided to go on with our plans. It was a very quiet trip. We hadn't recovered yet from the shock of the bulletin we had heard. It seemed so peaceful and quiet as we sat eating lunch in a tearoom in Santa Fe. As we drove through the rolling hills, it was hard to believe that we were at war. This was the quietest and most peaceful experience we would have for several years.

I found out the next day when I went to the base that an inventory had been taken the day before of the armaments available for defense of the base if needed. As I recall, there was a grand total of three dozen .45-caliber automatic revolvers, which are accurate up to about fifteen feet, and one old World War I machine gun.

When I returned home that evening, Millie had received a telegram from Lois, wanting to know if we had any news about Bill. Millie had written a letter to tell her we had heard nothing but not to worry because Bill had been gone only three days so he wouldn't have been anywhere near Pearl Harbor. Millie wanted to get the letter in the mail at once, so we drove to the main post office. She waited in the car while I took the letter in. I dropped it in the box and turned around. There stood an old sergeant from the hospital. He looked very sad. "Did you hear about Lieutenant Schick, Sir?" he asked. "No, what about Lieutenant Schick?" "He was killed at Pearl Harbor," was his reply. "I don't believe you, Sergeant. It's just a rumor." "No Sir, it's in tonight's *Denver Post*." I rushed to the car and told Millie the bad news. At first we were too shocked to speak. "I'm going to get a paper and see for myself before I believe it," I told Millie. We went to every newsstand in Albuquerque without finding a copy of the paper. Finally, one newsdealer said we might get one if we went to the home of the distributor. We got the last copy he had, and there in the middle of the front page was the list of those killed, and Bill Schick's name was there. He was the first doctor in our armed forces killed in World War II. We heard later that in all the confusion following the Pearl Harbor attack someone boxed up the clothes he was wearing when he was killed and sent them to Lois. She received his torn uniform riddled with bullet holes and stained by his blood.

I tried to find out how Bill was killed, and after several years I was able to piece together the information I had gotten from people who had been there. After leaving Albuquerque that Thursday morning, the group had flown to Hamilton Field, California, where they received orders to fly across the Pacific to Hickam Field, Hawaii. The flight departed Hamilton Field Saturday, arriving in Hawaii at the height of the Japanese attack. Our planes did not have their guns in place, and, in fact, the guns were still packed in Cosmoline in boxes. When the leader of the flight saw the Japanese planes, he at first thought they were our planes. Then he saw the rising sun on the wings and heard the gunfire and saw the smoke rising from the burning ships, planes, and buildings. The B-17s were almost out of fuel, so the pilots could not make a run for it. The formation split up, and it was everyone for himself. According to my information, the plane that Bill was riding was hit but not badly damaged. One crew member received a minor bullet wound. The pilot decided to make a wheels-up landing, which was successful. When the plane came to a rest, the door was opened, and Bill, among others, made a dash across the runway for shelter. It was then that a Japanese plane came in low, strafing him with bullets.

We never saw Lois again, but she and Millie corresponded for quite awhile. She went back to being a nurse, and she and her mother lived together. A few months later, we learned she had a baby boy born on Bill's birthday. Of course, he was named William. As far as we know,

Lois never remarried. We haven't heard from her in years. As a tribute to Bill, the government gave his name to a veteran's hospital.

Things tightened up immediately after Pearl Harbor. No more half days off—in fact, no days off at all. We were on duty seven days a week and were required to be in uniform at all times. There were no leaves granted.

A few days after Pearl Harbor, I was given another job. A soldier from another command had been injured in an automobile accident and was a patient in a civilian hospital in Holbrook, Arizona. Ours was the military installation nearest Holbrook so we had the job of retrieving the patient. My instructions from Major Tracey were to pick up orders from personnel and travel vouchers from transportation and proceed. I had no idea where Holbrook was, but I soon found out. I had reservations on the *California Limited* from Albuquerque to Holbrook and on the *Grand Canyon Limited* back to Belen, which is fifteen or twenty miles south of Albuquerque. The train was crowded, but I had a good meal in the diner and arrived at Holbrook about 8:30 P.M. When I got off the train, it was cold. I still wasn't able to afford an overcoat so I just shivered. I walked into the station and stood by the stove to get warm. I asked the station agent the location of the hospital. It was about four or five blocks away, so after getting warm, I started to leave, but first I checked on the time the *Grand Canyon* was expected. I was told it was late and running farther and farther behind schedule. I also asked the agent to confirm the return reservations for the patient and me and was told he had no reservations. "Sir, I'm an officer on official business. My orders are to transport the patient by train back to Albuquerque, and the train I'm to take is the *Grand Canyon Limited*. Furthermore, I'm to be back in Albuquerque in the morning," trying my best to speak in a voice full of authority. I succeeded because the old agent got on the wire and immediately had confirmation. We were to have two lower berths on the *Grand Canyon*.

Holbrook appeared to be a town of about one thousand population. The streets were dark and quiet. Following the directions of the station agent, I came to the hospital, a small one-story building near a large residence.

I was greeted by a nurse; in fact, she was the only person on duty. It was a very small private hospital. The doctor lived in the residence nearby, and he came over shortly after. He was very cordial, and I thought he must be competent. He took me in to see the patient, and there he was, wearing a cast from his toes to mid-thigh on one leg. A pin had been placed through his ankle, and the ends of the pin protruded through the sides of the cast. "Well, Doctor, I'll need an ambulance to get this man to the train," I said. "I'm sorry, we don't have an ambulance in town," was his answer. "How am I going to transport this man to the station? He can't walk, and he's too heavy to carry," I said. Then I spotted a gurney outside in the hall. "Doctor, could I borrow this to get this man to the train?" "Sure enough," he replied. I was in business. Back to the station.

The station agent told me the train was running late. Normally, it was due in at about 10:00 P.M., but now it wasn't expected until 1:00 A.M. Back to the hospital I went and asked the nurse whom I could get to help me down to the train. She told me that the night constable surely would help and that I could find him at the local restaurant drinking coffee. I went to the restaurant, sat at the counter, and ordered coffee and a sandwich. The counterman pointed out the constable, who assured me he would be glad to help. I told him I would keep him updated on the arrival time of the train. I shuttled back and forth between the station and the hospital, trying to time the operation so that I could get the patient there in time but not too early. Finally about 2:30 A.M., I notified the constable. We loaded the patient on the cart, covered him with several blankets, and started down the middle of the street. We pushed the cart into the waiting room close by the stove. My timing was accurate because the train arrived in about fifteen minutes. I could tell the crew was irritated because they were running late and had to make a stop at this little town. They were quite irritated when we came pushing the patient out on the cart and they realized he was going to have to be loaded through a Pullman car window.

We placed the stretcher up on top of a high, level, baggage cart, which brought the patient up just below the window. The porter had to use a window jack. We then brought the stretcher through the window across the aisle to the berth on the other side, squared it around, and laid him in the berth. I thanked the constable, and we took off. I was exhausted and ready for some sleep. I had the berth across the aisle from the patient. I asked the porter to look after him and showed the patient the call button in the berth next to the window. I went to sleep instantly but was awakened by the porter shaking me. "What's the matter?" I asked. "Doctor, your patient's got to pee. What'll I do?" he asked. Fortunately, I had experience riding Pullman cars, and I remembered that every men's lounge at the end of the car was equipped with spittoons. I told the porter to clean out a spittoon and let him use that and rolled over and went back to sleep. I had left a wake-up call with the porter, but before having breakfast in the diner, I asked the conductor what was the expected arrival time at Belen. I then asked him to drop a message at the next station to send to the hospital at the air base so an ambulance would be there to meet us. After breakfast, I checked on my patient, who was still asleep. The ambulance was there when we arrived at Belen, and unloading the patient from the train was a piece of cake with all of the help from the ambulance crew.

The following day Major Tracey again visited my office. "You did such a fine job getting that man back here in spite of all the difficulties, I want you to do one more thing," he said. "What is that?" I asked with some hesitation. It seemed every time the major visited me he had a tough job to do. "I have received a directive to transport the patient on down to the General Hospital at El Paso." "Well, here we go again," I thought. That time, however, it was an easy trip. The train to El Paso originated in Albuquerque, so we had plenty of time and help to get the patient aboard. It was an overnight trip so I could get a good night's sleep, and this time I took a urinal in a pillow slip. The next morning the ambulance from the hospital met the train and transported the patient to the hospital, which was many times larger than ours. That evening they furnished me with a staff car and driver, and I went back to El Paso, had a good dinner at a local hotel, boarded the train, and arrived well rested the next morning in Albuquerque.

I didn't know until Major Tracey told me to turn in my travel mileage to the finance office that I had earned about a hundred dollars' extra pay for my trouble. I had been worrying about where I was going to get the money for a decent Christmas present for Millie. I used the extra money to buy her a fine watch. I'll always believe that Major Tracey knew that our money supply was quite meager, and that was his way of helping to give us a merry Christmas. Unfortunately, Christmas was far from merry.

We were at war. Most of the Pacific Fleet had been put out of service. The coastal defense of the continental United States was practically nonexistent. The Japanese had invaded the Philippines and Southeast Asia and controlled the sea-lanes of the Pacific, South Pacific, and Indian oceans. We also were at war with Germany and Italy. That was one of the darkest hours in the history of our republic. The attack at Pearl Harbor united everyone in one of the most concerted efforts ever witnessed. The armed forces were deluged with volunteers. Our industrial complex immediately geared up to produce the mountains of war materiel needed, and everyone sacrificed in one way or another.

Major Tracey called me in about the end of January 1942 to tell me I was going to be ordered out. I wasn't surprised, since I knew that troops were being sent to overseas theaters of operation at a greatly accelerated pace, and with my time in service, I was most likely to be going soon. He told me he had requested the command surgeon to let me stay, but the reply he received was, "Hell, don't you know we are at war?" Major Tracey told me he had been grooming me for a more responsible position, perhaps eventually as a hospital commander. That was very flattering, and I appreciated his interest in me.

I received my orders but not to an overseas assignment. I was transferred to the Santa Ana Army Base in California. Millie and I were pleasantly surprised when the base quartermaster and his wife gave us a farewell party. We didn't realize we had made so many friends in the short time we had been in Albuquerque. That night at the party, the colonel talked about his friend Ernie Pyle, a well-known syndicated newspaper columnist who later became famous for the poignant columns he wrote about the American GIs in combat. He went into the trenches and the front lines, sharing the hardships with the men and writing about their experiences. He used their names and brought news that didn't make the front page back to their loved ones at home. Ernie was living in Albuquerque at that time. "Colonel, Millie and Ernie Pyle come from the same little town of Dana, Indiana. We have seen a man we thought was Ernie playing croquet up the street from where we live, but thought it surely wasn't him," I said. "In fact, I wanted to stop so Millie could ask him if he was Ernie Pyle." "That's Ernie, all right," replied the Colonel, "He plays there almost every day." If Millie had stopped to visit him, she would have been written up in his column, but it was too late. We never met Mr. Pyle. Toward the end of the war, he died at the front lines with his beloved GIs somewhere in the Pacific.

When we first arrived in Albuquerque, we didn't like it. The land was barren compared to the lush countryside back in the Midwest. You could drive for miles in New Mexico without seeing a town. Nothing but sagebrush. No corn or wheat fields, no orchards, not even any grass, but when we left, we were sad. The country had grown on us. There was a strange beauty in the vast open spaces and blue sky. We would miss it.

When we reached Williams, Arizona, we decided to take a short detour up to Grand Canyon. It was Sunday, and when we arrived at the hotel on the South Rim of the canyon, it was so quiet and peaceful that it seemed a different world. There was a deep snow on the ground, and it was cold. I still had no overcoat, but I couldn't resist walking through the snow. Just Millie and I, looking at the beautiful trees draped in their mantle of snow. We edged our way to the canyon rim to look down into the vastness of this great gorge, the tiny river winding far below like a silver ribbon. There were only a few people at the lodge, but the large rustic lounge was made cozy by a roaring fire in the fireplace. We had a leisurely lunch in an almost deserted dining room and lingered in the lounge for a few minutes to soak up the heat. Then we got back into the car to return to the real world—the world torn apart by the terrible conflict.

As we drove slowly back to Williams, I said to Millie, "I wish we could stay here in this beautiful place until the war is over. It is so peaceful and quiet." But that could not be. A few minutes later, we heard the bad news—Corregidor had fallen to the Japanese. We drove for miles, not uttering a word. When we arrived at the California border, we had to pass through a checkpoint manned by uniformed agents of the California Department of Agriculture. To protect the fruit and vegetable crops that contributed so much to the economy of the state, there were strict laws preventing the importation of plants, fruits, and vegetables.

Before we left Albuquerque, we had been warned that we should not attempt to take any such items with us. Millie was unhappy that she had to find new homes for her green things before we left. I informed the inspector that we were aware of the California laws and had made sure we had no contraband in our car and that I would appreciate it if we could go on through without delay because I was on orders and needed to keep moving. He ignored me completely and instructed me to open the trunk of the car. Everything we owned was in the car. The trunk was packed full, the space behind the front seat was packed almost to the roof, and other items were stacked on the seat and down on the floorboard. I was told to unpack the car and lay everything out on a long table under a shed nearby. I fumed and fussed, but he ignored me completely. He then ran his hands through everything, pulling clothing from our bags and strewing things all over the tables. He then turned and walked away without a word. We spent nearly a half hour repacking suitcases and trying to get everything back in the car as it was before. As we drove off, I was about ready to explode. "I hate California, and I hate everything in California," I huffed as we drove on toward Santa Ana. Fortunately, I had received a partial advance payment on next month's paycheck because we had hotel bills to pay and needed money to pay the rent when we found a place to live.

AFTER SPENDING THE NIGHT, I went looking for base headquarters. I discovered that the Santa Ana Army Air Base as such didn't yet exist. It was still under construction about seven or eight miles from Santa Ana on land that had until then been under cultivation, planted in sugar beets. The army had commandeered the city hall for use as temporary headquarters. I found the office of the hospital commanding officer located in the mayor's former office. Colonel Schroeder was behind his desk when I walked in. The colonel's head was bald except for a fringe of gray hair. I saluted. He finally condescended to salute and peered sternly through his steel-rimmed glasses. He was very stiff and formal, strictly military, not at all like Major Tracey. "Lieutenant Mitchell reporting for duty," I said and gave him my orders. He waved me to a chair and carefully read my orders. He told me that the base was still under construction and that it would be several days before we could open the hospital. The air base was a part of the Western Training Command, and command headquarters was being constructed in the city of Santa Ana simultaneously with the construction of the air base. The colonel told me to find a place to live and said preferably I should live in the beach area, since housing in the city was being saved for officers at headquarters.

Newport Beach, Balboa, Balboa Island, Lido Island, and Corona del Mar were all snuggled together on the shore of the Pacific. Approximately ten blocks long and two blocks wide, Balboa Island lies on Balboa Bay. Across a vehicular bridge at the south lies the small island approximately three blocks by two blocks. Off the north end of Balboa Island was Cagney Island, accessible only by a foot bridge. (In the 1940s the island was owned by actor James Cagney.) There was a large house surrounded by a number of guest cottages. During the war, the island and its buildings had been turned over to the Coast Guard. The buildings were painted battleship gray. The western side of the bay was bounded by a peninsula. The villages of Balboa and Newport Beach were located here. To the north was Lido Isle and to the south overlooking the ocean was Corona del Mar. We took a bridge to the island. The village, as the business district was called, consisted of a hardware store, grocery store, drugstore, filling station, restaurant and bar, real estate office, and post office. We entered the real estate office, and a man behind a desk came to his feet, walked over, and shook hands. We told him we were looking for a place to rent. It wasn't long before we were touring the island with Earl Stanley, the real estate agent.

A parkway ran down the center of the island with connecting streets at right angles east and west, ending at the bay, one long block from the parkway. A broad concrete walkway and seawall ran around the island. The streets were lined with beautiful homes. Most were vacation homes owned by people from other parts of California. Along the shores of the bay were many boat anchorages and marinas containing yachts and cruisers of all sizes. Sailboats scurried along, driven by the stiff breezes. It was truly a "picture postcard" scene. Mr. Stanley showed us home after home, all completely furnished. Before starting out, we had told him we were on a restricted budget. After inspecting several houses, we settled on a new three-bedroom house at 217 Pearl Street. It was a two-story house, set well back on the lot, screened on each side by a high hedge. The front lawn was planted with myriad varieties of flowers, and a low white picket fence ran across the front of the lot. Stairs ran up at one end of the house to a roofed balcony across the front. A trellis extending from the floor level of the balcony was covered by brightly blooming bougainvillea, the scarlet blooms falling down over the edge of the trellis. Under the trellis was a patio with lawn furniture and a barbecue grill. In front of the patio was a sand pit for sun bathing. Off the balcony on the top floor was the living room with a ship's bunk built in one corner and a gas fireplace, the master bedroom, bath, and kitchen. Entrance to the two guest bedrooms and bath on the lower level was off the patio. The garage was built into the house off the alley. The house was completely furnished and came with a rowboat tied up in the bay just down the street.

Mrs. Brown, one of the owners, was there checking on the house when we arrived. We learned that the house was their summer home, but with gasoline rationing, it was not possible for them to make the trip from Los Angeles on weekends. The rent was sixty dollars a month, but that was more than we felt we could afford. Millie asked if we could rent the upper floor only for thirty dollars a month, but Mrs. Brown didn't want to rent just a part of the house so Millie came back with another proposition. "Could we rent out the two spare bedrooms?" she asked. "I have no objections," said Mrs. Brown, so the deal was made. Mrs. Brown even offered us the use of the linens, but we declined. She was a lovely person. Mr. Stanley was so elated over renting us the property that he took us to dinner. At that time, there was no market for real estate on the island. The people along the coast were fearful of a Japanese invasion, and those who could, had moved to a safer place inland. Due to wartime restrictions, there was no market for vacation rentals. It wasn't long before there was a huge influx of military personnel into the area, and every house was occupied. Mr. Stanley prospered, and I learned that after the war he became a millionaire when the real estate boom hit California.

After dinner, we moved into our new home. It didn't take long because all we owned was packed in our Ford. We had hardly carried in the last of our belongings when there was a knock at the door and there stood Mrs. Springer from across the street. She had come to welcome us to Balboa Island and to bring us a gift of avocados from her own trees. Friendliness, we found, was the rule among the people on the island. The Turners, the Kennels, and all the others on the street called to get acquainted.

On Monday morning I reported back to the city hall in Santa Ana. For several days, I had nothing to do except sit around the office. Finally, Colonel Schroeder called me in to inform me that I was to be in charge of the dispensary, which was to become operational the next day. I drove to the base. The hospital was still under construction, but the medical supply office was open, and I surveyed the building. The dispensary was just a building with nothing in it—no water, no lights, no heat, and no telephone. Lieutenant Jesser and I had to be ready for sick call the next day. We visited the medical supply office and carted over some wooden boxes to serve as tables and chairs. Also, we met Lieutenant Ferguson, the supply officer, and made out a list of supplies. We ended up with a large jar of aspirin and another large jar of throat lozenges. The only surgical supplies he could furnish us were gauze dressings, bandages, and tape. He did have some surgical needles, those large curved "stay" needles used in abdominal surgery.

Early the next morning, we were on duty, ready to receive our first patients. We didn't have to wait long before they began flocking in. Men from squadron after squadron arrived, each led by a sergeant with a sick book. Two medical corpsmen and a nurse were assigned to help us in the dispensary, and it was evident that I needed to come up with a plan to keep things in order. The corpsmen were given the job of taking the temperature of each patient and recording it on a card, along with the patient's name, serial number, and organization. Those cards became the medical file on that patient. All patients were kept waiting outside on the ramp until they were called in, a squadron at a time. Jesser and I sat on small boxes behind the packing box table. The men lined up in front. We looked at each card, checked the temperature that was recorded, and took a brief history. If it was deemed necessary, we examined the patient as he stood there. If a private exam was required, we sent the man into an adjoining room to be examined after the others had been dismissed. Regardless of the diagnosis, each man got either aspirin or throat lozenges or both. One man came in with a laceration on his face. We most certainly couldn't use the huge stay needle to repair the laceration so ended up closing the wound with adhesive tape. What a way to practice medicine! When we had finished sick call that first day, almost 150 lucky souls had received the ultimate in medical diagnosis and treatment.

Shortly, furniture and equipment began to arrive. We had heat, electricity, water, and a telephone. Telephones were the last to be installed, and for nearly a month, our only communication was by runner. The hospital finally became operational and all four wards—a hundred beds—soon were filled.

It didn't take me long to discover that our two corpsmen were not trained. One was of Greek heritage, and the other was Polish. Before entering the military, one had worked in a steel mill in Gary, Indiana, and the other had worked as a lumberjack in the state of Washington. When I asked them where they had trained, they told me at Letterman General Hospital. "What did they have you doing?" I asked. "Washing windows," was their reply. They were both bright young men so I asked them if they really were interested in the medical field. When they replied in the affirmative, Jesser, the nurse, and I set about giving them a condensed course in the techniques required of a good corpsman. They learned quickly and in no time were doing an excellent job. They could do beautiful repair of a simple laceration and took pride in what they were doing. I wouldn't have traded either for any other corpsman in the Army.

Colonel Schroeder had informed me that I not only was in charge of the dispensary but also was attending surgeon, officer in charge of immunizations, receiving and disposition officer, officer in charge of the pharmacy, and officer in charge of the ambulances. Later, each position would be filled by a separate officer. Our day started early, sometimes as early as 6:00 A.M., and we finished late. Sick call came first, and the number of patients averaged about 150 per day. The majority were young aviation cadets eighteen to twenty years old. Like all young men of that age group, they were looking for ways to beat the system. We soon learned about "goldbricking." An unusually large number from a squadron would appear at sick call while the other squadrons had a normal number of around four or five. That aroused our curiosity; on taking a history, we would find each man had the same set of vague complaints with normal physical findings. The next day an abnormally high percentage of another squadron would appear at sick call. The word had gotten around. The time on sick call gave the men more time away from classes or drill. It was evident that the practice had to be nipped in the bud. Looking at the cards they presented, we noticed the temperature recorded. If the temperature was normal, and the complaints were vague, we walked down the line sticking our fists in each man's belly. If he didn't flinch, we felt pretty safe in assuming there was no inflamed appendix. We would then announce to the men that we had a pleasant surprise: cocktails would be served. As he walked past the corpsman, each man was handed a paper cup containing a mixture containing equal parts of Epsom salts and caster oil, flavored with a dash of quinine. The next day that squadron would have only two or three men on the sick book.

When sick call was over, we set up tables loaded with syringes and started giving immunizations. We scheduled a squadron of 180 men every fifteen minutes. Each man received an inoculation of typhoid, tetanus toxoid, and a smallpox vaccination. We used large glass syringes, each holding twenty doses of vaccine. As the men walked by, we gave a shot in each arm, followed by a vaccination for smallpox. The needles were changed and the syringes filled by the corpsmen. We developed a rhythm of picking up the syringe, giving the shot, tossing the syringe backhanded to the table, picking up another syringe, and repeating the procedure like an automatic machine. We never looked at the syringe we were picking up and looked only at the arm we were sticking. If the line didn't keep moving, it was sure to happen that a man could receive more than two shots. Usually nurses or corpsmen administered the immunizations, but at Santa Ana, Colonel Schroeder insisted on its being done only by medical officers. Each man's immunization record was in triplicate, and Colonel Schroeder also insisted that the medical officers initial each immunization with a signature at the bottom. Jesser and I took stacks of cards home with us each night, and I can still remember sitting with a board across the chair arms, signing and initialing cards for two or three hours every night.

After the daily immunization session, we changed scenery again and began conducting physical exams on civilian employees. Sometime during the afternoon, I performed my duties as attending surgeon, seeing the dependents of military personnel who were in need of medical attention. Somewhere tucked into our busy schedule was the time I spent filling prescriptions for the ward physicians. I had a small room fitted out as a pharmacy, where I stood with a "cookbook" containing the instructions for filling the prescriptions—grinding, mixing, pouring, labeling, and finally placing the products of my labor in a basket to be delivered to the wards. After several weeks, I lost the job to a civilian pharmacist. If I had a few minutes during the day, I checked the ambulances and on the work being done in receiving and disposition. At lunch, I usually had time for a quick bowl of soup in the mess hall. It was dark when I arrived home at night. We worked seven days a week.

One Saturday afternoon a runner from the front office brought me a message from the colonel. He informed me that the next day at 3:00 P.M. the colonel's driver would pick me up at the dispensary and drive me to the post theater, where I was to give Charlie McCarthy a shot. The colonel was a stickler for correct protocol and was never one to joke, but I thought he had flipped. Charlie McCarthy was a ventriloquist's dummy. Edgar Bergen, the ventriloquist, had an hour-long show heard nationwide on radio each Sunday. I assumed that the act I was to perform was for publicity purposes and decided that if that was the case I would do my best to ham it up. I went over to medical supply and asked Ferguson, the supply officer, for a surgical gown and the biggest syringe and the longest needle he had. He thought I had lost my wits until I told him what the colonel had ordered me to do. The next day, promptly at 3:00 P.M., the car arrived. I picked up my props and was driven to the theater. I was greeted by Edgar, holding Charlie, and the orchestra leader, Ray Noble. Charlie was wearing the uniform of an army private. I donned my gown, and with Edgar and the MPs holding Charlie, I rolled up his sleeve and gave him the shot. Charlie's mouth was wide open as if he were screaming. Cameras flashed several times as the photographers recorded that historic event for posterity. I shook hands all around and left. As I rode back to the dispensary, I thought, "Here we are engaged in the greatest conflict in the history of the world, and I had to take time out of my busy schedule to do something silly." Maybe that is why America is so great. Even in times of greatest peril, we can take a minute to laugh. The shows that were given by well-known performers for the GIs were great morale boosters.

I first met Maj. Russell V. Lee on a Sunday morning as I was walking down a corridor in the hospital. He was with Colonel Schroeder. As they approached, I took a look at the new major and thought to myself, "This is one of the saddest-looking men I have ever seen." He had a large angular nose and large ears. His face resembled that of a beagle. The sleeves of his uniform blouse and the legs of his trousers were short. The insignia fastened to the lapel of his blouse was not on straight. I wondered what rock he had crawled out from under. "Lieutenant," said Colonel Shroeder, "I would like you to meet Major Lee, the new Chief of Medicine." I thought to myself, "If this is what we are getting as Chief of Medical Services, we must really be in trouble."

It wasn't long until I realized I had completely misjudged the man. The first week he was there, he received a call from the White House. Mrs. Roosevelt wanted to talk to him about her brother, whom he had been treating before he came to Santa Ana. I started dropping around to visit with the major in his office, and we became good friends. He had founded Lee Clinic in Palo Alto, one of the largest medical clinics in the country. He hadn't been at Santa Ana long before he demonstrated his talents as a "wheeler-dealer." He talked the commanding officer into sending him to the annual meeting of the California State Medical Society to recruit additional doctors for the service. Lee showed me the material he was going to hand out to prospects. He promised that no one would come on active duty with a rank less than captain. Each man would be stationed permanently close to his home so he would be able to commute. Furthermore, each would receive a promotion every six months. I couldn't believe that he expected anyone to swallow that, but when he returned from his trip, he had a wide grin. The suckers had bought the deal. As I recall, he added approximately a hundred doctors to the ranks.

The war was going badly. The Philippines had fallen. The Japanese controlled the Pacific. Hitler had overrun Europe and North Africa and was rapidly destroying London and the industrial cities of England. It was hard for me to keep up my morale, but Lee seemed to be the eternal optimist. When I was especially low, a visit to his office was a shot in the arm. At times, it seemed as if he was clairvoyant. Once, after several days of nothing but bad news from the Pacific, I visited Major Lee. He seemed especially happy, and I couldn't understand why he was in such a good mood. I told him I thought things were going from bad to worse and that nothing we did seemed to have any effect on the Japanese war machine. After listening to me awhile, he said, "Just wait, we are going to come up with something that is going to begin to turn the thing around. It is big, and the Japanese are going to be taken by surprise." I thought to myself, "This man is nuts, but at least he makes me feel a lot better." A few days later, the entire base was put on round-the-clock alert. One half of all personnel had to be on the base at all times, and the rest had to be near a phone, ready to return to base immediately if called.

Slit trenches were dug all over the camp. No one knew what was going on. All sorts of rumors were floating around, the most logical one being that a Japanese invasion was imminent. Then the news broke: the Battle of Midway Island had occurred. It was true that the Japanese fleet was steaming toward our West Coast, but far out in the Pacific near Midway Island, our fleet lay in wait. Taken by surprise, the Japanese were mauled badly by our big guns and fighters and bombers from our few remaining aircraft carriers. The Japanese suffered tremendous losses of ships and men. Our losses were relatively minor. That was a major turning point in the war. After the good news arrived, I thought back to my conversation with Lee. That was what he knew was going to happen, but how did he know? Sometime later, he happened to mention he had a twin brother who was an admiral. Was that the source of his information?

Through his friendship with Mrs. Roosevelt, Lee had access to the White House. He also had been the personal physician of General Arnold, who was the Supreme Commander of the Air Corps. It was evident that he was a man with clout. He had no regard for military protocol, and it wasn't unusual for him to pick up the phone and call high-ranking persons in Washington. The local base commander later learned about that when a letter to Lee came back through channels referring to the phone conversation. The local commanding officer was burned up, but he couldn't do anything about it. Lee had the clout. Through his recruiting efforts, a good number of the doctors from the Lee Clinic were assigned to our hospital. They were all excellent doctors and helped to boost the quality of care we were giving.

Colonel Schroeder was given another command, and his place was taken by Col. Paul Gilliland. His personality was completely different from Colonel Schroeder's. Colonel Gilliland was all business, a commander who spoke with authority and who conducted himself in a manner that exuded confidence, yet a man who had the respect of all. Shortly after he took command, I received a promotion to captain.

One day while I was busy in the dispensary, a runner from the front office came and told me the colonel wanted to see me in his office immediately. I rapidly reviewed all that I had been doing and tried to figure out where I had screwed up as I hurried to his office. When I arrived, the sergeant major told me the colonel was busy and asked me to take a chair. I was too nervous to sit down. I stood awhile and paced awhile. Finally after about a half hour, the colonel buzzed the sergeant major, and I was directed to enter. I walked through the door, saluted, and stood at attention. The colonel smiled and waved me to a chair. I was certain that it was bad news and that he thought I could take it better sitting down. I just knew I was going to get my overseas orders.

The colonel began to speak. "I just received a message from Washington," he said. "Why is he telling me this?" I thought. He continued, "They have told me this hospital is to be expanded tremendously from the present hundred beds, and they also directed me to select the key personnel to operate the new hospital. The personnel I select, if they perform satisfactorily, will remain here for the duration of the war and will be promoted to the grade commensurate with their responsibilities." Before I could absorb all he had said, he continued, "I have selected you to be the executive officer of this hospital second in command to me." I almost fell out of my chair. Then I thought, "I don't know anything about administration. I can't do what the colonel is asking me to do." I finally took a deep breath and stated what I had been thinking. Looking me straight in the eye, without smiling, he said, "Young man, you are in the army. There is a war going on. You have no choice in the matter. You will do as you are ordered. You are the new executive officer."

"Yes, Sir," was my answer. I saluted and floated out of the room. I was given the opportunity to learn something about my new assignment by working with Colonel Anderson, who was the present executive officer. He was being transferred to another base to assume command of its hospital.

Along with learning the duties of executive officer, I continued as receiving and disposition officer, performed the duties of adjutant, and was in charge of all hospital records. My days continued to run from early morning to late night. I had to see that all hospital records were in order, listen to complaints from patients and staff, interpret regulations, and handle a mountain of correspondence. There were army regulations, air corps regulations, regulations from the Air Surgeon's office, plus directives from Command and Base Headquarters that had to be read and absorbed. In addition, every day's mail brought changes to be incorporated into all the regulations. I began to think I should have studied law.

After Colonel Anderson left for his new assignment, Colonel Gilliland asked me to move into his office. He thought that we could work closer together with the arrangement. A large desk was moved in and placed back to back with his desk. That was a good idea because it gave us the opportunity to discuss all matters concerning a given problem and work out a solution without the necessity of sending memos back and forth. It didn't take long for me to gain confidence and to begin to feel comfortable in my new job. My close association with the colonel gave me added insight into the tremendous ability he had to organize and implement the many projects necessary for a top medical facility.

Our primary mission was to give complete physical and psychological tests to each aviation cadet assigned to the base. We had a large staff of qualified specialists in internal medicine; cardiology; ear, nose, and throat; ophthalmology; surgery; psychiatry; and psychology. The standards for air crew members were the highest, and the "washout" rate was fairly high. If a cadet had a correctable surgical defect, he was hospitalized, and the defect corrected. A large number of operations were performed to correct muscle imbalance of the eyes. Each cadet also had to pass the high altitude test. The high altitude unit, as we called it, was equipped with huge cylindrical tanks similar in size to the fuselage of a bomber. After receiving instructions in the use of their equipment, the cadets were placed in the pressure chamber, and the pressure was reduced to simulate flight to high altitudes. Some were flunked after the test. After medical and academic tests were completed, a board classified the cadets as pilots, bombardiers, or navigators. The rest who didn't make the grade were reassigned to the ground forces.

Those who were going on to flight school had to pass an extensive course of study in academic subjects before being assigned to one of the basic training schools located in California, Arizona, New Mexico, Nevada, or Texas. The average stay at Santa Ana was about twelve weeks. Our secondary mission was to provide the best of medical care for all military personnel. We eventually became a regional hospital to which all problem cases were evacuated for specialized treatment.

I hadn't been in my job long before we received word that the expansion we had been promised was about to begin. The hospital was to be enlarged from a hundred to nearly two thousand beds, an expansion covering an area of about fifty acres. The contractors arrived and work began. The colonel assigned me as coordinator of the expansion. I spent considerable time looking at blueprints and talking to the various foremen. I did make sure that the colonel and I would each have a large office. No more cubbyholes. Our offices were isolated at one end of the administration building, and we had an exit to the rear where we could leave without being seen. Work progressed rapidly, and the new buildings, completely equipped, were in use in a matter of months. The wards rapidly filled with patients. The staff was expanded until we had between 110 and 115 doctors, 35 to 40 dentists, 125 nurses, several medical administrative officers, 1,000 enlisted personnel, and about 300 civilian employees. All of that increased the administrative load tremendously. I continued to put in long days, seven days a week, and the paperwork I carried home each night kept me busy until midnight. I had two phones on my desk, and it seemed they were ringing all the time. Calls from headquarters, other military bases, and occasional calls from Washington kept me busy. I had to make decisions quickly. Only the most important decisions were relayed to the colonel.

One day a letter came across my desk informing us that we had two patients diagnosed with active tuberculosis. I discussed the problem with the colonel. He did not know the procedure for handling such a problem so he gave it to me. Studying the regulations, I finally found the answer. The two patients would be transferred to a veterans' hospital for long-term care. They would be on active duty with the army until they entered the veterans' hospital. At that moment, they would revert to civilian status. The problem now was to proceed through the red tape to comply with the regulations. I sent a letter and complete records on both patients through channels requesting the designation of an appropriate veterans' hospital. After several weeks, I received authorization to transfer them to a hospital in Excelsior Springs, Missouri. Then I had to forward a request for honorable discharge for medical reasons. The orders had to read that they were discharged upon entry into the veterans' hospital. It was required that a medical officer escort the patients to the hospital. I informed the colonel that everything was in order and asked him to name the escorting officer. He looked at me and grinned. "You did all the work and did a good job. You haven't had any time off since you came on active duty back in July of 1941. I want you to go, and while you're at it, get a few days' delay en route and hop back to Illinois to see your mother." On the way home that night, I got to figuring. I would get additional per diem pay to and from Missouri plus six cents per mile over all land grant railroads both ways. Roughly, that came to between two hundred and three hundred dollars. With that extra money, I could afford a ticket for Millie. A tentative date was set for my departure, so I arranged to send Millie home a couple of weeks before I left. I had a close friend, a Maj. Clark Henkle, who was in charge of transportation, so I asked him the impossible. Could he get Millie Pullman reservations round-trip from Los Angeles to Terre Haute, Indiana? That he did. Millie had very little experience in train riding and had never taken a long trip on a Pullman. I explained to her how the seats used in the daytime were made into sleeping berths at night. The day came for her to leave. I took her to Union Station in Los Angeles to board the train due to leave at 9:00 P.M. We walked through the large waiting room filled with a milling mass of soldiers, sailors, and marines. On the platform going to the train, the traffic was just as heavy. I found her car, and the porter took her bags aboard. We only had a couple of minutes to talk before it was time to leave. I knew Millie was nervous and half scared to be embarking on such a long trip by herself. We kissed good-by, and she got on the train and disappeared from view. The train was starting to move slowly down the track when suddenly Millie reappeared on the steps of her car. Tears were streaming down her face. She screamed, "There's a sailor in my berth. What will I do?" By that time, the train was moving at a good speed. "You're on your own, Kid, you're on your own," I yelled as the train moved rapidly away. To this day, I've never gotten the whole story.

My orders finally came through. The trip to Excelsior Springs would require at least forty-eight hours if we had no delays. All passenger traffic during the war had low priority. Freights carrying war materiel had top priority. As a result, passenger trains spent a lot of time on sidings. My two patients had a bedroom, and I had a roomette. They were confined to the bedroom the entire trip. All their meals were served in their room. I checked on them several times a day, making sure that they had plenty of reading material and that they got their meals on time. I had made Pullman reservations to take the train from Kansas City, an overnight trip to St. Louis, and then on to Terre Haute for a three-day rest at home, but our train slowly plodded along, frequently moving onto a siding to make way for speeding freight to pass. I realized I wasn't going to make connections so I sent a telegram canceling my rail reservations and making a reservation to fly from Kansas City to Indianapolis. Being on a military mission, I had a certain degree of priority.

We were due in Excelsior Springs at 9:00 P.M. but were way behind schedule. I had the patients hit the sack, and I sat up watching the time and the schedule. Approximately three-quarters of an hour before my estimated time of arrival, I got them up and ready to go. At about 3:30 A.M., we pulled into Excelsior Springs. It was a typical small-town railroad station, dark except for a light in the station agent's office. The train stopped only long enough for us to hop off. It was quite chilly. I looked around for a car. I had been told a car from the hospital would meet us. Seeing no car, we went into the dark waiting room and up to the ticket window. I asked the agent if a car had come for us. He said someone had come about 9:00 P.M. when the train was due but had left and hadn't come back. I was put out because they hadn't made any attempt to find out when the train might arrive. I called the hospital, and they sent a car. To complete the discharge of the patients from the army and admission to the veterans' hospital, I first had to get a receipt from the officer in charge at the hospital with the date and time noted.

A copy of the orders and the receipt were placed in an envelope addressed to army headquarters and dropped in the mailbox at the hospital. The night duty personnel were very hospitable, but the officer of the day was quite the opposite. He was an older man, a typical VA career doctor. The nurse aroused him from his sleep, and he came stomping down the hall in pajamas and robe, hair standing up and a frown on his face. I introduced myself and asked him to sign the receipts and take charge of the patients. He grumped and sputtered while he signed the receipts; then I asked him if he could supply me with a car and driver to get me to the airport in Kansas City since I had a plane to catch in about three hours. He really sputtered then; "We don't furnish cars for anybody here," he said as he stalked off down the hall. The night staff asked me to come into the kitchen for coffee and told me they would work out something to get me to the airport. There was one taxi in town operated by a local garageman. One of the nurses called him, getting him out of bed, and soon we were on the way to the airport. Right then, I formed a lasting opinion of Veterans' Administration hospitals, and it wasn't favorable. I thought of the many times we had visitors at our base who needed transportation, and we never failed to provide whatever they needed.

14

At War

PENICILLIN CAME ON THE SCENE in the early 1940s. We now had the first of what would eventually be a long list of antibiotics. Antibiotics would be effective in combating many of the terrible infections that had plagued the human race since the beginning of time.

Producing penicillin was a laborious procedure. Only a small amount could be produced, and demand was far greater than supply. A national board was created to control distribution. The armed forces had first priority, and the drug could be used only for specific life-threatening infections. Injections were given every three to four hours. Penicillin is excreted in the urine so all urine was collected from the patient being treated. The excreted penicillin was recovered so that it could be used again.

The public was aware that the antibiotic that could save lives was being used by the military. One day a family came into my office to plead with me for some penicillin. A member of the family was dying, and penicillin could save his life. In tears, they begged for some, but I could only tell them none could be released to the civilian population.

HOLLYWOOD STARS WERE most generous in putting on shows for the troops—Bob Hope, Bing Crosby, Jerry Colona, Spike Jones, Edgar Bergen, Eddie Cantor, and many others. One day, a man walked into my office and began talking like Donald Duck. He introduced himself as the voice of that famous cartoon character; he had come to entertain our patients.

Frequently the Sunday night coast-to-coast radio broadcasts of those stars originated from our base. Many of the television shows so popular in the 1950s originated from army performances. All personnel involved with the show would arrive early Sunday morning. The technicians began assembling and testing the equipment; then the cast would start rehearsals. In the evening, the performers were ready for the show.

The commanding general had a party for the cast at the Officer's Club after the show. Millie and I were always invited, and we had the opportunity to become acquainted with the stars. One night I found Millie sitting with others at a table with Spike Jones. Millie and Spike were discussing their little daughters, both of whom were named Linda. Frances Langford, the singer with Bob Hope, started writing a syndicated newspaper column about her experiences visiting with the troops. She asked me for an interview and did a column on battle fatigue.

Bing Crosby was on the base to do a show and was busy rehearsing when a Red Cross woman came into my office and told me about a patient in the hospital who was dying of cancer. He was a longtime fan and told her that he would give anything if he could meet Bing. "Do you think he would take time to come see this man?" she asked. "I'm sure he would," I replied. "Why don't you go ask him?"

It wasn't long until she returned with Bing and his photographer. "Let's go see this man," said Bing. Down to the ward we went. Because of his critical condition, the patient was in a private room. "Hi, Sarge," Bing said. I thought the patient's eyes were going to pop out. "I heard you were laid up, and I thought I'd drop by to see you. I'm sure you'll be up in no time." All the time Bing was talking, the photographer was busy snapping pictures.

"Say," said Bing looking at the bedside table, "I see you are a pipe smoker. You know, I like a pipe and I'll tell you what I'm going to do. When I get back to Hollywood, I'm going to send you a new pipe and a jar of my favorite tobacco, along with these photos." The sergeant was smiling broadly, and his eyes were brimming with tears. "Well, I must run along now and you need to rest. So long." With that he left. That night at the party, after the show, I talked to Bing and thanked him for taking time from his busy schedule to come to the hospital. His answer was, "Any time I can do anything to spread a little cheer and make things a little better for someone, I'll do it." Two or three days later, a big package arrived for the sergeant. In it was the pipe, tobacco, and autographed pictures. The sergeant was so happy. A week later he died.

Betty Miller was a volunteer, a "gray lady." I didn't know who she was, but I often saw her as I walked through the wards during inspection. She usually was carrying a bedpan. As the ward personnel came to attention, she would do the same. I finally learned her name and discovered that she was the wife of Colonel Miller, who was on the general's staff at headquarters. Millie and I became well acquainted with her, and it was evident that she was really dedicated to doing her bit in helping around the hospital. I learned from others that Colonel Miller, as a civilian, was board chairman of Pacific Gas and Electric, which was the major power company in California. Betty's maiden name was Folger, of the Folger Coffee family. They lived across the bay in a huge mansion complete with servants.

Learning the date of Millie's birthday, Betty called and asked if we could come for dinner. When we arrived, we discovered she had invited other guests too. That was a surprise. We went to dinner in a large dining room, and Millie was seated as guest of honor to Betty's right. The entrée was prime rib, meat we rarely saw during the war years. One of the other guests was the former silent movie star, Billie Dove. Millie was awed to be in the presence of a movie star. "You know, Billie, you were always my favorite idol when you were in the movies. I named all of my dolls after you," she said, as I kicked her under the table.

It was not all fun and games. We were still at war and we still worked long hours, but things were improving. The war was going much better for the United States and our allies. We could begin to see that victory was not too far off.

It was known that there was an organization called the Office of Strategic Services, the OSS. The organization was involved in covert operations, and Gen. William ("Wild Bill") Donovan was its commander. Little else was known. It was rumored that those forces were involved in behind-the-lines missions, underwater demolition, and other secret operations.

One day a man in civilian clothes came to my office. He didn't identify himself. He produced a letter stating that we were to cooperate with him and give him whatever he wanted. He told me that from time to time there would be a need for medical supplies. A list would be presented, and we would be expected to furnish the supplies. Furthermore, there would be patients in need of medical treatment who would appear. They would be dressed as civilians but would have identification. Treatment should be furnished, but no questions were to be asked.

After our meeting, I never saw him again. We did get requests for supplies from time to time, however, and the supplies were furnished. Occasionally, we did receive a civilian for treatment. It wasn't until after the war was over that I found out the OSS had a secret training center on Catalina Island just off the coast.

Army regulations specifically stated that a hospital of our classification could have only the field-type ambulances. Those were the same heavy-duty ambulances used in combat zones. They could not be equipped with red lights or sirens. I received a call from headquarters that the commandant, Colonel Robertson, had obtained a metropolitan-type ambulance from a local undertaker and that a ceremony would take place the next day. At that time, the undertaker formally would present the ambulance to the hospital. A metropolitan-type ambulance came equipped with red lights and siren, and I knew if we accepted the ambulance we would be in violation of regulations. At the hospital we discussed the matter, but we knew we couldn't overrule Colonel Robertson. The ambulance had a lot of miles on the odometer; thus, I knew that we were likely heading for trouble. It had been completely reconditioned at the motor pool, including all new tires. The colonel was all smiles when he turned the vehicle over to the hospital, but my apprehension persisted.

The daughter of an enlisted man was a severe diabetic and had to be transported to Children's Hospital in Los Angeles. That was the first trip for our fancy ambulance. Not long after leaving the base, a tire blew, throwing the ambulance into the ditch. Fortunately, no one was injured. Sometime later, on a Sunday afternoon, I received a call from the officer of the day, who reported there had been a terrible accident on Highway 101 and our ambulance was involved. Later, I got the full report.

The ambulance had been dispatched to Los Angeles to pick up one of our Chinese cadets, who had come down with malarial meningitis. The patient was comatose, and the ambulance driver was speeding back to the base. He took a shortcut down through the country, driving wide open with the red lights flashing and the siren blaring. He was on a road flanked on both sides by orange groves. Suddenly he came to Highway 101, the major four-lane highway that ran north and south through the state. He made no effort to slow down but depended on the siren and the red lights to stop the traffic. He shot out across the highway. There was a terrible crash, and when the dust had settled, three automobiles plus the ambulance were totally destroyed, three people were killed, and several others were seriously injured. The physician riding with the patient received a fractured leg. The only one uninjured was the Chinese patient. The next day, I received a call from a local garage asking me what to do with the wrecked ambulance. "Junk it," I said. The matter of the fancy ambulance was laid to rest.

Millie kept busy working with Civil Defense down on the island. Of course, she was a member of the first aid team that responded to each air raid alarm. She was also an airplane spotter. There was no such thing as radar to detect enemy aircraft. The early detection of enemy aircraft was totally dependent upon the sharp eyes of those people scattered at posts around the countryside. All the volunteers had to be trained to identify the different types of aircraft. On the island, training sessions were held three nights a week. Cards with silhouettes of the planes were flashed, and the volunteers had to give the proper answer quickly. Millie's post was a sandbagged foxhole on a bluff above the bay. When a plane was seen, headquarters was notified by using a crank-style field telephone. The type of aircraft, estimated altitude, estimated speed, and the direction were reported immediately. The posts were manned around the clock. Each pair of observers spent three hours at their posts. Millie's partner was Jascha Heifetz, the renowned concert violinist. I questioned her about her teammate, but she assured me he did no fiddling!

According to regulations, all military personnel who were hospitalized had to return to full duty upon release from the hospital. As a result, the hospital always had a large number of patients who were ambulatory and had received maximum definitive treatment, but had not recuperated to the extent that they could return to the strenuous activity of soldiers. Lying around the wards with nothing to do was boring and hard on morale. What was needed was a change in environment and a rehabilitation program. I discussed my idea with Colonel Simpson, the Base Executive Officer, and he came up with a solution to the problem.

The Irvine Ranch totaled several hundred thousand acres of southern California land. The land was obtained by the Irvine family through a Spanish land grant. Old Mr. Irvine was fabulously wealthy. There were thousands of acres of orange groves and rangeland close to the base. Mr. Irvine jealously guarded his property. He maintained a large force of security guards, and anyone found trespassing was arrested immediately and prosecuted. Colonel Simpson, however, had a good relationship with the old gentleman. As a result, we were given access to a wooded area on the shore of one of the many lakes that had been created on the Irvine property, and a convalescent camp was constructed. The patients were housed in tents with wooden floors and furnished with good beds. There was a large mess tent where top quality food was served. The lake had a sand beach, and the swimming was great.

Mr. Irvine specified that there would be no fishing, although the clear water showed fish in such large numbers that they were nudging one another trying to find swimming room. The camp was staffed with physical training and recreational personnel who devised a complete reconditioning program. Fresh air, quiet surroundings, good food, and conditioning paid off. Boredom disappeared, morale soared, and the lost duty days were cut dramatically. The program was a huge success.

The medical personnel, medical officers, and nurses had little, if any, field training so we decided to set up such a program at the convalescent camp. The staff was divided up into small cadres of fifteen to twenty officers and nurses who spent a week living under field conditions. Various exercises were scheduled, such as setting up a battalion aid station and evacuation of patients under simulated battle conditions. We also discussed the art of camouflage, sanitation, and the proper method of establishing sanitary facilities in the field (how to construct a latrine). I slept in the first morning, which as CO, I felt was my prerogative. About 9:00 A.M., I wandered down to the mess tent to have a leisurely breakfast. Mess was closed so I walked into the kitchen to give the cook my order. About that time, the mess sergeant descended upon me breathing fire and brimstone. With his chin stuck out and his clenched fist in my face, he gave me orders to get out, and if I wanted to eat breakfast in the morning I should be on time. I backed away, waving the collar of my fatigues with the attached oak-leaf insignia of a major, but that made not a bit of difference to the sergeant. "Yes, Sir, Sergeant, I understand and tomorrow I'll be on time." Rank meant nothing to the sergeant.

It was customary for each group of officers and nurses who were bivouacked to produce a talent show for the entertainment of the patients. Capt. Paul LeVan, who was in our group, had been in show business before going into medicine. Naturally, I put him in charge of producing our show. One of the highlights was the Floradora Sextet, consisting of six high-stepping doctors. We needed costumes so we borrowed the necessary accoutrements from the nurses. On the night of the show those doctors with high-kicking, hairy legs brought down the house.

Jack Hall was a resident in internal medicine when I was at Methodist Hospital in Indianapolis. He and his wife, Pat, lived in the same apartment building where Millie lived. We all had been close friends while we were at Methodist. Shortly before we left Indianapolis, Pat discovered she was going to have twins. A year or so later, Jack reported to me for duty at Santa Ana. Millie and I were delighted to see them again. They moved into a house down on the island, and we got together often. The twins had become two beautiful little girls. Pete Treadwell, the obstetrician, and his wife also had twin daughters about the same age. The two mothers frequently took the girls for a stroll in their buggies around the island. Later, Jack was assigned to one of the other bases in our command. A year or so later, he was reassigned to Santa Ana. That time they were able to rent a house on the oceanfront across the bay at Balboa. Pat really loved living on the ocean. Jack came in the office one day and asked if we had any troop trains moving back east. He wanted to get back to Indianapolis to get his car, and if he could get a trip back as an escort, he could get free transportation. I was able to arrange that and also got him a delay en route so that he could have plenty of time to drive back.

While Jack was gone, Pat went to see Dr. Treadwell, who discovered that she had an ovarian cyst and advised surgery. The surgery was anticipated to be routine, and Pat decided to go ahead with it before Jack returned. As Pete came out of the operating room, the look on his face was enough to tell us something was wrong. "Pat has cancer," he said. "It's spread all over her abdomen." X-ray therapy was the only treatment to offer, and Pete didn't really think it would do any good. Arrangements were made for Pat to have the treatments at the hospital in Los Angeles administered by Major Jamison, head of the X-ray department. Jack wanted to get back closer to home in Indianapolis before the worst came. He discussed the situation with Colonel Gilliland and me. By pulling a lot of strings, we arranged a transfer back to Stout Field near Indianapolis. Pat lived only a few months after they returned.

AN IMPORTANT ORGANIZATION on any military base in wartime is the Officer's Club. Many officers on the base at Santa Ana were unmarried or didn't have their wives with them. They resided in the bachelor's quarters, which were very spartan. The rooms were small and furnished with a bed, a chair, and a small bedside table. The Officer's Club offered a place for fellowship, good food, and entertainment. We had an Officer's Club with a large comfortable lounge, dining room, bar, and ballroom. It was my privilege to serve on the Board of Governors. The food was good and the prices were reasonable, since the object was not to make a profit. Our chefs were GIs who had staffed some of the best restaurants in the country.

Every Friday was special. Officers were encouraged to bring their families for dinner. The food was served buffet style. Usually there was a huge centerpiece carved from ice by our talented chefs. There were all kinds of appetizers, shrimp, prime rib, lamb chops, as well as a selection of salads and vegetables. The price for adults was $1.50, and for children the cost was $.75. After dinner there was entertainment in the ballroom, followed by a dance.

The members of our resident sixteen-piece dance band were all members of big-name bands before entering the service. Officially, they were assigned to the post military band but performed also in the dance band. The stage was arranged so that it could be opened out onto the central courtyard during good weather. That meant that in good weather there was dancing both in the ballroom and in the courtyard. At least once a year, we held a stag for the officers. We had approximately a thousand officers, and we allocated fifteen thousand dollars from the club funds for the big bash. We had big-name entertainment from Hollywood, except on one occasion, when we brought the entire cast from a Los Angeles burlesque house in for the evening.

The major source of revenue for the club was the slot machines. We had twelve slot machines, which were adjusted for the maximum payoff. We still made a tremendous amount of money. All club funds had to be expended for the good of the officers. No matter how much we spent, we could never get close to the bottom of our pocket of money. We had board meetings monthly and, after the treasurer's report, we would start discussing ways of spending money. If the furniture in the lounge hadn't been replaced for two months, that would be done. Once I remember that we had run out of anything to buy so we had mother-of-pearl toilet seats installed in the ladies lounge. When the war ended, there was still about $250,000 in the treasury. According to regulations, the money was to be sent to Washington and placed in a fund for the relief of widows and orphans.

Orders from Washington arrived in my office for Lieutenant Colonel Lee (he had been promoted to lieutenant colonel and made Chief of Professional Services). I called and told him he had orders. "It's about time," he said. "I've been looking for those orders for several days." No one in our office or base headquarters knew that Colonel Lee was getting orders, but he did. The orders specified he was to report to Hamilton Field in San Francisco, where secret orders would be issued. We found out later that everything had been arranged by Colonel Lee himself, through his request to his old friend and former patient General Arnold, commander in chief of the Army Air Corps. We didn't see Colonel Lee for three or four months. When he returned, he was promoted to full colonel. I asked where he had been, and he told me that he had visited every theater of operations in the world. The reason given for the trip was to study malarial conditions. I guess that included Alaska and all the other cold spots where we had fighting men. He had traveled VIP all the way, just as a four-star general would.

I asked Colonel Lee why he had arranged such a trip. "I was bored and I wanted to go where the action was," was his answer. He hadn't been back long when he got new orders to report to the Air Surgeon's Office headquarters in Washington. He was also given a two-week delay en route to his new assignment, which allowed him to be at home over Christmas. Instead of packing and shipping his belongings home and riding the train to Palo Alto, he did what we expected—he requested the pilot and plane of Major General Cousins, the commander in chief of the Western Flying Training Command.

On Saturday morning Colonel Lee came to say good-by. Colonel Gilliland was going to accompany him to get in some flying time. I asked Colonel Gilliland if there was anything special he wanted me to do while he was gone. "Not a thing," he said. "Everything is pretty quiet." He walked from my office and then turned and said, "Get out of that chair and come along. You need a change."

I gave Millie a call and casually remarked that I might be late for supper because I was flying to San Francisco and back. We drove over to the flight line and when we got out of the car, the crew was lined up as if they were expecting the general. We loaded aboard. Colonel Lee seated himself in the general's seat, the telephone hanging on the wall next to his left elbow. We took off and flew without incident to Moffet Field. About forty-five minutes before arriving, Colonel Lee had the pilot radio ahead to instruct headquarters to notify his wife to meet us at the gate.

When we taxied up to the hangar, a jeep-load of sailors (Moffet Field was a naval base) came up, opened the cabin door, put the steps in place, and stood at attention as we disembarked. We needed a staff car and two jeeps to get to the main gate. We rode in the staff car, and Colonel Lee's luggage was carried in the jeeps. Along the way, a flight bag fell off one of the jeeps, and the driver didn't notice. Colonel Lee counted all the luggage when we arrived at the gate and discovered a bag missing. The poor driver took off at full speed and was back shortly with the missing bag. "Damn," yelled Colonel Lee, "that's the bag my 1812 Napoleon Brandy was packed in." I thought the driver was going to faint. Colonel Lee carefully checked through the bag and suddenly stood, a big smile on his face, cradling the precious bottle in his hands.

We drove to the Lee Mansion, which was located on the Stanford campus. I had doubted the colonel before about his Stanford connections, but that doubt was now laid to rest. We were ushered into a large, sunken living room and later into the beautiful dining room for lunch. He noted that the large game room in the basement had been decorated for him by the cartoonist of the *San Francisco Chronicle*. There was no question that the colonel had power and knew all the right people. After lunch, Colonel Gilliland and I were driven back to Moffet Field. We bade the Lees good-by. That was the last time I saw him, although I followed his career after the war. He went back to the Palo Alto Clinic, which he had founded. It had grown to be one of the largest medical clinics in the country. One of Colonel Lee's sons, who was in school then, later became under secretary of Health, Education, and Welfare in the administration of President Johnson.

When General Arnold died, the newspaper article I read gave the cause of death and stated that the information had been received from Dr. Russell V. Lee, the general's personal physician. I wrote to Colonel Lee once after the war and received a very cordial reply. I'm sure he has passed on now, but he was one of the most unusual characters I have ever met.

After months of struggling with the enemy on many fronts, the might of America began to slowly make itself felt. The millions of civilians laboring around the clock to produce the tools of war and the millions of raw recruits who had been turned into top combat soldiers swiftly and skillfully began to turn the tide against our enemies. With our success against the enemy continuing to mount, the need for training of additional combat personnel decreased.

At that time, early in 1944, the mission of the base was changed from training for combat to demobilization of personnel. The official name was "redistribution center." A considerable number of those returnees had physical or psychological problems as a result of their war service. It was the policy that those men receive the maximum definitive treatment and rehabilitation before final disposition of their cases.

The keystone of the entire operation was the convalescent hospital. Those convalescent centers were outgrowths of the convalescent program we developed earlier, but instead of having the ambulatory patients in the same hospital as those who were bed patients, the convalescent hospital was located at a separate site.

Col. Howard Rusk was the "father" of the convalescent program. He was in charge of the program for the entire Air Corps. The facilities were strategically located over the entire United States. Our convalescent hospital had a capacity of a thousand beds. No new buildings were built. Instead, we remodeled a group of unused barracks. The bare studs of the barracks were covered and painted in attractive pastels. Bunks were replaced by regular hotel beds. Desk lamps, lounge chairs, and drapes were placed in the rooms and the dormitories.

Colonel Gilliland asked me to take over the command of the new convalescent hospital. I had been an enthusiastic supporter of the convalescent program, but the new operation was much more elaborate. Most of our patients had psychological problems. They required not only specialized care but also—maybe more important—plenty of empathy. Our plan was to assign to each barracks or ward a family physician who could exude warmth and confidence. The men learned that their assigned "Doc" was there to answer questions, give advice, and listen. As a backup for the family physician, we had a staff of psychiatrists and psychologists. Good food was in ample supply. The mess hall was open around the clock. The selection was almost unlimited: fresh eggs, bacon, ham, sausage, hot cakes, hot biscuits, hot cereal, and more for breakfast; prime rib, lamb chops, steak, fresh shrimp, fresh fish as entrées, fresh salads and vegetables, plus fruit, ice cream, and French pastry for lunch and dinner. Patients could raid the refrigerator any time they liked. Fresh milk and ice cream were the two items they enjoyed the most. It wasn't unusual for a man to gain thirty to forty pounds during his stay with us.

Many patients had their education interrupted by the war. Some had never finished grammar school, while others still had their high school diplomas to earn. To fill their needs, we had grade and high schools with complete curricula. The schools were certified by the California Department of Education. We had both an academic and a vocational curriculum. There was a machine shop, a sheet metal shop, an automobile repair shop, photography, architectural drafting, home planning, and an agricultural department.

Our staff consisted of fifty officers and several hundred enlisted men. Most of the personnel had been college professors or instructors at the grade or high school level in civilian life. We also had a large staff involved in physical education and conditioning. Commencement ceremonies were held every three months. All graduates wore caps and gowns and were presented with diplomas.

A broad range of recreational activities was available. Golf, baseball, football, basketball, bowling, tennis, and swimming were offered. If a man's interest was directed toward less strenuous activities, there was trout fishing in the mountains or deep sea fishing in the Pacific.

We had a fleet of two 55-foot cruisers and a 105-foot cruiser berthed at our dock in Balboa Bay. Full crews were on duty around the clock. If the men wanted to go deep sea fishing or maybe just take a cruise to Catalina, a call was made to alert the crew, and the bus was dispatched to take the men the five or six miles to the bay.

There never was a lack of entertainment. Hollywood was only a few miles away, and the stars of stage and screen went all out to entertain the men. There was no formality. Performances were impromptu, often just sitting and having a bull session. It felt good to see the expressions on the faces of the men. Sometimes the stars invited the patients to Hollywood. Buddy Rogers and Mary Pickford often entertained at Pickfair, their huge estate. Atwater Kent, a millionaire industrialist and inventor, also entertained at his estate. I feel sure that those patients probably spent more time telling their families and friends about being with the stars than they did relating their war experiences.

Our whole program was designed to get the men back to normalcy as quickly as possible so that they could return to civilian life. There was no way that any of us who hadn't been there could know what psychological trauma they had incurred. The brutality of war, killing and maiming, horrible living conditions, dirt, vermin, insects, and smell of death—all inflicted permanent scars on the psyche of the men. Though no two men have the same breaking point, every man can reach a point where the spring gets wound too tightly. If that happens, the spring can break, a condition we called operational fatigue.

We attempted to unwind the spring before it snapped. The family physician in each ward was always available. Patients were encouraged, but not coerced, to discuss their problems—a process we called "ventilation." The more they talked, the more relieved they would feel. The men needed assurance; in talking with their doctors, they could get the feedback necessary to help understand their problems. The doctors attempted to assure their patients that they had nothing to regret or feel sad about.

I remember two of our men. The first was a member of a B-17 bomber crew who had flown several missions over Europe. He was scheduled to fly a mission one day but became ill the night before and was grounded by the flight surgeon. Another man took his place. In the course of the mission, the man who had substituted was struck in the head by a piece of shrapnel and died. Our patient blamed himself. He had terrible nightmares.

The second man, also a gunner, was on a bombing raid over the English Channel when his plane was hit. The crew parachuted safely, but one man was without a life vest. He panicked and started struggling with our patient, pulling him under. Our patient struck the man a blow, and he disappeared under the water and never came up. Our patient had lived a constant nightmare because of guilt connected with the death of his friend. We got amazing results in our efforts at recuperation. Very few required a medical discharge or a longer stay in a veterans' hospital.

One day I received a visit from the provost marshal and an FBI agent. A bank had been robbed in Los Angeles, and the employees and customers had been trussed up and gagged with adhesive tape. The weapons used were Colt .45-calibre revolvers. A few weeks earlier several of that type had been stolen from the firing range at the base. The FBI was trying to tie the stolen revolvers to the bank robbery and also to match the tape used in the robbery to tape from our hospital.

A few weeks later I was again visited by an FBI agent. The agent told me that the FBI had been involved in an investigation of a pornography ring in southern California. The trail had led them to the convalescent hospital. I was shocked. The man who was suspected of being the ringleader was a lieutenant. A fighter pilot, he had returned from combat and had been assigned to head our photography program. He was also the personal pilot for General Easterbrook, the commandant.

I suggested we pay the lieutenant a visit. When we arrived at the photography building, I went in alone. I found the lieutenant giving a lecture in one of the classrooms. I called him into the hall and proceeded to confront him with the charges. His face blanched, and he began to stammer that he was innocent. I asked him to dismiss his class. On my way outside to the agent, I saw a sergeant lighting a fire in a metal wastebasket. Quickly we dumped the basket and extinguished the flames. That was an attempt to destroy evidence.

The lieutenant's car was parked nearby, and we asked for the keys. He complied without protest. The car was searched thoroughly, and a huge pile of pornographic pictures was found. The FBI went through the building with a fine-tooth comb and found other items in a false ceiling. The lieutenant had obtained the models by inviting some of the attractive female clerks from the PX to come to the photography building late at night for a sitting. Of course, the women quickly found out they had been duped. We later learned that we had uncovered one of the largest pornography operations in the country.

The war was rapidly approaching a climax. In May 1945, the Germans surrendered and the war in Europe was over. Although the Japanese continued to fight, there was no doubt about the outcome. The chief concern was that before the Japanese would surrender it would be necessary to occupy their homeland. Such an invasion would result in horrible loss of life for our soldiers. It was then that the world was introduced to nuclear warfare. The dropping of the atomic bomb from the B-29, the *Enola Gay*, on the city of Hiroshima brought the Japanese to their knees.

The surrender of Japan in August ended the war. Our mission at Santa Ana was finished, and the time had come to shut things down. I had enough points to be relieved from duty, but I volunteered to remain to help finish the job, which lasted until the middle of November. Colonel Gilliland wanted me to make a career of the army, but all I wanted to do was to get back home, pick up the pieces, and get into private practice.

My last day on the base was spent wandering around taking a last look. The place was like a ghost city. I went through all the buildings in the hospital complex. There was deathly silence. The furniture and equipment had been moved out and left behind were dust and piles of debris. I stepped into the building that had housed the architecture and home planning units. In the corner was a set of drawings rendering some GI's dream house. In what had been our art section, I found a charcoal painting lying on top of a pile of debris. I studied the painting, trying to analyze what the artist had been trying to communicate. A piece of wheel from an artillery piece was partially turned in an upright position. A single army shoe lay nearby, a large hole in the sole. Further away was a rifle, bayonet in place, stuck in the ground. In the background were trees, their naked limbs starkly outlined against a sky filled with ominous, black, low-lying clouds. There was one break in the clouds where rays of the sun were filtering through.

I decided that the unknown GI artist must have been through some terrible experiences. He had attempted to put his feelings into the painting. The terrible war had been there but now had rolled on. The broken wheel, the shoe, the rifle stuck into the ground, the trees that had been all but destroyed by artillery fire were left, but the black clouds of war were starting to break away and the sunlight of peace was beginning to filter through. The storms of war were over. I picked up the painting and the set of house plans and brought them along with me as souvenirs. Later, I had the painting framed and hung in my den. I still wonder who the artist was and what happened to him.

I had mixed feelings as I checked out of the base and drove through the gate for the last time. I had been there before the base had been completed over three years ago, and now I was one of the last to leave. So much had happened. Thousands of cadets had been processed through here and later had gone into combat. How many of those young men had made the supreme sacrifice? How many had survived but would remain cripples for life? For those unscathed, what would be the impact of the war years on their future life?

The members of the hospital staff had been like a family. Most of them had been there for a long time, and we had become good friends. Now we were scattering to the four winds. Would we ever see each other again? It was doubtful.

Our neighbors on Pearl Street gave us a surprise farewell dinner the night before we started back to Illinois. Such good friends! They had welcomed us to their neighborhood with love. We had so many good times, even though we were at war. When we had block parties, we barricaded the street and set up tables loaded with food, tubs of cold drinks, and watermelons. The street dance would start after the tables were cleared away. Now they were bidding us good-by. Grandpa and Grandma, Little Cap, Terry and his wife, Harriet Kennel and her husband, the master of the ferry we had ridden so many times—all were there. We knew we would never see them again, but we also knew that we would never forget all the love and kindness they had bestowed on us.

15

Starting a Practice

WE LEFT CALIFORNIA almost as we had come, with everything we owned in the old Ford. We had two possessions now that we didn't have when we arrived on Balboa Island—a sweet little daughter, Linda, and Millie's dog Cinderella.

We traveled through Indio and across the desert our first day and spent the night in Arizona. The second day we made it to Albuquerque, the city where we had begun housekeeping. The next night we planned on staying in Oklahoma City, where I had made reservations at the Black Hotel. Everything was going nicely. We had passed by the Sandia Mountains and were rolling along on Route 66. We crossed into Texas heading toward Amarillo. Suddenly, there was a loud noise, and we knew we had blown a tire. I pulled to the side of the road and found a huge hole in the right rear tire. The wind was blowing about forty miles an hour, and as far as we could see in any direction there was nothing but blowing dust and sagebrush. I was really disgusted because I had started with four new tires.

I unloaded everything we had carefully packed into the trunk, starting with the dog in her portable kennel at the rear. Finally, I got down to the jack, tire tool, and spare tire. After the tire was changed and all the luggage and the dog were put back in place, I stuffed the blown tire in the trunk and started on to Amarillo.

I found a tire shop and inquired about getting a new tire. The owner, a typical Texan wearing a cowboy hat, said I would need a ration stamp but would have no trouble getting one at the courthouse since I was in the service. I asked him how long the office would be open. "Oh, they don't close until five o'clock," he drawled. It was about ten minutes until four when we started to the courthouse. As I ran up the stairs to the ration office, the clock struck four; but when I reached the door of the office, it was shut in my face. I was furious. Back to the tire shop we went. To the Texan with the cowboy hat I said, "For your information the ration office closes at 4:00 P.M." He just grinned. I didn't want to spend the night in Amarillo. I wanted to get home, and we had reservations in Oklahoma City. "Tell you what I'll do. I'll sell you a tire that has been rebuilt and I'll make it cheap," said the friendly Texan. So we got the tire that had a huge patch vulcanized into one side, roped it on top of the trunk, and resumed the trip.

It was midnight when we pulled into the old Black Hotel in Oklahoma City. We must have looked a sight. The desk clerk said: "It's a good thing you have a reservation. There is a convention in town, and there isn't a room available anywhere." He furnished a baby bed for Linda, and it wasn't long before we were asleep.

We finally arrived in Marshall, home to stay at last. I hung my uniform in the closet, never to be worn again. The next day I traveled around town visiting my old friends and looking things over. The war hadn't seemed to touch our town except for the faces that were missing, those who had made the ultimate sacrifice in the war and others who had finally passed on because of various infirmities.

We had no definite plans for the future. I had always had the desire to specialize in orthopedic surgery. Millie supported me, and we both thought Indianapolis would be where we would locate. We made several trips to Indianapolis, visiting friends and looking into the residency possibilities.

On one of those visits, I contacted a friend who had been chief resident in surgery when I was at Methodist. He was associated with a group of orthopedic surgeons. After we talked, he took me to see the head of the group, Dr. Mumford, who offered me a position with the group on a salary. One half of my time would be devoted to handling the group's patients; the other half of my time was mine to devote to my own patients. I would receive training in the field of orthopedics from my associates. That didn't sound too bad, but I realized the training I would receive would not be recognized by the specialty board so I declined the offer. Later, I contacted the chief of orthopedic surgery at the Indiana University School of Medicine, Dr. Garceau, whom I had assisted while interning. He invited me to meet him for lunch at St. Vincent's Hospital. He told me that there was a great deal of competition for residencies, but that if I wanted one, I could have it. He said that I could start any time. I also asked about salary. "Seventy dollars a month," was his answer. I told him I would think it over and give him an answer shortly.

Although we had tried to save during my army career, we didn't have a lot. We had bought war bonds every month and had a small savings account. Our total resources were about two thousand dollars. There was no way we could live for three years on what we had. The only alternative would be for Millie to go back to nursing, but we had Linda. She needed her mother. We finally gave up our dream of my becoming a specialist.

Mom hadn't taken part in any of our deliberations, but we knew that down deep she was hoping I would locate in Marshall and pick up where Dad had left off. That was the last thing in the world I had in mind. I knew that Millie was disappointed, but she never raised her voice in opposition. The decision was made that we would live in Marshall and I would be a country doctor.

I was licensed in Indiana, not Illinois. I found that even though there was reciprocity between the two states, Illinois required that I take a practical examination in radiology, laboratory, ear, nose, and throat, medicine, and surgery before I could be licensed. The next exam was not to be given until February. I made my application and was instructed to report to Cook County Hospital in Chicago to take the examination. I hadn't treated a patient for nearly three years. I had been involved in administration totally, and my only contact with patients was seeing them as I passed through the wards on inspection.

I thought myself probably the worst-prepared doctor to enter the private practice of medicine. I learned of a monthlong refresher course at Indiana University School of Medicine. I enrolled and was given a fast review of obstetrics, medicine, surgery, and pediatrics. Most of my time was spent in walking around with the staff and observing their methods of diagnosis and treatment. I also spent considerable time at Paris Hospital reviewing X-rays. One of the doctors there lent me a large number of pathological slides, and I spent hours reviewing them under Dad's microscope.

The day before the exam Millie began having abdominal cramping and vaginal bleeding. We knew that she was pregnant, but she hadn't had an examination yet. I had to make a decision. I didn't want to leave and have something happen to her. Yet, if I missed the exam, it would be another three months before it would be given again. Millie insisted that I go, so I got her to a specialist who examined her and assured me he would take good care of her.

I took the train to Chicago and spent the night with Millie's sister and her husband. I was to report to Cook County Hospital at 8:00 A.M. When I arrived, I was told the exam wouldn't be given until 1:00 P.M. There was a fairly large group to take the exam, and we were all furious. There was nothing to do but wait. We spent most of our time drinking coffee in a restaurant across from the hospital. The exam wasn't particularly difficult, but you never know how you have done until you get the grades.

I took the night train home and found that Millie was still having trouble, but her condition hadn't worsened. She was admitted to the hospital and was found to have had an incomplete miscarriage. After the D&C she made a speedy recovery. It would be six to eight weeks before I heard my examination results.

Dad's old office was located on the west side of the Courthouse Square. My uncle had continued to practice there for awhile but eventually had moved to a new location. Mom had rented the building to the Department of Welfare, but it was now vacant. There was a total of ten rooms, plus an apartment on the second floor. Mom had stored all the equipment from the office in the apartment. The office had to be cleaned thoroughly, and all the equipment had to be brought down and reassembled. I couldn't afford to pay for any help (I had only $1.31 in the bank), but my friend Gene Spotts volunteered to help. We worked for days sweeping, mopping, carrying out debris, washing windows, and reinstalling equipment.

There were three other doctors in town, including my uncle and old Dr. Weir. Dr. Illyes, the youngest of the three, was very busy. People began calling the house asking me to see them, but I had to tell them I couldn't because I didn't have my license yet.

Dr. Highsmith from the neighboring town of West Union was a member of the State Medical Examining Board. One night he called to tell me I had passed the exam, but I still couldn't practice medicine until I received my certificate.

Millie and I discussed how we were going to run the practice. Neither of us had any experience in the business world, so we had to devise our own system. Millie would function both as a nurse and bookkeeper and as my chief advisor. We had inserted a small notice in the local paper announcing the opening of our practice. When we went to the office the first day, Millie was all decked out in her white uniform and nurse's cap. I carried my new doctor's bag. We parked in front, unlocked the door, and went inside. We sat all morning with no patients, not even a phone call. At last, the door opened and a distinguished looking man came in. Millie, with a big smile, asked what she could do for him. Speaking slowly and using very proper English, he said, "I desire to consult with the doctor." OUR FIRST PATIENT! I knew the man. He had formerly been a neighbor. I also knew he was an executive of a large corporation and was quite particular. I used my best bedside manner and gave him a good examination.

He had a simple case of gastroenteritis. I wondered after he left if I had made the correct diagnosis and if my treatment was correct. The next day I received a call from him telling me he had recovered. What a relief! My fee for the visit was $1.50. As days went on, Millie and I began to get discouraged. Few patients darkened our door.

ONE MORNING I received a frantic call from a man telling me he had an emergency. His daughter had swallowed a bobby pin. She was in no pain, but he wanted something done immediately. I met him at the office and took an X-ray. Sure enough, there it was lying in the stomach. "What are you going to do?" asked the anxious father. "Nothing," I answered. "It will eventually pass. Just feed her a soft diet, and if she does have any severe pain, let me know immediately." The following day I received another call. "It hasn't passed yet. I want another X-ray." There was the bobby pin, but now it had moved to the small bowel. That went on for several days, and I began to wonder if the damned thing would ever come through. Finally, I received a call from the jubilant father. "It passed, it passed!" He had the bobby pin, and I had what was probably the most complete set of X-rays ever taken recording the journey of a bobby pin through the gastrointestinal tract.

DR. WEIR asked me if I would do a delivery for him. He was approaching eighty years of age and felt he was getting too old to deliver babies. Besides, I suspect he thought that by giving me the job it would help me get started. Dr. Weir was a true horse-and-buggy doctor. He was serious and dignified.

He asked me to come to his office at 10:00 A.M. on Sunday so that I could examine the patient with him. I arrived promptly. He introduced me to the patient, and we proceeded with the examination. She was almost at term. This was her first baby, and it was to be a home delivery. She lived in the south part of town, about seven or eight blocks from where we were living with my mother.

It was only a few days later when she went into labor. The husband came to our house to get me. They had no telephone. Millie and I packed a large suitcase with sterile supplies and instruments for deliveries, the same kind of bag I had used as a student in Washington. I also had a small portable surgical operating lamp, which I thought would come in handy. We picked up the bag, operating light, and rushed to the patient's home.

After I examined the patient, I told the family I thought it would be some time before she delivered. I instructed them on the signs to look for as the time of delivery approached and at that time they were to notify me.

Millie and I went back home and stretched out on the couch with our clothes on, thinking we could catch a few winks. We had just dozed off when a banging at the front door awoke us. The time had come. When we got back to the patient's house, we discovered the baby already had arrived. It had delivered breech—rear end first. Mother and baby were doing well, but the mother had sustained a laceration. I delivered the afterbirth, tied and cut the cord, and repaired the laceration. There were no postpartum complications. My fee was twenty-five dollars, which, incidentally, I don't believe I ever collected.

ONE SUNDAY AFTERNOON IN August, as we were sitting on Mom's front porch, one of the local undertakers drove up in his ambulance. He said he had someone in the ambulance who was quite sick. Could I come to the office?

When I arrived, the ambulance was parked in the alley by the side entrance to the office. The ambulance attendants carried the stretcher in, and I observed the patient was sitting up with the sheet draped around him. I thought to myself, I'll bet the patient is sitting on a bedpan. He must have diarrhea, perhaps from food poisoning.

When I pulled back the sheet, I was right. He not only had diarrhea but about then started to vomit. I immediately gave him a hypo of morphine and atropine. In between gags, he told me he had been attending a family reunion at the local fairgrounds and had eaten a lot of potato salad. Potato salad left sitting for any time in hot weather can be extremely dangerous to the gastrointestinal system. In a short time he began to improve, but then others began to arrive, all with the same symptoms. I soon had all the examining tables full and then began laying them out on the floor. Having only one bathroom didn't help matters any. I realized that I needed help and called Millie.

We kept giving hypos and tried to clean up the mess, but the people kept coming. When we finally got everything under control, we had treated about thirty-five people. I didn't know any of the people, but they were most appreciative. After their symptoms were controlled, they wanted to know what my fee was. I had no idea. Finally, I came up with a fee of three dollars for each patient. It was nearly 9:00 P.M. when the last one went on his way.

We were both exhausted. Looking at the mess that had been left behind, soiled linens and floors that were going to require a good mopping, and adding to that the hours we spent treating the patients, we decided that financially we had come out in the hole. We soon found out that most of those people became our patients. Not only that, but they told their friends about us and we added them to our list of patients.

THE WIFE OF ONE of my high school classmates had an uncle living with her. He developed problems breathing, and I was asked to make a house call. After examining the man, I determined he had congestive heart failure. I never really had treated a patient with the condition before. In those days, we had no specific medications for relieving the lung congestion caused by the heart failure. Digitalis, of course, was the drug used to improve the heart condition. Cardiac asthma was the immediate problem.

I knew that morphine oftentimes would relieve the symptoms, but there was some risk involved. His condition was so bad that I decided on morphine along with digitalis. The problem was that I didn't as yet have my narcotics license. I called on Dr. Weir, and he let me have some morphine. The morphine worked and the patient began to breathe easier. He recovered and went on to live many more years.

I WAS SMART ENOUGH to know my limitations and vowed that whenever there was any doubt I would ask for consultation. I was determined to think everything out carefully before making a diagnosis. Furthermore, I would treat a patient as I would want a member of my family or myself to be treated. I felt that I had a good basic knowledge of anatomy, physiology, and neurology and that by using good common sense and through careful examination, I could arrive most of the time at the right diagnosis.

Early in my practice, I had a young lady with a pain in her right side. That was a challenge. What was the history? What symptoms did she have? After getting all the information, I began to review the organs in the region of the pain and then I examined her. After I had put all the information together, I made a diagnosis of a right ovarian cyst. I referred her to a gynecologist, who came up with the same diagnosis. At surgery, the diagnosis was confirmed. I found that although my formal training was minimal, I could learn much by just keeping my head, by observing, and by consulting with others more knowledgeable.

ONE OF THE OTHER DOCTORS was away when one of his patients developed acute congestive heart failure. The family called me, and when I arrived, the patient was almost black and gasping for breath. I had learned since my first case of congestive heart failure that the drug aminophylline, when diluted and given slowly intravenously, often would have a dramatic effect on the patient. I had known the woman since I was a small boy; in fact, the family knew me and perhaps that was not to my advantage. I filled the syringe, placed a tourniquet around the patient's arm, and inserted the needle into the vein. Releasing the tourniquet, I slowly injected the medication. Almost as if by magic, the woman's breathing became normal and the skin became a normal pink color. It was then she was able to talk and she thanked me. I listened to her chest and the lungs were clear and the heart action was normal. What had been a room full of skeptics now was filled with believers. I said a little prayer as I left. What if the results had been different?

The first few months of practice were rough. We both became

disheartened at times and wondered if we had been wise in deciding to go into practice in Marshall. Gradually, the volume of patients increased until we could afford a bookkeeper, thus relieving Millie of the chore. We still weren't rolling in money. I had accumulated the maximum amount of terminal leave (120 days) when I was released from active duty. Because of that I was able to continue receiving my monthly paycheck from the army. That money is what we lived on until the income from my practice began to build.

We had been living with Mom for eight or nine months and, although we had no problems, we decided we needed a home of our own. There was a nice, relatively new, three-bedroom house on North Eighth Street for sale, but we wondered how we could finance it. Mom arranged to purchase the house, and we rented it from her. That was our first real home since Millie and I were married. Millie had the house redecorated before we moved in, but we had little furniture. The living room was bare except for a small set of unfinished bookshelves, which I purchased at a ten-cent store and varnished myself. Sitting on the top shelf was Millie's radio from nurse's training. Our only new purchases were a stove, a refrigerator, and a Duncan Phyfe table that Millie had insisted upon and for which we scraped the bottom of the barrel. But if we wanted to sit down, we sat on the floor. We borrowed a bed and dresser from Mom and a dining room table and chairs, a kitchen table, and a beautiful oriental rug for the dining room floor from Millie's Aunt Nellie and Uncle Ward. The two guest rooms were unfurnished. The big day arrived, and we were finally in our own home.

My practice kept building until I could afford a nurse. Ada Catherine Tucker, a recent graduate from nurse's training, was a good worker and fit right in. Millie now had time to fix up the house and be with Linda. As we had the money, we slowly added things we needed in the house.

We had a great group of neighbors. Most were older people, and it had been some time since a young couple had lived there. Linda became the sweetheart of the neighborhood. They all came to visit or would have her to their houses. Millie spent a lot of time making pretty little dresses for Linda.

With my practice growing, I had less time to spend at home. I'd leave early in the morning, and it often was late at night before I returned. I felt I had two obligations: first, to have an adequate income to support my family; and, second, to give my patients the best care possible. Those two things kept me stimulated. I had office hours starting in the morning and running through until all patients were seen. Eventually, we worked in the office as late as midnight and sometimes later. I assisted on all my surgeries and did deliveries.

A typical day might be surgery or house calls in the early part of the morning, in the office through the rest of the day, and then maybe more house calls or a delivery after leaving the office at night. I tried to take Thursday afternoons out of the office but usually would get caught and stay most of the afternoon. Frequently, I was called out at night to take care of an emergency. Sunday was like every other day, except I had no scheduled office hours, but I was usually in and out of the office several times and I always had the usual house calls. On Thursday and Sunday afternoons I tried to visit the patients I had referred to the hospital. Those were about the only times the family would be together, so I had them ride along. I know they were boring times for the family, but at least I could visit with them without any interruptions as we drove along.

As a result of working straight through the lunch and dinner hour, I didn't get to have meals with my family. In fact, I estimate I ate 95 percent of my meals (late supper) at a local restaurant—not what could be called a wholesome family life. Without Millie's love, dedication, and patience, we never could have succeeded. Our children, now grown with families of their own, have told me many times they never knew me when they were growing up. That is what I missed during those years. It is what I never will have the opportunity to experience. Millie raised our girls by herself and did a beautiful job.

A DOCTOR FROM A neighboring town was away when one of his patients went into labor. I was at a meeting, and Millie called to tell me I was needed. I picked up my OB bag and drove to the address she had given me. The head was showing, so I hurried to get things ready. My instruments weren't sterile so I asked for a pan of hot water and poured some Lysol in the pan. The Lysol splashed back in my face, with some of it hitting my left eye. My eye burned like fury but I didn't have time to do anything about it since the baby was coming. As soon as I had completed the delivery, I washed my eye thoroughly with cold water, but the damage had already been done. I developed a corneal ulcer, which I treated with ophthalmic ointment, and I kept my eye covered with an eye patch. My eye didn't return to normal for six weeks. It was surprising how having only one good eye distorts the depth of perception. It was difficult to put in sutures or deliver a baby with only one eye.

IT WAS New Year's Eve—and Millie and I had planned a rare night out, nothing fancy, just a midnight show in Terre Haute. When we returned about 2:00 A.M., Mom, who had been baby-sitting, told us that I had a patient in labor. This was to be a home delivery northwest of town. It was a cold night, and I wasn't looking forward to the long wait. I drove to the patient's home, a two-room house set back quite a distance from the road. The patient was lying in bed, with a child next to her. The room was rather small and lit by only a single kerosene lamp. Heat came from a woodburning stove. The husband came out from the other room, stayed a short time and went back. I didn't see him again. I managed to examine the patient without waking the sleeping child. It was going to be awhile, so I settled down to wait. The only chair in the room had once been an overstuffed easy chair, but now all that remained was a seat cushion and several wooden slats across the back. The room was cold in spite of the stove. The only fuel was green wood. I wrapped up in my overcoat, put on my gloves and hat, and sat with my feet against the stove. The cold kept me awake. Periodically, I checked the progress of the patient. Finally, about 10:00 A.M. she was ready to deliver. I tucked the mother and new baby in bed with the older sister, washed up, and went home.

We had New Year's dinner with Mom, but I was almost too tired to eat. I lay on the couch after dinner to take a nap. Millie let me sleep about three hours before she awakened me to tell me I had several house calls. When I went out to the car, I saw that there had been a freezing rain. The windshield and windows were covered by a layer of ice. I took a scraper to the windshield and started around the rear of the car when my feet slipped. I came down hard, my left chest hitting the bumper guard with full force. The pain was terrible, and for a minute or so I couldn't breathe. I went back in the house and lay down for a while. I knew I had broken some ribs. After I took some aspirin, the pain eased a little. I finally got up and made my house calls. That night Millie strapped my chest with a roll of three-inch adhesive tape. Two or three weeks later, while awaiting a delivery at the hospital, I had my ribs X-rayed and found I had two fractures.

EARLY ONE MORNING I received a call from a patient several miles south of town. From the information I was given, it was evident the patient was having a miscarriage. I had just gotten my clothes on when I received another call from a patient in town who was having abdominal cramping. I decided to run by and see the patient in town on my way to the country. I found that the lady with the cramps was also pregnant. I couldn't find anything too unusual, so I left instructions and hurried out to the country to take care of the miscarriage. I had breakfast when I returned home and was going to the office to do a circumcision. The nurse was standing at the curb when I pulled up. She told me she had received an urgent call from the husband of the first woman I had seen here in town. I raced to her home and dashed into the house, where I found the patient unconscious and breathing her last. I tried to revive her, but she was gone. I looked around and there was her husband, tears streaming down his face, with his arms around four little boys crying their hearts out. That was the worst experience I ever had. I frankly didn't know what to do. As I drove back home, I tried to second guess. Where did I slip up? What didn't I do that I should have done? I couldn't come up with any answers. I must have looked like a ghost when I walked into the house. I told Millie what had happened and she did her best to console me, but I was crushed. I called the office and canceled the circumcision. Then, for the first and last time, I took a nerve pill and went to bed.

BEFORE DAYLIGHT ONE MORNING I received a call from a woman who said her husband was having severe chest pain. They lived some fifteen miles away on a country road, two or three miles off the main highway. She told me she would have a neighbor waiting at the highway to guide me to their house. I hurriedly got dressed and drove off in the dark. I found my guide, and we hastened to the farmhouse, where I found the patient in extreme pain. There was no question he was having a coronary. He was holding his hands to his chest, his face contorted in pain, and sweating profusely. I immediately gave him a large dose of morphine and proceeded with a quick examination. After I called an ambulance, I asked the wife where she wanted her husband hospitalized. She named a hospital, about fifteen miles away, a small private hospital owned and operated by a doctor. I was not particularly pleased with the wife's selection, but I had no right to argue.

I called the hospital and told them I was sending in a patient with a coronary occlusion. The ambulance arrived, and the patient was placed inside. On my way home, I kept wondering if the patient would die en route to the hospital and if I should have insisted he be sent to a better equipped hospital. A day or so later I received a call from the patient's wife, asking me to pay her husband a visit in the hospital. She was not pleased with the care he was receiving. Her request put me in an awkward position. Not being a member of the staff, I just couldn't barge into a private hospital. I advised her that medical ethics wouldn't permit me to visit her husband unless the doctor invited me. I thought that the problem was resolved, but it wasn't long until I received another call from the lady. She had talked to the doctor, and he told her he would be happy for me to visit the patient and he would cooperate fully. Reluctantly, I agreed to make the visit.

It was on Saturday night after I had finished office hours that I drove to the hospital. When I stepped through the front entrance into the main corridor, I found people sitting on benches in the hallway. I introduced myself to the receptionist and asked to see the doctor. I learned from the man sitting next to me that they were outpatients waiting to see the doctor. After about thirty minutes, I was ushered into the doctor's office. He was cordial and apologized for the delay. He told me the patient was progressing nicely and was happy that I had come to see him. He didn't offer to go with me to see the patient but asked me if I wanted a stethoscope and assured me that I was welcome to examine the patient and to review all the records. When I arrived at the nurse's station, I asked for the chart. Except for the nurse's notes, I could find little else on the chart. Laboratory work consisted of one urinalysis and one blood count. I found the patient in a small room not much larger than a closet. It was obvious he was not doing well. I knew that what advice I might offer the doctor would be ignored. I stopped by and thanked the doctor and left the hospital. I had accomplished nothing that might help the patient's recovery, but maybe I'd made his wife feel a little better. It was about midnight when I started home.

A railroad ran parallel to the highway most of the way home. Just as I was leaving town, the midnight passenger train was pulling in. I knew somewhere along the way I would see the train again. I had to pass by a small town about halfway home. Just before I got there, I heard the train whistling for the main street crossing, and then I heard a squealing as the emergency brakes were applied. I just knew the train had hit something. I went around a curve in the highway and saw the train stopped. At that point it was only about a hundred feet from the highway to the track. I pulled to the side of the road and could see the train crew's lanterns swinging alongside the train. I stepped out of the car and yelled out to the crew. "What's happened?" "We hit a man," was the answer. I ran back to a tavern located on the curve. It was closed, but the proprietor was still there. I identified myself and asked him to let me call an ambulance. I called the local undertaker and notified the county sheriff. I went on over to the railroad track to talk to the crew. The engineer said he was going about sixty miles per hour when, just beyond the crossing, he could see something on the track. He applied the emergency brakes and pulled the whistle cord. Now in the glaring beam of the locomotive headlight, he could see a man lying across the rails, but there was no stopping that train in such a short distance. Finally, about a half mile up the track, the train ground to a halt. The undertaker arrived with his ambulance, and shortly after, the sheriff arrived.

We started at the point where the man was lying and found the remains of a sack of groceries and a bottle of whiskey, unbroken. Proceeding slowly up the track we flashed our lights from side to side. We gathered up pieces of body all the way to the train up the track. We looked under the entire train and found one more piece, an arm wedged under the brake beam of one of the cars. It was nearly five in the morning when I returned home. After the sheriff finished his investigation, it was revealed that the man who was lying on the track had spent the evening at the nearby tavern. After leaving the tavern, he lay down on the track. Whether it was suicide or not was never determined.

WHEN I WENT INTO PRACTICE, I became the fourth Dr. Mitchell in town. There was my Uncle Earl, who was in general practice, and my Uncle C. D. and my cousin Frank, who were dentists. It was confusing to people as to which Dr. Mitchell was the one being discussed, so they solved the problem by referring to us by our first names. To this day, I'm known by everyone as Dr. George—not Dr. Mitchell.

When I opened my office, I became the sixteenth doctor in Clark County, a county with a total population of sixteen thousand. Every town in the county had at least one doctor. Several of the doctors had been in practice many years and were most helpful to a young doctor just getting started. It was the custom for the county medical society to meet once a month in one of the member's offices. The meetings were informal, but the older doctors in particular took them seriously. All items presented were discussed thoroughly.

When addressing one another, they did not say "Charlie," "Frank," or "John." It was "Doctor." The first meeting I attended was in a neighboring town. I was the new kid on the block and kept my mouth shut most of the time, just listening to my peers who had been in the business so many years. The discussion moved from one subject to another until we came to constipation. Our host had a speech impediment. When he got excited, he stammered. He also prefaced most of his remarks with "By God." "B-B-By G-G-God. I have a t-t-treatment that n-n-never fails," he stuttered. "I g-g-gave the p-p-patient a big c-c-coal oil enema." I couldn't hold myself. "Doctor, I have a question." "What's your question, young man?" he said, scowling over the rim of his glasses. "How far do you have to chase the patient to catch him after giving the enema?" I realized that I had violated a cardinal rule. Never poke fun at a colleague.

Later, it was my turn to host the monthly meeting, and we had hardly begun when I received a call from the wife of a farmer living several miles out of town. While the man was lying under a piece of farm equipment making repairs, the heavy machine slipped off the supporting blocks. A piece of sheet metal attached to the equipment caught the farmer across the throat, and he was bleeding profusely. I told my guests I had an emergency, but for them to go on with the meeting.

I arrived to find the man lying in bed and the bleeding had been controlled by pressure. It was a clean laceration extending across the throat and I thought if the patient was to have a thyroidectomy, this was the incision that would be made. I injected a local anesthetic, cleaned the wound and surrounding skin, and repaired the laceration. I applied a dressing and gave the patient an injection of tetanus antitoxin and went back to the meeting. I had to give a report to my colleagues detailing the accident, the injury, and the treatment. When I mentioned the patient's name, an old doctor from the west side of the county said, "That's my patient. I have taken care of that family many years." He then laughed and told me that he knew they had recently moved here. "They are fine people, and I am glad you now have them for patients."

WE HAD NO ANTIBIOTICS when I first started. Although penicillin had been developed, there wasn't enough available for use outside of the armed services. Sulfanilamide, the first antibacterial that we had, was fairly effective against some infections, but its use could cause some rather severe side effects, including kidney damage. The mildest reaction was a rash. The most serious was anaphylactic shock and death. We used a lot of aspirin and cough medicine. Really, we didn't have much in the way of specific medications for any of the diseases. Recovery depended on the patient's own body defenses, good nursing care, and a lot of prayer.

Lobar pneumonia was one of the dreaded diseases. All of the patients wore a pneumonia jacket. The jacket was made of outing flannel and was liberally doped with some kind of liniment that acted as a counterirritant to the skin, making the skin hot. All cases ran a high fever, sometimes for several days, followed by the "crisis." The patient either died or made a dramatic recovery. Those who recovered had a break in the fever, a return to a normal temperature, and heavy perspiration. The convalescence was prolonged, and occasionally an empyema developed.

Empyema is a collection of pus in the pleural cavity, and the pus must be removed if the patient is to recover. Sometimes that could be accomplished by sticking a large needle between the ribs over the site of the abscess and sucking the pus out with a large syringe. If the pus was too thick or the abscess was too large, chest surgery was required. After antibiotics became available, empyema became a rarity.

It seemed as if the seasons of the year could be marked by the epidemics. The only immunizations available were typhoid vaccine, smallpox vaccine, tetanus antitoxin, and diphtheria antitoxin. All contagious diseases—chicken pox, mumps, old-fashioned measles, three-day measles, whooping cough, scarlet fever, and the dreaded poliomyelitis—were quarantined by the board of health. A large red card with the name of the disease imprinted in large letters was fastened to the front of the house to warn all visitors away. The breadwinner of the family, after being examined and found to be free of the disease, moved out for the duration of the quarantine. Groceries and the necessities were left on the steps by the delivery man. For most diseases the quarantine lasted from two to six weeks. Of course, if another member of the family contracted the disease, the quarantine was extended. It could mean that the quarantine might be in effect for weeks. Sulfanilamide was effective against the hemolytic streptococci of scarlet fever but had no effect against viruses or bacilli.

Typhoid is contracted by consuming contaminated food or drink. With improvements in sanitation, the disease had become rare, but upon my return to Marshall I began seeing some cases caused by drinking water from a shallow well located close to an outdoor privy. Typhoid carriers are another source of the disease, but fortunately those are rare. The carrier is not ill, shows no signs of any disease, but can transmit the disease through handling food. The gall bladder of the carrier is loaded with typhoid bacilli. I had several people with typhoid in a nearby town. They all lived in the same area. All possible sources of contamination were checked and found to be negative. In quizzing the victims, I found that they had eaten fairly regularly at a certain restaurant. Stool specimens of the employees were checked, and we finally found the source—the cook. She underwent a cholecystectomy, and the diseased gall bladder was removed. She was a carrier no more.

A TEN-YEAR-OLD girl had a high fever and was coughing almost continuously. Her eyes were red and watery, and I could hear some bronchial rales in both lungs. Her ears were clear, and then I looked at the throat, her tongue, and oral cavity. I saw the clue for which I had been searching. Turning with a smile on my face, I announced to the parents, "She has the measles." "But, Doctor, that can't be," said her father, the skeptic. "She has no rash. All people have a rash when they have the measles." I explained that at the onset there is no rash but there is a clue that makes the diagnosis. I had seen the white spots with a red ring on the mucous membrane between the gums and the side of the mouth. They are called Koplik spots and are only present in measles. I had stuck my neck out, but I knew I was right. I left instructions with the parents on the proper care of the patient and asked for a report the next day. As I got into the car, I felt pretty proud of myself.

The next day they reported that the child's condition hadn't changed much, "and, Doctor, she hasn't broken out yet." "Don't worry, she will." I got the same report the next day and the next. But my confidence had eroded considerably, and I could tell that the parents were anxious. "Please be patient," I told the mother. "I know this is difficult, but I promise you the measles will break out, and when the rash appears, she will feel better almost at once." After giving that speech, I felt like the boy whistling through the cemetery at midnight. The next morning I got an excited call from the mother. "Doctor, the measles have broken out. She's covered and her temperature is almost normal. The coughing has stopped. It's just like you said it would be. You certainly know your business."

I WAS SEEING a considerable number of children with the croup during the winter and spring. The diagnosis wasn't hard to make. They all looked sick, had considerable fever, and a harsh cough that sounded almost like a frog croaking. Some bronchial rales were apparent with the stethoscope. In severe cases the inflammation and swelling in the vocal cords, trachea, and bronchial tubes were so great that the child could hardly breathe. Sometimes it seemed each time the child tried to take in a breath the abdomen would be drawn almost back to the spine. This was becoming an emergency situation. When our Linda was a baby, she had frequent rounds of croup. I was advised by a pediatrician to make a croup tent with a vaporizer pouring steam into the tent. Nobody around Marshall had ever used one. I still had Linda's vaporizer, so I loaned it to the family with the croup case. I showed them how to put a sheet over the head and both sides of the crib. Leaving the down side open for ventilation and then placing the vaporizer on a chair next to the crib, the parent directed the spout under the sheet. The child was lying in a cloud of steam. Almost immediately, the child would begin breathing easier and the coughing would cease. It wasn't long before the local druggist began stocking vaporizers.

I was called to the country to see an elderly woman one night. She had a severe respiratory infection. After I had examined her I thought to myself, "She has the croup." I had thought croup was reserved for youngsters, but this apparently wasn't true. I told her daughter and son-in-law that I would go back to town and get something that would help her. I remembered that I had last loaned my trusty vaporizer to a family in the north part of town and that they hadn't returned it after their child had recovered.

Arriving back down in the country, I sat the woman in a chair in the dining room, filled the vaporizer with water, and placed it on the dining room table. After the steam started rolling out, I threw a sheet over her, making a big croup tent. All the time, the daughter and her husband stood looking at me as if they thought I had lost my mind.

Almost immediately, the patient stopped coughing and started breathing normally. I told the family I wanted the vaporizer running continuously. We got the patient in bed, covered the head of the bed with a sheet, and restarted the vaporizer. When I next checked on the patient, I was treated coolly by the family. The patient was doing well, but when I pulled the sheet from the head of the bed I could see the reason for the cool reception. The steam had removed all the varnish from the headboard.

WITH THE RETURN of the men from the war, I began to see patients who had served in parts of the world where malaria was prevalent. The men had recovered from their original illness but now occasionally suffered chills, high fever, and aching. A round of quinine brought them back to normal. Finally, the malaria burned itself out, and they had no more relapses.

I once heard loud laughter coming from the waiting room and opened the door. There on top of the floor lamp sat a monkey. The creature belonged to one of the patients who had just returned home after serving in the Philippines. He came into my consultation room leading the monkey by a leash. He sat down and wrapped the leash around the leg of the chair. I was taking a history from the patient when suddenly there was a loud scream from the back of the office. Both the patient and I went running to the back hallway. There stood Ada Catherine, the nurse, jumping up and down clutching her upper thigh. Hanging from the bottom of her dress was the leash. The monkey had gotten loose from the chair and slipped to the back hallway and up the leg of the nurse.

We were finally able to get penicillin, but only for the most severe cases. Each dose had to be mixed just before it was given. An injection was administered every three hours around the clock. That meant either the nurse or I had to visit the patient at home or teach a member of the family to give the injections, which is what I eventually did. It was miraculous the way the medication took care of the infection for which we formerly had no specific treatment. Vaccines were developed for the prevention of tetanus, diphtheria, and whooping cough. All babies received those inoculations within a few weeks after birth. We eventually established a regular immunization program in the schools. All the doctors in the county cooperated.

POLIO WAS STILL uncontrolled. The spring and summer months were the polio season. Every patient I saw with symptoms and signs of a respiratory infection was suspect. I was worried that I might miss diagnosing a case of polio. I checked for stiff neck and absences of reflexes in all those patients.

On a Saturday morning in early fall a member of the local football team came in complaining of headache and backache. He had played in a rough game the night before and was pretty well beat-up. I checked his temperature, and he had a fever. I found that he hadn't felt well for a week. Earlier in the week, he had had symptoms of the flu, but the symptoms had cleared up. I discovered that he had a stiff neck and some of his reflexes were absent. I immediately hospitalized him, and a spinal tap confirmed my diagnosis. He recovered without any residual paralysis.

One Saturday night the wife of one of my patients came into the office for some pain pills for her husband. I asked her what the problem was. "He has the backache and just wanted to get some pain pills." She then told me he was waiting for her in their truck in front of the office. "Tell him to come in. I won't give him any medication without checking him out." "I doubt if he will. You know how stubborn he is," she answered. Shortly she returned with her husband, who was upset with both of us. "This is ridiculous, Doc. All I've got is a little backache." I put him on the table and found he had a fever. He not only had a backache, but he also had a stiff neck and the absent reflexes. My diagnosis was confirmed by a spinal tap. He, too, made an uneventful recovery with no paralysis.

Finally, a polio vaccine was developed. Massive polio immunization programs were started and by the next year the incidence of poliomyelitis had dropped to near zero. I haven't seen a case since. Later, vaccines were developed for mumps, measles, and three-day measles. It was wonderful not to have the worry of treating those childhood diseases and their complications.

16

General Practice

MY OBSTETRICAL PRACTICE began to build. Although I had decided that the specialty was not one to which I wanted to devote myself full-time, I did get a feeling of having accomplished something important when I delivered a fine healthy baby without complications. The joy of the parents at the time of delivery was contagious, and I was happy to be able to play a part.

Sharing the experience with the family seemed to bring everyone closer; the bond between doctor and patient grew to mean so much through the years. As the tiny babies grew, they, too, looked to the doctor as a trusted friend. After several years, the walls of my office were covered with school pictures and drawings brought to me by my children. No higher compliment could have been paid me.

One of my early patients was a young woman who had lost her first baby. According to her history, she had toxemia throughout her pregnancy. The pregnancy was interrupted before term by Caesarean section. With her past history, I decided to see her at least weekly throughout her pregnancy. She was placed on a strict salt-free diet, and each week her weight, blood pressure, and urine were checked. Fortunately, she didn't develop toxemia.

I had been taught that once a section, always a section—because of the danger of rupture of the uterus at the site of the scar from the previous section when labor contractions became severe.

My patient had selected the hospital for her delivery, but I could find no surgeon who agreed with me that an elective section should be performed before she went into labor. That put me between a rock and a hard place. Later in my career, I simply would have told the patient I didn't want to endanger her or the baby and instead would have referred her to a surgeon who would perform an elective section at a different hospital.

The problem was resolved quickly one morning when the woman suddenly went into hard labor and was rushed to the hospital. I arrived only a few minutes later. The patient was in the preparation room, and the nurse was in the process of completing the surgical prep when she called me to hurry. The patient was lying on the prep table, her legs apart, and I could see the head beginning to show. I just had time to grab a towel and complete the delivery—a fine redheaded boy. The problem I had been agonizing over had been resolved quickly. Mother and child were fine. No ruptured uterus. I whispered a little prayer. The woman had several more children, but I didn't let myself get boxed in again. She went to a different hospital and had Caesarean sections for the rest of her pregnancies.

The closest hospital to Marshall was nearly twenty miles away, a distance that posed a problem when a patient was ready to deliver. Most women were hospitalized well in advance of time of delivery, but even then it was difficult to predict accurately when delivery would occur. Occasionally, a patient would wait until labor was well advanced before calling. I was on staff of both hospitals in Terre Haute, twenty miles to the east, and Paris Hospital, sixteen miles to the north. On several occasions, I traveled at speeds up to a hundred miles an hour to make it to the hospital in time. I never took chances, but when I had clear pavement ahead, I went at top speed.

I bought a new car and, shortly afterward, made a high-speed trip to the hospital. The following day a state trooper asked me if I would please let him know the next time I traded cars. He had chased me all the way to Terre Haute the night before and couldn't catch me. I didn't even know he was after me.

One afternoon I received a call that my patient was in the delivery room. I was running nearly ninety miles an hour down through a creek bottom. Just beyond was a curve and a hill. As I rounded the curve, about two hundred yards ahead were two trucks coming down the hill side by side. The driver of the truck being passed had his brakes set down hard, smoke coming from the brakes. I had to make a split-second decision. To my right was a narrow shoulder about five feet wide and next to that running upward at a 45-degree angle was a solid embankment. I swerved the car onto the shoulder and literally tightroped my way past the trucks. If my hand had been extended out of the window, I would have lost it. My immediate reaction was not fright. I was furious. I wanted to turn around and chase the truck that was passing and grab the driver, but I had to get on to the hospital. I arrived just in time.

One of our daughters was graduating from high school. I had missed many of the school events she had been involved in over the years, but this was one time I was going to be there, regardless. The whole day had been uneventful, and I was looking forward to being with the family. Late in the afternoon, one of my patients came to the office in labor. After I had examined her, I sent her to the hospital. I knew her previous labors had been rather short, but I thought she wouldn't deliver until later that night.

There was no telephone in the high school gymnasium so I had to arrange for some other means of communication. My car was equipped with two-way radio with the base station at my office. My nurse, Clara Norton, stayed by the phone in the office and kept in touch with the delivery room. I left the gym and checked in by radio every few minutes. I got to stay for the entire program, but when I got to my car and called in, Clara told me she had just received a call and the patient was in the delivery room. My mother took the family home, and I headed for the hospital at high speed.

As I approached Terre Haute, I saw flashing red lights far to the rear. I kept on driving but finally pulled up in front of a drugstore in West Terre Haute. The Indiana state trooper got out of his car and came over. "Do you know how fast you were going?" he asked. "Yes, I do, Officer, but I'm a doctor and I have to get to the hospital. My patient is ready to deliver," I answered. "Let's see your driver's license." I searched in my shirt pocket for the license, but it wasn't there. I had changed shirts before going to the commencement and failed to transfer the driver's license. The only identification I had was a Shrine Club membership card. "OK, Doctor, go on, but some day you're going to kill yourself." I walked into the delivery room to be greeted by the nurse. "Hello, jailbird." "What do you mean?" I asked as I hurriedly delivered the baby. "Oh, the policeman called to check on you. He asked if Dr. Mitchell was expected." The nurse answered, "Yes, he is and if he doesn't get here soon, it will be too late." The local police kidded me the next day. The policeman also had contacted them to see if I really was a doctor from Marshall.

One cold night, as I was leaving the office, a man came in with his wife, who thought she was in labor. I examined her and determined she was in active labor. About that time, I received a call concerning a patient with a possible appendicitis. The patient lived in an apartment across the square from the office. I hurried over to check on him, leaving the woman in labor in my office with her husband. I returned about twenty minutes later in my mother's car, which I was driving while mine was being repaired.

During the short time I was gone, the patient's contractions had become much closer and much harder. Her husband was so agitated that I put her in my car and raced for the hospital. I was driving about ninety miles an hour, my left hand on the wheel with my right arm holding the patient's legs together and telling her to breathe through her mouth. The pains became almost continuous. She had her legs extended out straight, with both feet almost pushing through the floorboards. Next she leaned her upper body over until she was in between me and the seat back, pressing me forward over the steering wheel. About ten miles down the road, just as we drove onto a bridge over a small creek, she screamed, "Doc, it's coming!" I released my grip on her legs and reached down with my right hand, keeping my eyes on the road and trying to get stopped. She was right. I could feel the head starting to come through.

Backhanded, I gently brought the head on out along with the body. The delivery was completed just as I finally stopped on the shoulder along the highway. Looking back, I could see the father jump from his car and, in the headlights from his car, could see him coming up the highway, peeling off his overcoat and jacket. The baby was lying on his wife's lap crying lustily. We wrapped the baby and mother in his coat and went on to the hospital, where I completed the job. There were no lacerations, and the baby didn't even develop the sniffles. The following day, my mother came into the office. "Mom, you'll never guess what happened in your car last night." "You delivered a baby," she said. Having been many years a nurse and the wife of a country doctor, nothing ever surprised her.

IT WAS PAST MIDNIGHT when I received a call to come to the office. When I pulled up, I could see two men sitting in a car. The head of one was completely covered with blood. After cleaning away some of the blood, I found a long, deep laceration of the scalp. In fact, the scalp was laid back about halfway. I knew neither of the men but judged the patient to be past seventy years of age.

Working without a nurse, it took me quite a long time to get the bleeding controlled and the laceration repaired. It was obvious that the man was under the influence. He was feeling no pain, laughing and talking most of the time. He continued to move his head, making me miss my mark. Finally, I yelled that I was going to clobber him if he didn't lie still. That threat got through to him, and he peacefully went to sleep. I wondered how he got into that mess and learned he had been to town on Saturday night and had spent the evening in a local tavern. Driving home, he ran off the road on a long hill and rolled the car over in a deep ditch. No one had seen the accident, and he lay there until he could finally work his way out from under the car. Instead of looking for help, he started walking home, nearly three miles. He slipped into bed quietly, and when his wife awoke, she felt a wet pillow. That was when she called a neighbor, who brought the man back to town. It was difficult to determine the blood loss, although his vital signs were all normal. I sent him back home wearing a huge dressing.

On Monday he returned, and I inspected my handiwork. It looked fine and there was no sign of infection. The patient was now sober and still happy, joking and laughing, particularly when I told him I felt like killing him for being so boisterous the last time I had seen him. He and I became good friends, and I took care of him and his family from then on.

WE HADN'T HAD ANY time off since I had been in practice. I was afraid to leave for fear of missing a call, but we finally decided we needed to get away, if only for overnight. Millie's aunt and uncle lived at Dana across the line in Indiana. We made big plans to spend Saturday night with them. On Friday night I had a home delivery in the country and, as usual, Millie assisted me. The delivery was routine, but we were up most of the night. I worked all day Saturday, finishing up late in the evening. Before we left for our "vacation," I had to make a house call to check in on the delivery of the night before. It was 10:00 P.M. before we got off.

When we arrived at Dana, it was almost midnight. After breakfast the next morning, I began to squirm. I just had to get back before I was missed, so we said our good-bys and we were back home before noon. We later made other trips to Dana to spend the day or occasionally to spend the night. With all of the experience she'd had over the years as a doctor's wife, my mother knew exactly how to handle phone calls. It was a comfort to know she was in charge when we were out of town.

I had been treating a young mother suffering from Addison's disease. At that time, there was no cure. As the disease progressed, the patient became weaker and weaker. Both the patient and her husband knew she couldn't live much longer. They had several small children, and it tore at my heart each time I made a house call. Medicine had nothing to offer the doomed lady, and all I could do was offer feeble words of encouragement. Finally one night I received a call from the husband. As I parked in front of the house in the dark, I could hear the children crying and I knew the end had come. I walked slowly to the porch and on into the house. The father and children were gathered around the bed where the white-faced slip of a woman lay, a look of peace on her face. Those left behind were in tears. I remember I stayed for a long time, sitting on the front porch in a rocking chair, holding the youngest daughter in my lap as I attempted to console her in her sorrow.

I SOON FOUND that no matter how hard I tried to be a good doctor and give the best service, I couldn't satisfy everyone. One young woman was going to have her first baby. My father and her parents had been very good friends, and Dad had brought the woman into the world. I had met the patient's husband only once before the night she delivered. I had no trouble with the delivery and came out to tell the father he had a nice healthy boy. In order to save on expenses for the patients, I usually kept mother and child in the hospital for only two or three days if they had no complications. Because I thought circumcising a day-old baby was a little too soon, I did most of the circumcisions in the office a week or so later. That also saved money for the patient.

I had signed the order for release from the hospital when I received a visit from the husband, who told me he wanted to have a talk. I took him into an empty examining room and shut the door. He began raking me over the coals because I hadn't circumcised the baby. I tried to explain but couldn't get through to him. Finally, I said, "All right, I'll cancel the discharge order. We'll go to the hospital and circumcise the baby and keep your wife another day." I was furious, but I kept my temper. Then he started in again. "I don't like you, and I've been wanting to tell you that." "What have I done to make you not like me?" I asked. "Nothing," was the reply. "I don't like you because you were a doctor in the army during the war and I hate army doctors." That lit my fuse. I couldn't stand to be nice any longer. "You mean if I had dodged going into the service of my country, you would think I was a great doctor and a great person?" "Yes," was his answer. He never knew how close he came to getting punched. He went on to tell me his wife had a right to choose her own doctor and he wouldn't interfere, but as for himself, he would never let me treat him. I replied, "You couldn't be a patient of mine for any amount of money. I wouldn't touch you unless you were dying and I was the only doctor around." With that he stomped out. From then on, I avoided him. Neither his wife nor I ever mentioned the encounter.

A year or so later, there was an explosion early in the morning at the local refinery. An ambulance pulled up in front of my house, and the driver came to the door to tell me that he had a patient for me. I asked him why he didn't take the patient to the company doctor. "He made a specific request to be brought to you," the driver replied. I walked to the ambulance and looked in. There lying on the ambulance cart with a broken leg was the man who swore he would never let me treat him. We became good friends, and he never had another doctor but me from then on.

I received an emergency call that there had been a serious accident on a farm several miles in the country. When I arrived, it was almost dark and I was directed down a lane back to a field. It was early spring and the dirt surface of the lane was quite soft. As I approached the end of the lane, through the dim light, I could see a farm tractor turned upside down. I grabbed my bag and hurried toward the tractor. A man ran to meet me. He was almost hysterical. "It's my wife!" he was screaming. I was horrified to see the crushed body of the victim. She had died instantly. The tractor she was driving had flipped over backward while she was attempting to dislodge a plow that was stuck in the mud. She was the woman whose husband had berated me because I hadn't circumcised their son in the hospital.

WHEN I FIRST went into practice, I discovered that the telephone service left much to be desired. The telephone office was on the second floor of a building on the east side of the square, the same location since I had been a small boy. Each call had to be placed through the local operator, a time-consuming process. The phone was an old pedestal type. Later a dial system was installed, but all long-distance calls were operator-assisted.

Rural phone customers, and many of those in town, were still on a party line. In some cases, as many as six customers were on one line. It was very frustrating to try to call a patient, only to get the busy signal because someone else was on the line. There was no such thing as privacy. All a neighbor had to do to eavesdrop was to pick up the phone and listen. In the country, some people lived as much as a mile from their nearest neighbor. The elderly especially were at risk if the phone didn't work. It wasn't unusual for a phone to be out of service for several days. A fire or medical emergency couldn't be reported if there was no phone.

I was called out several miles in the country on another tractor accident. An elderly man was plowing on a slope, and as he made a turn, the tractor rolled over, partially pinning him underneath. When I arrived, the neighbors already had lifted the tractor up far enough to get him loose and had carried him to the house. It was difficult to determine the full extent of his injuries, but I knew he had a fractured femur and possibly a fractured pelvis. Despite his age, he was in pretty good shape, and his vital signs were good. I had to call for an ambulance and also wanted to call to alert the hospital that the patient would be arriving before long. The phone system was one that hadn't been improved on since its inception. There were several customers on each party line.

I took the receiver off the hook and listened. Not hearing anyone talking, I gave the crank several vigorous turns. The switchboard for the telephone system was manned by an elderly man, Sylvester, and his wife. When he answered, I told him I needed to make a long distance call. He could tell where I was calling from by looking at the switchboard. He knew by my voice I was not a member of the family, so I gave him my name.

"What's the matter, Doc?" "I need an ambulance." "Well, who is sick?" "It's Bruce," I answered. "Is it bad?" "Yes, he was pinned under a tractor," I answered. With that he plugged into the switchboard and yelled, "Everybody off the line, everybody off the line! I've got an emergency." Then someone came on the line and asked, "What's the trouble?" "It's Bruce. He got pinned by his tractor." Finally, after the news broadcast was finished, the call went through, and an ambulance was dispatched and the hospital notified.

I complained many times, and I finally called my attorney, who arranged a meeting with the district manager of the phone company. I received a promise that he would see that the service was improved. Service did improve for a while but then began to deteriorate.

Telephones became an obsession with me. I hated them. If it rained, the wires got wet and shorted out. Lightning knocked out the lines, and the transmission wires were downed by wind, snow, and ice. I finally decided the only solution to the problem was to write directly to the president of the entire phone system. I poured out all my troubles in that letter, insisting that something had to be done.

It wasn't long until I heard from him. He was sending one of his top executives to investigate. I arranged a meeting at my office. I had asked several people from Marshall and the surrounding community to attend. The man from the phone company was very diplomatic. He sat quietly, holding a clipboard, and listened as we made our complaints for nearly two hours. He recorded all of our comments, and then he said: "You people really do have problems with your telephone service. These are all legitimate complaints, and the company is going to have to correct these things or they will be in trouble with the commerce commission. I have just taken over this position with the company; as an ex-Marine, I mean to see that we get action and that your service is improved."

Within a few days, a number of trucks from the telephone company were seen around town. Linemen were busy climbing poles and working on the lines. A friend who was having coffee in a local restaurant overheard a conversation at a nearby table, where a group of telephone employees were eating. "We wouldn't be here having to do all this work if it wasn't for some doctor by the name of Mitchell." I received a number of telephone calls from that ex-Marine telephone executive over the next several weeks. He was asking if the telephone service was improving. It wasn't long before the telephones lines were rebuilt, party lines were eliminated, and the service was excellent most of the time.

TWO ELDERLY WOMEN entered my consultation room together to discuss their medical problems. I had a job to finish up in the next room so I excused myself. After I left the room, they began a discussion of their successes and failures in raising flowers. I was halfway listening to their conversation when one woman said, "I'm having trouble with my everyday bloomers. They keep falling." I just couldn't resist. I stuck my head through the open door and asked, "Why don't you put some new elastic in them?" Neither one of the women laughed. The only response I received was a cold stare.

I enjoyed my patients most of the time. I got to know them well and also got to know the other members of the families I treated. These people were all good, honest, and hard-working. They sized you up quickly, and if you met their standards, they not only accepted you as a doctor but also as a friend.

Trust in the doctor was essential in treating the patient, I felt. These people also appreciated what was done for them, even though sometimes the outcome was unfavorable. Many times it has been said to me, "Doc, you did all you could. Nobody could have done more and we appreciate it." These words helped to ease the pain I felt because I had failed to keep a patient alive. We have always received many cards at Christmas and even for my birthday. Gifts of cookies, homemade sweet rolls, candy, apples from a patient's orchard, or fresh butchered meat have been brought to the office many times over the years.

DR. HIGHSMITH, my West Union friend, had instructed all his patients to call me if he was not available. Usually, he would let me know if he was going to be out of town for more than a day. It was in late fall and the nights were quite nippy. I was called to see one of the Doc's patients.

He had told me previously about an elderly man who was not expected to live. Millie decided to ride along with me, and when we arrived, I told her I shouldn't be long. She bundled up in her coat, and I went in to see the patient. It was a large Victorian house occupied only by an elderly couple. A nurse met me at the door and took me upstairs to the bedroom, where the man lay in a huge antique bed. The color of his face blended in with the white sheets. He was unconscious, and there was no question after I examined him that he was dying. Occasionally, using a large asepto syringe, the nurse sucked the mucus from the patient's throat. It was obvious to me there was nothing I could do. I sat down and talked to his wife as gently as I could and tried to explain what was going on. I attempted to prepare her to accept the inevitable. It was quite evident she didn't believe everything I had told her. I just wasn't old "Doc."

Nearly two hours passed. I was thinking of Millie sitting in that cold car. I wanted to bring her in but was too timid to ask. I kept walking in to check the patient, wondering to myself, "How long can this go on?" Finally, about five in the morning, the nurse called to me. I walked into the room as the man took his last gasp.

I pronounced him dead, consoled his wife, thanked the nurse, and started out. I turned to the nurse and said, "My wife may be frozen by this time. She has been sitting in the car all night." Both the woman and the nurse exclaimed, "Why in the world didn't you bring her in here where it's warm?" "I don't know," was my answer. When I got to the car, Millie was rolled up in her coat lying in the seat, shivering. I apologized all the way home, but she was sweet about the whole thing. I already knew I had a wonderful wife, but now I knew I had the best wife in the world.

EARLY ONE Sunday morning I received an urgent call to come to a farm north of town. An old man had a severe nosebleed. I knew the patient was very frail and couldn't stand to lose very much blood. I was just going out the door when the phone rang again. It was the husband of an OB patient who lived in the country south of town, telling me his wife was in labor. "How long has she been in labor?" "She just started, Doc," was the answer. I told the husband I couldn't come then because I had an emergency that I had to take care of. "Take her on in to the hospital, and I'll meet her there later." The husband in a slow drawl said, "Won't be able to, Doc. She's going fast." I could visualize the man standing at the crank telephone hanging on the wall. He continued slowly, giving me a play-by-play account.

"It's comin, it's comin. It's here." I could hear the baby cry. "I'll get another doctor for you. Who do you want?" "Doc Highsmith," was his reply. I knew the doctor was out of town so I told him I'd have to get someone else.

As I hung up the phone, I thought of old Dr. Weir. I hurriedly called him and asked him if he would take care of the case for me. "I would be delighted," was his answer. I drove as fast as I could, worrying all the way that I had been delayed too long and the man was already dead. I ran into the house and found him lying in a pool of blood and in shock. I had the family call an ambulance. By the time the ambulance arrived, the bleeding had stopped. I could hardly get any blood pressure, and his pulse was racing. He was sweating profusely, he was cold, and he had lost consciousness. It was nearly fifteen miles to the hospital, and I was sure we wouldn't make it in time. I followed the racing ambulance, and to my surprise and relief he was still alive, but just barely.

We started a blood transfusion as soon as he arrived and, after several pints of blood, he began to perk up. The color came back to his cheeks, his blood pressure rose to normal, and he was out of shock and talking. He lived several years after that incident and never had another nosebleed.

I called Dr. Weir later that day to thank him. "Doctor, it was my pleasure," was the old doctor's reply. "Mother and baby are doing well and, you know, it's such a nice feeling to know you still can be of service."

I CONTINUED TO GAIN confidence in my ability to diagnose and treat, but I never ceased to learn over the years, not only from reading but from my colleagues with many more years of experience. It gave me a good feeling to know that if I needed advice I could call on these men anytime and they would be happy to oblige. I discovered, too, that what I learned from the textbook was not necessarily the way it was in actual practice. I picked up a lot of clues on my own just by observing—things that would help me in making a correct diagnosis. When I saw these same things again, I would remember that I had seen them before in some other patient, and that would help make a quicker diagnosis.

One day at the hospital I was going to assist in surgery on one of my patients. The surgeon had to see a little fellow on the children's ward who had been referred by one of the pediatricians with a diagnosis of appendicitis. The pediatrician had an excellent reputation and had helped me many times when I had a problem case. The surgeon asked me to go with him to see the patient. I stood at the foot of the bed while he was conducting his examination. The boy was lying on his back and the surgeon was gently pressing on his abdomen. Just a slight touch of the surgeon's fingers caused the child to flinch and cry out. His abdomen was extremely tender. As I watched, I noted the way he was breathing. The light coming through the window shone across his chest, and I noticed there was a difference in the chest expansion between the two sides. One side lagged behind the other. I had noticed that before in a case of pneumonia. "Doctor, have you checked the chest?" I asked the surgeon. "Yes, I have, but the breathing sounds were normal," was his answer. "Anyhow, I would suggest a chest X-ray before you operate," I said. He wasn't offended but instead immediately ordered the X-ray. A large area of pneumonia was seen on the side where I had observed the lag in expansion of the chest. The surgery on the boy was canceled, and he was treated for pneumonia.

I thought of a boy I had seen in my office with a history of an onset of abdominal pain twenty-four hours before. The pain had gotten worse and was accompanied by repeated vomiting. When I saw him, he was quite ill with a high temperature and an extremely tender belly. The maximum tenderness was right over the appendix, and the abdomen was rigid. The white blood count was quite high, and I was sure he had a ruptured appendix with peritonitis. I noticed, however, that there was a slight difference in expansion between the two sides of his chest. The breathing sounds, though, were normal. Before sending him to the hospital with a diagnosis of a ruptured appendix, I took him across the hall for a chest X-ray. Sure enough, he had a large patch of pneumonia. I gave him a large injection of penicillin and followed with oral penicillin and fluids. I saw him in the office again the next day, and he was improved. A week later, he appeared normal. I repeated the X-ray, and the pneumonia had completely cleared. After a few more days of antibiotics, he was released.

BEFORE BEING IN PRACTICE long, I concluded that many patients had psychological problems along with their physical complaints. In some cases, the psychological problems were entirely the basis of their illnesses. Those things I hadn't learned in school. I had no formal training in psychiatry but found that by simply sitting and listening to the patient, I was involved in therapy. A lot of people can benefit simply by the doctor's lending a sympathetic ear.

One elderly man made frequent trips to my office complaining of backache. Although he had arthritis, I was convinced he was not suffering any more than many others who had the same complaint and controlled the discomfort by taking aspirin. Although he complained constantly, his affliction didn't interfere with his caring for the livestock he had or with his job as a highway maintenance worker. I was just leaving the office to go to supper when he walked in all bent over. I thought, here comes "old backache" again. I was a bit upset because I could see I wasn't going to get any supper.

"Well, Charley, you got the backache again?" I asked with a hint of sarcasm in my voice. "This time I got hit across the back." "Tell me about it, Charley." "Well, I was working on the highway east of town on the bridge at Big Creek. We had a flagman up the hill around the curve to slow down traffic and send the cars over into the left lane. I was standing in the back of the truck and had started to swing a ladder around to set it off the truck, when a big bus came roaring down the hill past the flagman and hit the end of the ladder. The ladder hit me in the back and knocked me clear over the cab, and I landed in the creek." "When did this happen, Charley?" "Oh, about two this afternoon." "Where in the devil have you been?" "Well, Doc, this shook me up good so I went home, and when I went out to feed the stock, I had to make water. When my water came out, it was pure blood." I immediately began an examination. The man was very tender over the right kidney, and a urinalysis verified what he had told me. The urine was nothing but blood. "I've got to get you into a hospital right now." "Can't you give me some pills and let me go home to rest?" "No, your kidney has been badly damaged. If you lose it, you'll only have one left." "Doc, I've got only one kidney. They had to take the other one out years ago." I called the ambulance, and within minutes he was on his way.

I referred him to a urologist who, after performing X-rays, determined that the remaining kidney had been split in two and was just barely being held together by the capsule. The patient's temperature went to 105 degrees right after admission to the hospital, and he remained in critical condition for several days. The urologist considered an attempt to repair the kidney but was afraid the trauma from the surgery might worsen the situation and cause more bleeding that he wouldn't be able to control. His decision to leave well enough alone was wise because, after several weeks, the kidney healed and the patient's kidney function was back to normal.

A NEW PATIENT, Mrs. Kemper, was going to have a baby and wanted me to be her doctor. I did not know her but discovered that her mother was a patient of mine. In taking her history, I learned that she lived in Union Center. I had never heard of Union Center but found it to be a wide place in the road about twenty-eight miles west of Marshall. I told her I didn't do home deliveries anymore. I also told her that if she wanted me to be her doctor she was going to have her baby in the hospital. She agreed to move in with her mother in Marshall for the last month of her pregnancy. She had an uneventful prenatal course, coming regularly on schedule for her examinations.

The night was very cold, and I was snuggled deeply under the blankets, enjoying a good night's rest when the phone rang. A voice on the other end said, "I'm calling for Mrs. Kemper. She's having labor pains. We'd like you to come check her first." "All right. I'll be there shortly. What's the address?" There was a bit of hesitation, and the voice on the other end said, rather apologetically, "She's at her home at Union Center." I was thinking real fast, "What a mess. It's too far to race the stork and I'd probably get lost on the way."

Then I had a brilliant idea. "I'll tell you what I'll do. I'm going to call Dr. Johnson in Casey, which is not too far from where you are, and ask him to take care of the delivery." After I hung up, I had a guilty feeling, but not too guilty. I gave Dr. Johnson a call, and after several rings a sleepy voice answered. "Hello, Howard. This is George. How are you? Say, Howard, could you do a favor for me? I have a patient at Union Center. Incidentally, where the hell is Union Center?" Then I proceeded to give him the details. Good old Howard said he would be glad to do this for me. "I owe you one, Howard. Thanks a lot." I thought, "This is going to work out after all," as I rolled over, pulled the blankets under my chin and settled down to continue my snooze.

The phone began ringing again. When I answered, it was Howard on the other end. "George, I checked your patient, and I'm back home now.

She's doing okay, but she's moving pretty fast. I think you can make it in time if you hurry." He gave me the directions to Union Center and hung up. I had been boomeranged! I hurriedly dressed and finally got the car started. I drove as fast as I could and finally found the village of Union Center—only three or four houses and a general store.

It wasn't daylight yet, and there was only a kerosene lamp to furnish light. The light was almost too dim to see the patient. She was ready to deliver. I gave my flashlight to her husband and told him to hold it steady. The head began to show, and I carefully brought it through and completed the delivery. It was so cold in the house that steam came off the wet infant. I began to lecture the mother. "Why didn't you do what I told you to do? You were to live with your mother in Marshall during the last month of your pregnancy." She grinned at me as she answered, "Well, you know I didn't want to go to the hospital. I wanted my baby born at home. I guess I just told you a fib." (Recently, while on a Sunday drive through the country, I revisited Union Center—the first time since that cold night nearly forty years ago. The house was abandoned and surrounded by tall weeds and brush. I sat for a moment and relived that event of many years ago.)

ONE WINTER STANDS OUT in my mind during the early years of my practice because all the roads became nearly impassable. When one of my patients died, the undertaker couldn't get his hearse through so the body was brought out in a farm wagon pulled by a team of horses. My car was stuck many times. I got through deep mudholes by what I called "bulldozing"—lining up the car with the mudhole, then accelerating and hitting the mud full force so I could skid on through. Although the maneuver usually worked, sometimes the car would be shoved sideways in the process.

One of our prominent citizens asked if I would make a house call to his mother, who lived far in the country and was near death. The family was opposed to hospitalizing her, and they didn't expect any miracles. The man offered to accompany me. We started about noon, and as soon as we left the city limits, we hit bad roads. I told my companion that I would be "bulldozing" most of the way. I hit my first mudhole head-on at high speed, and the car bounced and swerved and almost went sideways into a field but finally straightened out. It was comical to see my passenger with the butt of a cigar clamped between his teeth, trying to hang in the seat and keep his hat on at the same time. He wasn't easily excited, but after we had gone through several good-sized mudholes, he looked over at me and asked, "Don't you think we are going to end upside down in the ditch if we don't turn around and get out of here?" I just laughed and told him that it wasn't bad compared to some of the roads I had traveled.

After two hours, we had gone only about seven miles. We finally arrived, where we were met with the supreme challenge. His brother's house was at the top of a steep hill. I didn't know if we could make it to the top, but there at the bottom of the hill was a big farm tractor with the hired hand sitting in the seat. He had been waiting for us. As soon as we stopped, he backed the tractor around and hooked a cable to the front axle of my car. Then he slowly pulled us up the hill to the house.

I examined the women and found that she had a severe heart problem. I knew the end was near and told the family so. They were quite satisfied and thanked me for making the trip. We made the trip back, finally arriving about 6:00 P.M. It had taken us six hours to travel about thirty miles round-trip. He asked me what my bill was. I hadn't even thought about what my fee should be. My only concern had been getting back without getting hung up in the boondocks. "Oh, I don't really know what I should charge. Would thirty-five dollars be all right?" He pulled out his billfold, which was stuffed with money. I noticed the next day the car didn't drive properly. It seemed to lean to one side. I took it to the garage and the mechanic found I had some broken springs. The repair bill came to fifty dollars.

I WAS CALLED to see a patient who lived not far from the river some seven or eight miles from town. I found that she was pregnant and was losing blood. I urged her to go to the hospital because I knew that mild bleeding could rapidly become a severe hemorrhage. I tried to convince her husband that it was important that she be in the hospital where she could be observed and any emergency could be dealt with promptly. Both his mother and her mother were there, and they assured me they would take good care of her and would call me immediately if there was any change. Reluctantly, I drove back home, but I was worried and upset because I couldn't convince the family of the danger that was involved.

I had just gotten into bed when the phone rang. When I answered, all I could hear was a humming on the line. After hanging up, I got to thinking I'll bet that girl is bleeding and they can't get through to me on the phone. I gave the operator a call and asked her who might have tried to call me. "I don't know who it was, but it was somewhere on the 620." "Where does the 620 line run?" I asked. "Oh, it goes down southeast of town quite a ways." "Thanks. I'm sure I know who it was."

I jumped into my clothes and went bouncing down the country roads. When I arrived at the patient's house, I saw all the lights on. I hurried in and found the patient losing much blood and three frantic people by the side of the bed. I proceeded to give some injections to slow down the bleeding. Soon she was on her way to the hospital. The bleeding had slowed, and she arrived at the hospital in fairly good condition. The miscarriage was taken care of by a gynecologist, and she made an uneventful recovery only to become pregnant again later.

The second pregnancy ended no better than the first. She went near full term and, while she was in labor in the hospital, suddenly had an *abruptio placenta*, which occurs when the placenta suddenly tears completely loose from the inside of the uterus. That causes massive intrauterine bleeding, and the patient immediately goes into shock. The only way the bleeding can be controlled is by removing the uterus quickly. We started transfusing her immediately and then went on to surgery, where a complete hysterectomy was performed. As soon as the uterine arteries were clamped, the bleeding stopped. Of course, there was no way the baby could be salvaged, since it was dead as soon as the placenta had pulled away from the lining of the uterus.

WE WERE BUSY with patients in the office when I was called to the phone. The voice on the other end said, "Oh, George, this is Nellie. Please come right away. Carl is real badly burned." I yelled for burn dressings, and I checked my bag for supplies. My nurse and I were on our way in less than five minutes. I passed everything on the highway, including another car that was making the same turn off the highway onto a gravel road that I was. At one point I went over a culvert and was airborne for about a hundred feet. We found our patient calmly sitting on the couch with his hands in a pan of water. All of his clothes were burned off, and strips of burned flesh were hanging from his arms. "How's the pain?" I asked. "Well, it does hurt some," was the answer. While I administered morphine, the nurse set up a card table and made dressings with Vaseline and gauze. We quickly covered his entire body with the Vaseline and gauze and added heavy padding. We wrapped gauze bandages around his arms, legs, torso, and head. When we were finished, he looked like a mummy.

I started IV fluids, and by then the ambulance had arrived. I rode to the hospital with the patient, but I doubted very much if he would live more than a few hours. Well over 50 percent of his body was covered with second- and third-degree burns. He had been filling his tractor with gasoline when it exploded and he was showered with flaming gasoline.

During the first twenty-four hours in the hospital, he received thirty units of plasma. He continued to hang on and then gradually began to improve. After about four months, he was able to come home. Considerable skin grafting had been done, but he had horrible scarring, and there were severe contractures of his hands. However, he was still alive.

He had been home two or three weeks when I received an urgent call to come to his house. When I arrived, I found him on the living room floor unconscious and convulsing. I examined him, but when I finished I hadn't the slightest idea why he was having convulsions. I gave him an injection of an anticonvulsant, but it did not phase him. I was trying to think of what I could do next. I was afraid to try to move him to the hospital. In fact, I didn't move him off the living room floor to a bed for fear that he would stop breathing. Soon the priest arrived and administered the last rites. I sat and watched him for what seemed to be an eternity when finally the convulsions stopped. I got some help and moved him into bed. He was breathing normally and had not even a twitch. I walked to the kitchen, where the family had gathered and told them I was worn out and was going home to rest. I had been there almost ten hours. I told them to call if they needed me but that I would be back later. I walked through the living room and peeked in the door of the bedroom. As I stood there, Carl opened his eyes, looked at me, and said, "Well, hello, Doc. What are you doing here?" I didn't feel tired or sleepy anymore. We never did figure out what had caused the convulsions, but he never had any more. Carl lived a number of years and even had a hernia repair. He always had his contractures and his scars but otherwise lived a normal life.

IT WAS A WARM spring evening. The trees were beginning to bud and the frogs could be heard croaking down in the old brick pond near the cemetery. I was called down to the railroad southeast of town. The caller was unable to tell me what had happened. She had just been told to call a doctor. When I got to the railroad crossing, I saw nothing unusual. At a distance I could see the back end of a stopped freight train.

At first I thought the train had stopped for a red block signal, but looking down the track, I could see the green light of the signal. "This is strange," I thought. A green signal means a clear track and the train would not have stopped. The train must have hit something or someone, and it must be at the next crossing a mile on down the track. I turned and drove back to the main highway, drove south a mile, then drove east to the crossing. There was a big steam locomotive with the engineer sitting up in the cab.

The locomotive had been disconnected from the train and brought on to the crossing. I identified myself and asked what the problem was. "We hit a man back there," he said. "How far back?" "Oh, almost to the end of the train." I pulled out my bag and started stumbling along the right-of-way. "Wait a minute," yelled the engineer. "Come up on the engine and I'll back you down as far as I can. It beats walking." I shinnied up the steps with my bag, and the engineer reversed the engine and we went chugging in reverse until we came to the front of the train. About fifty car lengths back, I came to the victim.

The ambulance crew and the rest of the train crew were there. They were discussing how they were going to remove the victim, who was still alive but unconscious. It was evident that he had a severe head injury. The ambulance couldn't be brought any closer than a quarter of a mile, and the thick brush growing along the right-of-way made it impossible to bring in the ambulance cart. I suggested that the crew break the train where the man was lying and pull the long string of cars to a nearby siding, then back the locomotive down to where we were and hook onto the short string of cars in the rear of the train. We would place the ambulance cart on the back platform of the caboose, then pull the caboose up to where the patient lay. That done, the patient was loaded on the cart and placed on the back platform of the caboose. The ambulance attendant stood on the steps, hanging onto the handrail, and I did the same on the other side. We steadied the cart with our bellies. That protection kept the cart from falling off the train as the engineer backed down to the crossing where the ambulance was parked.

As soon as the patient was loaded, I started an IV and rode with the patient to the hospital. We had just gotten him into the operating room when he died. According to the train crew, the man had been lying along the outside rail apparently asleep. It was well known that he liked to tipple and also that he always hunted mushrooms along the railroad tracks in the spring. It was speculated that he had a few drinks, went out to look for mushrooms, got sleepy, lay down along the rail, and dropped off to sleep. The train woke him and, when he sat up, he was hit in the head by the under part of the railroad car.

17

Patients and Patience

I HAD BEEN working seven days a week for well over a year and needed a vacation. Millie needed one worse. We often talked about our days in California and our friends from the service. We had decided to take a three-week vacation. Our plan was to take the train from Terre Haute to Chicago and from there to Seattle. Then we would travel down the coast to Los Angeles, where we would visit about ten days with our good friends, Lois and Kenny Long, Linda's godparents. I got everything worked out in advance, including scheduling and reservations. I had to be sure I had coverage for my practice and was hoping to get all my babies delivered before leaving.

It was only a few days until we were supposed to leave, and I still had one baby due. Early in the morning, I got a call that the last pregnant patient was in labor. I asked her husband to bring her to the office so I could check her before sending her on to the hospital. I hopped out of bed and drove to the office. It was a pleasant summer day, so I sat in my car in front of the office listening to the birds sing and watching the sunrise. I felt great! I was almost ready to go on my dream vacation. Pretty soon I looked at my watch. I had been sitting there for nearly forty-five minutes, and the patient only had a five-mile trip to town. I began to worry. Finally, a half hour later, they pulled up. "Where have you been?" "Well, I had to take a shower before I left home," answered the patient, who by that time was having almost continuous contractions. "Get in my car. We can't waste any more time." Breaking all the speed laws, I just barely made it in time to deliver the baby. When we left a few days later, I felt as if a heavy load had been lifted from my shoulders. I didn't realize I was so tired.

We had a delightful trip, and it was so good to see old friends from our days at Santa Ana. We visited Balboa Island, Newport Beach, and Laguna. In just two short years everything had changed. No more military to be seen. The base was being converted into a junior college, and the real estate boom had just begun. There was traffic everywhere, even on quiet Balboa Island.

IT WAS NEARING the end of office hours on a Saturday night when an ambulance pulled up in front of the office. Lying on the cot was a woman whose face was horribly mutilated. By her side was a small girl about seven years of age who had several deep lacerations on her face. They had been driving in a convertible when they were sideswiped by an oncoming car.

The woman was still alive but was unconscious and in shock. One eye was on her cheek, and the rest of her face was almost pulverized. I covered her face with a dressing and sent the ambulance on to the hospital. I alerted the hospital and the surgeon and then went to the hospital. We had a team of five doctors working on the two patients. The woman's skull was fractured, and spinal fluid was draining from her nose. An internist furnished medical support, taking care of the heart and lung situation. The anesthetist handled the anesthesia. The surgeon and an ear, nose, and throat specialist worked to repair the face. They covered the areas with skin that had been left bare, put the eye back in place, and sutured tissue over the eye to protect it. At that time there were no blood banks so I had the job of drawing blood from donors and transfusing. I also repaired the little girl's lacerations. It was 5:00 A.M. before we finished. A week later the patients had recovered sufficiently to be transferred to Barnes Hospital in St. Louis, where the mother underwent extensive plastic surgery. She made a complete recovery.

The patient was well known in literary circles and wrote extensively for a number of top magazines. Her mother later complained that our bill was too high—one thousand dollars total—for the five doctors who worked all night and continued to care for her until she was transferred a week later. She said that the surgeons at Barnes had fixed up what we hadn't done right; their bill was around eight thousand dollars. All we did was save her life so that the frosting could be applied later.

THE FIRST TIME I SAW Sarah was when her mother brought her in because she wasn't feeling well. She looked pitiful. Her face was pockmarked from acne. She was wearing a heavy scarf around her head and down over her ears. She must have been around twenty years old. When the scarf was removed, I saw a wad of cotton in each ear. She was coughing up large amounts of sputum. The mother told me that Sarah had always been sickly and had been under the care of a specialist for a long time. I talked to the specialist, whom I knew well as an excellent man in his field. He couldn't help me much in deciding what I ought to do that had not already been done. Nevertheless, I began treating her with various antibiotics. Much to my surprise, she began to improve. As I got to know her better, I started kidding her a little. I found out that she had never had a date with a boy. She lived on a farm way off the beaten path, and it was evident that she and her mother lived like people did a hundred years ago. But as her health improved she began to blossom. She dressed in more modern clothes and had a smile and a snappy comeback to my teasing. It was just as if she had emerged from her shell. One day I said, "Sarah, don't you think it's time you found a man and got married?" "Oh, Doc, what are you saying? You know that I've never even had a boyfriend." "Well, I'll tell you what I'll do. You get the man, and I'll give you premarital exams for nothing."

I didn't see Sarah again for several months, until one night I opened the the waiting room door and there she sat with a strange man. They both stood grinning for a minute, and then Sarah said, "I want you to meet John, my fiance. We want our examinations so we can get a marriage license."

A year or so later, Sarah and her husband paid me a visit. "What's the problem?" I asked. "Well, I don't know exactly, but something is not right. I thought I might be going through the change because I quit menstruating." After I completed my examination, I made my announcement. "You are going to have a baby." I thought they were both going to faint. They wouldn't believe it. I gave her strict instruction on diet and exercise and told her she must come for an examination on the schedule I gave her. She was faithful in keeping her appointments, but she still couldn't believe she was pregnant. Knowing well her past history and that she was nearing the end of her childbearing years, I was concerned about her labor and delivery. I had prepared myself for a long, difficult labor and delivery and all the complications that could arise.

It was a raw, cold, damp evening when Sarah and her husband arrived. "I think I've got the flu," said Sarah. "I have cramping in my stomach and I've got diarrhea." I got her up on the table and listened to the fetal heart. It was clicking right along. While I was listening, she had several fairly hard contractions. Then I did a rectal examination, and I was surprised to find the head well down in the birth canal and the cervix already starting to dilate. "Sarah, you are in labor and you must get to the hospital right now." I called the hospital, and they took off. I followed in a few minutes.

When I arrived, she was in bed in the labor room, and the contractions were becoming quite severe. The cervix was almost completely dilated. We soon moved her to the delivery room, and I delivered a beautiful baby girl.

My office began receiving calls from her family when she didn't return home from the visit to the doctor for treatment of the flu. The family couldn't believe it when my nurse told them Sarah was at the hospital having a baby. Sarah had convinced not only herself but all of her family that she wasn't pregnant. There had been no baby showers, and Sarah herself hadn't bought even a diaper to put on the new baby. Sarah's baby grew into a fine young woman, got a good education, and is quite successful in her chosen profession. I still see Sarah and John occasionally. They have had a happy and successful marriage. It makes me feel good to think I might have had a tiny bit to do with it.

ONE QUIET SUNDAY afternoon I received a call from one of my patients, telling me that she was in labor. Her previous pregnancies and deliveries had been free from complications so I didn't anticipate any trouble with the delivery. I sent her to a hospital I had never used before. When I arrived, she was ready to go to the delivery room. Everything was quiet in the obstetrical department. No other patients were in labor. The supervising nurse wheeled the patient into the delivery room and placed her on the table. Only the nurse and I were in the delivery room. The patient was relaxed, and the pains weren't causing her much discomfort. The nurse gave her some ether, and after three or four contractions, she delivered the baby. Then trouble began.

A huge gush of blood came from the vaginal opening, and it didn't stop. I had never seen anything like this before. I didn't know what had happened. I quickly packed the vagina with gauze sponges. I lost count of the number of sponges I poked into the cavity until it was tightly packed. Then I pushed my fist in against the packing to stop the hemorrhage. I had an idea of how the boy with his finger in the hole in the dike must have felt. I told the nurse to start intravenous fluids quickly and to check the patient's vital signs. Fortunately, I had controlled the hemorrhage before the patient had lost enough blood to cause shock. Now that the immediate emergency was under control, I had to figure out what had happened. I finally decided that the head had been forced through a cervix that hadn't completely dilated and the sudden extreme pressure had split the cervix. I wondered how I was going to repair the damage without any help.

I didn't know any of the specialists on the staff of this hospital so I called on the nurse for help. "Dr. Spigler is a good surgeon and he only lives a block away." "Ask him to come over, please." She came back in a minute and said he was home taking a nap but he would come to the hospital immediately. My arm was getting tired, but I continued to keep my fist firmly against the packing. It wasn't long before the tall portly man came into the room. We didn't take time for formal introductions. He put on a gown, laid out his instruments, and asked the nurse to give the patient more ether. When he was ready, he asked me to remove the packing. When the packing was removed, there was hardly a trickle of blood. Luckily, I had made the correct diagnosis, and the emergency measures I had taken prevented much loss of blood. He then quickly sutured the lacerated cervix and the crisis passed.

A WOMAN I HAD KNOWN all my life came in with abdominal pain and vomiting. She had the classic symptoms of acute appendicitis. I quickly had her admitted to the hospital. When we got into the abdomen, we found a large swollen appendix covered with pus. We removed the appendix and then took another look around. When we exposed the right ovary, we found it was actually falling apart. We removed it and when the pathology report was received the next day, the diagnosis was ovarian carcinoma. A few days later we reoperated, removing the uterus, the tubes, and the other ovary. Later she received a course of deep X-ray therapy and made a complete recovery. She never had a recurrence of the cancer—the acute appendicitis had saved her life.

THE PATIENT WAS LYING on a couch, and there was no question she was seriously ill. Her face was flushed with fever, and her abdomen was distended. She was rolling from side to side, moaning. When I touched her belly, she let out a scream and almost rolled off the couch. I found that she had been sick for a week and finally got so bad that she traveled from her country home to her father-in-law's place in town. As soon as he saw her condition, he called me. She was in such poor condition that she couldn't answer my questions. I knew she had peritonitis and didn't waste any time getting her in for surgery. When the surgeon made the incision through the peritoneum into the peritoneal cavity, pus shot nearly three feet in the air. We must have drained nearly a gallon of pus from her abdomen. It was impossible to explore the abdomen because of her poor condition. Drains were inserted, and the abdomen was closed. I didn't think she would live.

That was before the advent of antibiotics so all we could do was give supportive treatment and pray. She gradually began to improve over a period of several weeks, but her weight steadily dropped from 160 pounds to 100 pounds. Then she began to get worse.

We called in more consultants and finally discovered she had developed empyema of the right lung cavity. The infection in the abdomen had spread up over the liver, forming a liver abscess. Then the infection had extended through the right diaphragm and into the lower right chest. More surgery was performed, and the abscesses were drained. In spite of the odds, she slowly improved until she finally went home after nearly four months. Her convalescence was quite prolonged, but she recovered fully and regained her former weight. She never has had a serious medical problem since. We finally decided the culprit was an abscess of the right fallopian tube, which ruptured, causing the general peritonitis.

A CALL CAME from an anxious mother one night, telling me something serious had happened to her son. When I arrived, I found the eighteen-year-old boy lying unconscious on the floor. I quickly examined him and found he had a high fever and a stiff neck. He had been in reasonably good health until that day, when he began complaining of a headache, fever, and chills. He had vomited but had no other evidence of any abdominal problem. Just before I had received the call, he suddenly had lost consciousness and had collapsed on the floor. My preliminary diagnosis was meningitis. I hurriedly had him admitted to the hospital. A spinal tap was immediately performed, and malarial parasites were found in the spinal fluid. The final diagnosis was malarial meningitis, a serious disease with a high mortality rate. He remained unconscious for several days but gradually improved and finally recovered completely. Although we had seen a number of cases of recurrent malaria in military personnel stationed in the tropics, a case of primary malaria hadn't been seen in the area for many years, since the eradication of the *Anopheles* mosquito. The patient hadn't been away from the immediate vicinity of his home, so the source of the infection was a mystery. The public health department conducted an exhaustive investigation of all possible breeding places for the mosquito but didn't find any of the *Anopheles*. No other cases of malaria developed.

I HAD NEVER seen a case of diphtheria but was constantly on the alert for one. Every patient with tonsillitis was suspect and carefully examined for the dirty grayish membrane described in the textbooks. With patients about whom I was uncertain, I gave injections of diphtheria antitoxin, just to play it safe.

One day a woman came in, complaining of a severe sore throat. She had been sick for several days and appeared to be toxic. I looked in her throat, and there was a heavy dirty gray membrane spreading over the tonsils and over the soft palate. There was no question. She had diphtheria. As soon as she was in the hospital, an attempt was made to get some of the membrane stripped from the tonsils. The membrane came away, leaving small bleeding points on the mucous membrane. The specimen was sent to the laboratory and was found to contain large numbers of the diphtheria bacillus. It was the first case of diphtheria diagnosed in Marshall in many years. The pathologist was so taken with his findings that he carried a piece of the membrane around with him in a test tube for a few days to display to other doctors. The patient was observed for several days for signs of the most serious complication of diphtheria, myocarditis. She made an uneventful recovery, and no other cases occurred.

JUST AS I WAS LEAVING the office one evening, a mother came running in dragging her son by his arm. Blood was flowing from his nose in a steady stream. I was a bit irritated because I was afraid I was going to miss the opportunity to have dinner with my family. Without removing my coat or hat, I got the boy, who was quite large for his age, up on the table and started packing his nose with cotton saturated with adrenaline. Suddenly he started struggling. He knocked the packing forceps from my hand, and blood flew in all directions. Most of it hit me in the face and splattered over my coat. I was infuriated, and the next thing I remembered I was sitting astraddle the boy, stuffing packing into his nose. He was so shocked that he lay motionless, his eyes opened wide in amazement. I got the bleeding controlled, and he climbed off the table and meekly left the office. Several weeks later, he was in the office with his mother. She told me that she had to take him to the dentist, who happened to be my cousin, and that she was dreading the visit because he was so unruly. In fact, on some occasions, the father had used his belt on the boy when he was in the dentist's office. I gave the boy a mean look and told him that if he thought I was tough, my cousin was twice as tough, and that if he didn't behave, he would get worse treatment than I had given him when I packed his nose. Later the mother told me how surprised the father had been when his son walked into the dentist's office, hopped into the dentist's chair without protesting, and sat quietly while my cousin worked on his teeth.

I'D HAD A LONG, HARD DAY before I arrived home about midnight. I had just settled into my easy chair with the paper to relax before going to bed, when the phone rang. There had been a truck accident near West Union and I was needed. As I arrived I noticed that there were no wrecked vehicles on the pavement, but then I saw a large tank truck lying in a deep ditch. The wrecker was standing crossways in the road, and an ambulance was parked nearby. The driver was pinned down, with his legs entangled in the levers on the floor and the steering column. There was water in the ditch, and he was cold and wet. By flashlight, I was able to check his vital signs and to examine his legs, abdomen, and chest. I couldn't determine if he had any fractures, but he appeared to be in fairly good condition, except for the effects of exposure.

The tanker was empty, but the use of a cutting torch to free the man was ruled out for fear of causing an explosion. The wrecker was not powerful enough to lift the truck, but a heavy-duty wrecker was on its way from Terre Haute, thirty miles away.

I had given the man a hypodermic as soon as I had completed my examination, and he relaxed after the medication took effect. The rescuers continued to discuss how they were going to extricate the victim, but no one seemed to have a solution. One suggestion was to place cables around the truck and use the heavy-duty wrecker to lift the wrecked truck up so that the victim could be released. The idea was abandoned when it was pointed out that if the cable slipped or broke, the whole thing could come back down, crushing the man. The debate continued.

Suddenly a large man, Harry Baker, arrived on the scene and made his way down the steep side of the embankment to the cab. Taking a flashlight, he surveyed the inside of the cab, the twisted levers, and the bent steering column. After looking things over for a few minutes, he said, "Get me a hack saw." He squeezed his huge frame into the cab and in his cramped position began methodically to saw through the steel rods. Some he sawed all the way through and others he sawed only partially through. With his powerful hands and arms, he bent them away from the driver's body. Finally, he sawed through the steering column, the last restraint. Then he lifted the victim out gently. Others carried the driver up to the highway, where he was placed on the cot and loaded into the ambulance. The big man handed the saw to the driver of the wrecker and left.

I asked one of the ambulance attendants to drive my car back to Marshall, and I rode in the ambulance. On the way, I was able to make a more thorough examination, and I could find no evidence of any serious injuries. However, I admitted the patient to the hospital for further tests. When I arrived home, I had been gone over five hours. The patient was released from the hospital the next day. A few weeks later, I read an account of a break-in at a school south of Terre Haute. One of the thieves was the man who had been rescued from the wrecked tanker.

LATE ONE HOT SUMMER NIGHT I received a call that a small child had been injured. I met the family at the office and found a frightened two-year-old boy bleeding from his mouth. His mother said that he had been eating ice cream, using a small tin spoon. He had the spoon in his mouth when he jumped from the chair, falling on his face. The tin spoon had been driven into his throat. When I examined him, I saw that the spoon had severed the anterior tonsillar pillar at the base of his tongue on the right side. I had no nurse so his mother, who was a large woman, held his head steady on the table. (I had delivered her baby only a few weeks earlier.) His aunt held his feet. She, also, was a large woman, and I was to deliver her baby in a few weeks. I had taped together several tongue blades to make a retractor to hold his mouth open and his tongue down. In spite of being restrained by his mother and his aunt, he continued to squirm. I managed to inject the back of his throat with Novocain. I had just gotten the suture needle through one side of the laceration and was starting to bring the needle through the other side when the lights went out. I was terrified. That was before we had suture needles that were permanently fastened to the suture. I was sure that the suture had slipped out of the eye of the needle and the needle had slipped into his throat. With my left hand, I fumbled around on a nearby table for my flashlight and luckily was able to find it. The aunt held the light, and I saw the needle, fortunately, was still fastened to the suture.

The aunt continued to hold the light steady and I went on with my work, holding the boy's mouth open with the tongue blades with one hand and suturing with the other until the repair was completed. Just as I finished, the lights came back on. We were all covered with sweat, and I was exhausted. The boy made an uneventful recovery.

ABOUT MIDNIGHT, I received a call from a man who lived about seven miles in the country. He said that his wife had died a suicide victim. We were having a violent thunderstorm at the time. I slipped on my raincoat and hat and went out to my car. As I drove down the highway, I could barely see because of the driving rain and the blinding flashes of lightning. The house sat back from the highway and was surrounded by large trees. I drove to the back of the house and made a run for the back door, hoping that lightning wouldn't strike as I ran past all the trees. A transformer had been struck and only the dim light of a candle illuminated the room when I walked inside. A good night for a murder, I thought.

The husband took me into the bedroom. The lifeless body of his wife was lying on the bed. Her white face and staring eyes were illuminated by the light of a candle. On the bedside table was an empty vial that had contained sleeping pills. After completing the routine of listening for a heartbeat, I questioned her husband. He told me that she had been quite depressed and had visited several doctors without telling any one of them she had been to another doctor. Each doctor had prescribed sedatives for her condition; apparently, she had waited until she had an ample supply, then took her life. She had gone to bed early, and he had no idea what was going on until he went to bed and found her. I told him that this was a coroner's case and that I had to notify the coroner as soon as I returned to town. Normally, in such cases, if the doctor uncovered no evidence of foul play, the body could be removed to a funeral home. However, I discovered that the husband wanted her taken to a funeral home in an adjoining county. I told him the body could not be removed until I had permission from the coroner.

Returning to Marshall, I notified the sheriff, who contacted the coroner. The coroner ordered an undertaker to bring the body to Marshall, and a coroner's jury was assembled at the police station. At four o'clock in the morning the sleepy-eyed jurors viewed the body in the hearse and returned to the police station, where they rendered a verdict of death by suicide.

IT WAS A COLD winter day. A freezing rain covered everything, making driving hazardous. I was called to see a sick baby girl whom I had delivered only a month before. She had a high temperature and signs of respiratory infection, but she also had a rigid neck. I was sure I was dealing with meningitis and it was imperative to get her to the hospital at once. The mortality rate among infants with meningitis was high. I drove my car up to the front door of the house and bundled the mother, the baby, and a friend of the mother in the car beside me. It was sixteen miles to the hospital, and the highway was covered with ice. I bent over the wheel and kept my eyes on the road, trying to go as fast as I could without sliding into the ditch or an oncoming car. I didn't look at the speedometer but kept alert for the slightest twitch of the car, which would tell me that we were about to skid. Arriving at the hospital I looked at my watch. It had taken only twenty minutes to make the trip. Later I talked to people who had taken an hour to make the same trip that day. A pediatrician examined the baby and did a spinal tap, confirming my diagnosis. After several days in the hospital, the baby made a complete recovery.

ONE SUNDAY AFTERNOON as I was doing yard work, a woman drove up the driveway. She had a large towel wrapped around one of her thighs. "What's the problem?" I asked. "I was attacked by a hog," was her reply. I followed in my car as she drove to the office. After getting her on the table, I unwrapped the towel. The flesh had been torn from just above the knee nearly halfway up the thigh.

The woman had gone into the pigpen alone to check on a sow and baby pigs. The sow attacked her and had her down in the mud tearing at her leg with its tusks. Her screams were heard by her dog, which came running and drove off the sow. The woman dragged herself from the pen and into the house and, after wrapping the towel around her leg, drove herself into town.

The leg was a mess, with mud and hog manure all through the gaping wound. I worked nearly two hours washing the filth out of the wound, irrigating with copious amounts of sterile water, cutting away damaged tissue, and then repairing the damage. I had given her antitoxin for both tetanus and gas gangrene and put on the dressing. She went out to her car and drove home. No infection developed and she recovered completely.

A WOMAN CAME INTO MY OFFICE holding her screaming young son. Blood was coming from his mouth. He had been riding his tricycle down the sidewalk while holding the handle of a toy hammer in his mouth. The front wheel of the tricycle hit an elevated slab, throwing him over the handle bars. He came down on his face, driving the tip of the hammer handle through the roof of his mouth. Upon examination, I could see the soft palate in the back of the mouth had been split. With my nurse holding his head and his mother at his feet, I managed to anesthetize the injury site and repaired the damage. For a long time afterwards when I had to examine the boy, he refused to open his mouth.

IT WAS A THURSDAY AFTERNOON when I was called to see an elderly woman who lived alone in the south part of town. She was toothless and had been eating meat when a large piece became lodged in her esophagus. She had tried to drink, but the water came right back up. I had never been confronted with that problem before. I helped her into the car and took her to my office. Since it was my afternoon out of the office, my nurse wasn't there to help me. I kept trying to think of a way of dislodging the meat. Then I remembered a large stomach tube that had belonged to my Dad. The plan was to grease the tube and pass it through the mouth and down the esophagus and to poke the meat on down into the stomach.

I explained what I was going to do and asked her to cooperate. With her lying on her back on the table, I started to slip the greased tube through her mouth and into her esophagus. As the tip of the tube hit the back of her throat, she began to gag and struggle and grabbed both of my hands. I pulled the tube back and held both her hands with one of mine and pushed the tube through her mouth and down the esophagus with my free hand. Then I wondered if I had the tube in the trachea instead of the esophagus. I held my ear to the end of the tube sticking out of her mouth and listened. I didn't hear any breath sounds so I gave the tube a push on down the esophagus and into the stomach. I removed the tube and gave the exhausted woman a drink. The water went down fine so I knew I had removed the obstruction. I took her home and she thanked me for getting rid of her problem. As I drove off, I began to think of the complications I could have had. I had been treating her for a bad heart. She could have died, or I could have punched a hole through her esophagus. It was then I began to sweat and resolved never to try that again.

One hot sunday evening, as we were entertaining another couple, there was a knock at the door. The man was quite excited. "Doc, can you come quick? Something has happened to my sister," he said. I followed him in my car to a church in the east part of town. The congregation was crowded on the porch outside. Lying on the floor just inside the church was an obese young woman.

She was not moving and appeared to be unconscious. I knew that Janie was often highly emotional and that this was probably a case of hysteria. I examined her heart and lungs and took her blood pressure. Everything was normal. "Okay, Janie, let's wake up now and get up off the floor. There's nothing wrong with you. You've made your point." She still didn't open her eyes or move a muscle. I decided it was time to lower the curtain so the spectators outside couldn't watch anymore. I asked her brother to close the doors. Then I got down to serious business. I slapped her on one side of her face and then on the other, but she didn't respond. Next, I pressed as hard as I could on the angle of her jaws just below the ears. That causes great pain, but I still got no response. Then I pinched both Achilles tendons in her ankles, which is also painful. I kept repeating the procedures and all the time was pleading with Janie to wake up. Finally, after about twenty minutes, Janie began to roll her head from side to side and her eyelids began to flutter. At last she opened her eyes.

"It's about time, Janie," I said. "Let's get up and get out of here. The show is over." I had sweated until my clothes were wet through. As I helped to pull Janie to her feet, one of the good ladies of the church said to me, "Doctor, you know the Lord laid his hand on Janie tonight." "Yes, sister. Yes, he sure did," was the answer of the exhausted doctor as he stumbled down the steps.

Janie was basically an intelligent young woman. After graduating from high school, she went on to nurse's training and had no trouble making good grades. On several occasions she helped me in the delivery room. She eventually became a registered nurse, married, and had a child. She gave up nursing and began work on a production line at a local factory when she learned that her child had Down's syndrome. Later, she had a second child who was normal. Janie had been urged by her family and friends to place her first child in an institution, but she stubbornly refused. One day she came to my office, distraught. She poured out her problems. She blamed herself for having a retarded child and therefore had dedicated her life to caring for her. The Down's child was past six years of age and had become combative. Janie said the child had threatened her with a knife several times, and she was afraid of her. She therefore had decided to petition the court to place the child in an institution. She had come to ask if I could expedite the court procedure. I called the judge and explained the emotional problems that Janie was having and asked him to get the child committed at once. That he agreed to do.

I tried to reassure Janie and told her that within the next day or so the child would be placed in an institution. My assurances seemed to relax her. When she left my office, she appeared to be perfectly calm. The next day was my day out of the office. That afternoon I was sitting in the kitchen talking to Millie when we heard sirens off in the distance. Then the phone rang. It was the sheriff's office asking me to come to an address in the south part of town. When I arrived I saw police cars and an ambulance in front of a small cottage. A policeman explained what had happened. Janie had taken the younger child to a neighbor's house and then returned home. She stabbed her Down's child with a butcher knife, killing her. Then she stabbed herself. I walked through the door into the house and there lay Janie on the floor on her back, fully conscious, with a large butcher knife sticking in her chest. The knife had been driven in up to the handle. "Janie, why did you do this?" I asked. There was no answer. I gave her a hypo and had the ambulance crew place her gently on the cot without touching the knife and sent her to the hospital. Using my car radio, I called through to alert the surgeon that the ambulance would arrive shortly. She was alive when she arrived in surgery, but in spite of the heroic attempts of the surgical team, she died.

I learned later that she had stuck the knife in her chest once but withdrew it and drove it home for the second time in a different spot. The second time the blade sliced through the wall of a major vessel at its juncture with the heart.

THE PATIENT WAS a hardworking woman nearly forty years of age. When I examined her, I found she was pregnant. The risk of complications increase greatly when a woman reaches that age so I watched her closely through the course of her pregnancy. The night she delivered was hot and muggy. She was in a small hospital, and the delivery room was not air-conditioned. Her labor was rapid and uneventful. She was taken to the delivery room about midnight, and I had only one nurse to assist me. After only a few contractions, the head could be seen, and it wasn't long until the baby was delivered. Immediately, blood began gushing from the vaginal opening. The memory of my previous experience with a lacerated cervix came rushing back. I knew I had a cervical laceration. I immediately put in packing to stop the flow, and I had the nurse start intravenous fluids and check the blood pressure. There was no evidence of shock, but I wondered what I was going to do if the patient needed blood. There was no blood bank, and trying to find a donor and getting the necessary laboratory work done at this time of night would be impossible.

The delivery room had no operating light and was equipped with only the bare essentials. Furthermore, I had no one to assist me. The nurse had to administer the anesthetic and monitor the vital signs. I got the instruments arranged and my suture ready; then holding my breath, I took out the packing. Without any light, I had to use my fingers to find the laceration high up in the vaginal vault. It felt like the laceration extended up nearly three inches. Using my finger on my left hand as a guide, I began to suture. All the time blood was oozing from the site of the tear. After what seemed an eternity, the bleeding stopped. I firmly tied and cut the suture. Then I ran my fingers along the suture line and it was firm. The patient's blood pressure had dropped only slightly, and she appeared to be in good shape. She was taken to her room, and I finally relaxed. I was soaked to the skin with sweat and completely exhausted. A blood count the next day was within normal limits, and she didn't require a transfusion. Two days later, she and the baby went home.

THE WOMAN WAS in pain and I could see why. A thick piece of rusty wire was sticking out of the top of her foot. Immediately, I gave her a hypodermic to reduce the pain. She had been mowing with a power lawn mower, and she was barefoot. The mower had picked up the piece of wire and had driven it into her foot. The X-ray showed the wire buried in the largest bone of the foot. In fact, the wire had been driven almost through the bone. I wondered how I was going to remove the wire without snapping it. I had never seen anything like this before. After studying the X-rays, I decided to dissect through the soft tissue down to the point where the wire entered the bone.

After preparing the operative site, I injected a local anesthetic and made an incision. I carefully dissected down along the wire, being careful not to cut any tendons, major blood vessels, or nerves. Finally, the bone was exposed, and I was ready to try the most difficult part of the operation. I had sterilized an ordinary pair of pliers. With the X-rays on the view box, I gingerly grasped the wire right at the entry site into the bone. Firmly but gently, I began to pull, making sure I was pulling straight out. Nothing happened, so I pulled a bit harder. The wire began to move slowly. Gently, I continued to pull. Finally, I had the wire, and it was all in one piece. I irrigated the wound with copious amounts of sterile water, then inserted a rubber drain. Once the wound was closed, we took another X-ray. This confirmed that the wire was out. Tetanus antitoxin was given and the patient placed on antibiotics. She was on crutches for a while but was completely recovered in about two weeks.

Lawn mower accidents were fairly common right after the rotary mower was introduced. The early mowers had no safety features. Not only was the mower operator in danger of being struck by flying objects, but bystanders were perhaps in more danger. A five-year-old girl was brought in with a laceration of the lower right jaw. The laceration ran parallel to and just below the lip. She had been playing in front of the house while a family member was mowing, and she had been hit by a flying object. Even if the foreign body couldn't be seen, it was routine to get X-rays. They showed a metallic foreign body about 3/8 inch long buried deep in the base of the tongue. Obviously, it was a piece of wire. Examination of the mouth revealed that the right lower molars were shattered at the gum line and there was a small puncture wound at the base of the tongue. I thought this was too big a job to do in the office but decided to give it a try.

After injecting a local anesthetic, I made a small nick at the site of the puncture wound and gently stuck the tip of a small hemostat into the opening. Looking at the X-ray, it appeared that the foreign body was buried almost three-quarters of an inch deep inside the base of the tongue. I slowly worked the hemostat in until I felt the tip hit something solid. I opened the hemostat a little wider and then closed it. I had it! Gently I pulled out the wire. Follow-up X-rays showed no evidence of a foreign body. The laceration of the jaw was repaired, and the little girl was referred to her dentist for her tooth problem.

A FARMER'S WIFE came in with a puncture wound in her left breast. She had been mowing when she felt a stinging sensation and blood began oozing through her shirt. An X-ray showed a metallic foreign body deep in the chest wall just over the heart. She was hospitalized and taken to surgery. We found a piece of metal lodged below a rib. After entering the breast, the metal had struck a rib, which deflected it. Otherwise, it would have pierced her heart and been fatal.

I WAS DEEP IN SLEEP when the phone rang. I hadn't had a good night's sleep for ages, it seemed. The caller was an anxious mother whose daughter had stepped on a needle. "Well, pull it out," I said. "I can't, Doc. It's in her heel." "Well, this isn't an emergency. It will still be there in the morning. Besides, there is no way I can remove it tonight without help." By this time I was really upset. What was a teenage girl doing parading around at midnight on bare feet? She should have been in bed. The mother was persistent that I see her daughter right away. I was wide awake by this time and I knew I wouldn't be able to go back to sleep, so I dragged out of bed and put on my clothes.

The mother and daughter were waiting when I pulled up in front of the office. I merely grunted when she greeted me. After getting the patient on the table, I examined the foot and could see a small puncture wound. X-rays showed the needle was buried deep in the heel. I explained to the mother that it would be necessary to take her daughter to the hospital but that there was no hurry. She instead informed me she knew that I could do the job and she wanted it done now. I was ready to explode. I had been browbeaten by this woman enough. I decided to prove to her that I was right. I injected local anesthetic around the site of entry and made a small incision. I told the mother I was only going to try one time and then we would do it my way the next day at the hospital.

Looking at the X-rays, I slowly worked the tip of a small hemostat down at what I thought was the proper angle. I knew that that was like looking for a needle in a haystack; I could work all night and never find the needle. Suddenly, I felt a grating on the tip of the hemostat deep down in the heel. I opened the end of the hemostat and then closed it and slowly pulled out the hemostat. To my surprise, there was the needle. "I knew you could do it!" said the jubilant mother.

Another X-ray was taken and what did I see? A needle, or more correctly, a part of a needle. Apparently, when the needle went into the foot it broke into two pieces, but the break didn't show up in the X-ray. I had gotten half the needle, but the other half was still embedded in the heel. "There's no way I can get the rest of the needle," I told the mother. "I was lucky the first time, but I'm sure that my luck has run out."

She insisted that I repeat the procedure. Again I felt the grating on the tip of the hemostat; to my surprise the rest of the needle was pulled out. Putting the two pieces together, I had a perfect fit and a whole needle. A follow-up X-ray confirmed my success. I gave the girl a tetanus injection, wrapped the foot, and sent the mother and daughter home to bed. As they were leaving, the mother said with a grin, "I told you that you could do it, Doc." It had taken only thirty minutes to complete the job, but I still didn't believe I'd done it.

IT WAS ALMOST MIDNIGHT when the phone rang. I didn't recognize the woman's voice on the other end of the line. "Doctor," she said, "I live at Auburn, and we need a doctor." Auburn is about five miles west of Marshall. "These men came to my door with an injured man." At that point, a strange voice cut in. "I need you out here right now. This man is bleeding. He has a big cut in his arm."

I was very suspicious. Who were these people? What were they up to? "I'll tell you what to do. Bring this man to my office and I'll meet you there." "Do you mean you're not coming and you're going to let him bleed to death?" he growled. "No, I didn't say that. Put pressure on the wound to control the bleeding and bring him to my office where I can give him the proper treatment. I'll meet you there. Will you be there?" "Ya," he growled again. I gave him directions to my office and hung up. "That was a strange call," Millie said. She had overhead the conversation. "Yes, something doesn't add up." "You're not going up there by yourself to meet those people, are you? It's too dangerous." "No, I'm calling the sheriff," I answered. I dialed the sheriff while getting out of bed.

When I arrived at the office, the sheriff and a city policeman were already there. A Volkswagon was parked at the curb, and four big men were standing in front of the office. One man had a towel wrapped around his arm. It was obvious he had been drinking. He was loud, and he kept spitting obscenities.

I was told he had gotten drunk and eventually driven his fist through the windshield. (This I didn't believe.) I told the men to take him to the Paris Hospital. I could have just as easily sent him to the hospital in Terre Haute, but I wanted to keep him within the state in case the police would become involved. I put a dressing on the arm, and they went out to the Volkswagon. I noted the windshield was intact. There wasn't even a crack. They were given directions to the hospital and drove off.

The sheriff and I were standing in front of the office discussing the situation when a state patrolman drove up. "Did you just treat a patient who had been injured?" he asked. "Yes, and I sent him on to the Paris Hospital." The patrolman told us that he had received a call from Casey, sixteen miles west of Marshall, that a filling station had been broken into. A glass in the door was broken, and there was blood splattered over the station driveway. I told him that the likely culprits were no more than five minutes on the road to Paris, sixteen miles north of Marshall.

Another patrolman confirmed seeing the Volkswagon headed north. The state trooper and the sheriff took off in pursuit, going one hundred miles an hour, with me along for the ride. When we reached the hospital, we saw several police cars in the driveway.

What actually had happened was that the injured man had insisted on driving even though he was drunk. The driver pulled into the driveway of a closed filling station to settle the argument. The drunk became enraged, jumped from the car, ran to the front of the filling station, and rammed his fist through the window. He was arrested and taken back to Marshall to jail. He continued to rave and told the police that his father was an attorney in Michigan and had connections. He could buy the two-bit town of Marshall. He was completely ignored by the police, spent the weekend in jail, and then was released after paying all damages plus a five-hundred-dollar fine. The four men were all karate experts on their way to a karate competition.

The ringing of the phone awoke me. The voice on the other end was that of a scared mother. "Doctor, my son has been in a wreck and is trapped in the car. Will you go help him?" "Where is he?" I asked. "On the gravel road north of Livingston. Turn right at the Y," was her answer. "I'm on my way," I told her and hung up the phone. Crawling out of bed at 2:00 A.M. is no fun, but I had been doing it for years.

It was a hot, humid, foggy night. After turning at the "Y," I drove on as fast as I could through the fog, and suddenly ahead I saw a fire truck and a wrecker parked near the wrecked car. The boy and his girlfriend were traveling down the narrow road in the fog and had struck the low concrete abutment of a narrow bridge. The car was sitting astraddle the left bridge abutment. The boy was hanging out the door on the driver's side. His dad was squatting on the ground supporting him. The front seat had been driven back almost to the backseat, and in some way or another his left leg was tangled in the spring and steel supports of the backseat. Taking a look with my flashlight, I could see that he had a compound fracture of both bones in the lower leg. I gave him a hypodermic of morphine and then began to figure how we were going to get his leg loose from that wire and steel. Fortunately, he still had good circulation. The firemen and the wrecker crew hadn't been able to get him loose. They were afraid that anything they did would do further damage to his leg. After studying the problem, I asked for a hacksaw. I began trying to saw through the coil springs. The steel in springs is very hard. It wasn't long before I was soaked with sweat from all that exertion. I kept on and finally had loosened the grip that the springs had on his leg. Next the firemen and wrecker people rigged a cable around the rear of the body of the car. The cable attached to the winch on the wrecker gradually tightened. I carefully watched the leg to see that the pulling by the cable didn't put additional pressure on it. Finally, the pieces of metal holding the leg began to pull away and the leg was free. The circulation was still good and the leg was splinted and the patient was moved to the hospital. The next day I was told that when I asked for a hacksaw the bystanders thought I was going to amputate the leg.

ANOTHER TIME, the patient had had a long stay in the hospital with a serious illness and was recuperating at home in a nearby town. He and his father-in-law were the local undertakers and lived in the second-floor apartment of the funeral home. About midnight the patient's wife called. She asked for a house call.

The weather was bad. We had a recent heavy snow, and the highway was icy. I arrived to find that the patient and his wife just needed reassurance. They offered me a cup of coffee before I started my trip back. While we were drinking coffee, the doorbell rang. They looked at each other and said, "I wonder who that can be? No one ever rings our doorbell at night." The father-in-law went down to answer the door. Soon he yelled, "Doc, come down here."

There in the doorway stood a man. His face was covered with blood. He was wearing a suit but no overcoat, and it was evident he was half frozen. We got him into the kitchen and began washing his face. He was shivering and shaking so that he could hardly talk, but it was obvious he was drunk. After we had gotten the blood off his face, we recognized him as Jake, a patient of mine. When he had warmed up, we got his story. He, another man, and a woman were in a car out in the country and had gotten stuck in a snowdrift. They all had had plenty to drink and weren't having any luck getting out of the drift. They started arguing, and blows were exchanged. Jake, badly beaten, struck out on his own. As soon as he finished telling us his story, he fell asleep.

The undertaker said, "What are we going to do with him?" "Well, he looks comfortable here. Why don't you make a pallet on the floor here in the kitchen and let him stay the rest of the night?" was my suggestion. "Oh, I couldn't do that," answered the undertaker. "I think you should take him back to Marshall with you and let them put him in a cell at the police station." That solution didn't appeal to me at all, so I tried a different approach. "You know, we don't know just what happened and the other man and woman could still be out there in the snow and could freeze to death. Don't you have a law officer here?" "Yes, a deputy sheriff," replied the undertaker. "Well, call him and get him up here." He roused the deputy, who was most unhappy. I could see right then that I was stuck. The undertaker told me that he really appreciated my help and would call the police department to alert them I was bringing in a "guest" to spend the night in lock up. I got Jake to the car and started back to Marshall. I had to drive very carefully because of the ice on the road. Jake was very comfortable sitting there in front of the heater. I was puffing away on my cigar, keeping a close watch on the road ahead. Jake, meanwhile, was trying to light a cigarette. He couldn't get the match and the tip of the cigarette together. My first thought was that he would drop the match on his clothes and we would have a fire.

I reached over and took the match and put it in the ashtray. "Jake, you let me do the smoking for both of us. I'll keep blowing smoke in your face." "Okay, Doc," he said. Before he dozed off he said, "Doc, you know that undertaker is the finest man in the world. He would do anything to help a person." "Yep," I thought, "he sure would." I drove up in front of the police station, and a policeman escorted Jake to bed for the night in his own private cell. "Thanks, Doc," I heard him say as he went through the door. "Yes," I thought, "and to all a good night."

Millie became pregnant and was getting along all right until about the end of her third month, when she almost miscarried. It was during the middle of the night, and I was at the hospital in Terre Haute awaiting a delivery, when I received an urgent call from Millie. She was having severe cramps. I drove the sixteen miles home at a high speed. As soon as I arrived, I gave her a hypo of morphine to stop the cramping. No sooner than I had the needle out, she started retching and vomiting. I hadn't known she was sensitive to morphine. The cramping stopped, but now I had a new problem. I was afraid the strain of retching might cause her to miscarry. Then the phone rang. It was the delivery room—my patient was ready for delivery. I called Mom to come stay with Millie and I rushed back to the hospital. It was nearly twenty-four hours before Millie was back to normal. Fortunately, she did not lose the baby.

I was busy in the office one night when Millie called to tell me she thought she might be in labor. She was at term so I called Dr. Cavins in Terre Haute, who was to deliver her. He drove to Marshall and, after examining her, called to tell me he thought she should go to the hospital. I loaded her in the car after Mom arrived to stay with Linda. Dr. Cavins left orders for Millie to walk up and down the corridors when we arrived at the OB floor. The idea was to keep the contractions going. After she walked all night, the pains stopped, and I brought my exhausted wife back home. Two weeks later Millie awoke me during the night. "I'm really in labor this time," she told me. "Are you sure?" I asked. "No doubt about it," was her answer. So off to the hospital we went again. On the way she gave me a lecture on the proper conduct for an expectant father. None of that stuff of delivering her to the hospital and not showing up again until she was in the delivery room, as had been the case when Linda was born.

She was admitted and placed in the labor room. I meekly pulled a chair to the side of her bed and sat there holding her hand. The next thing I knew, she was shaking me awake. "You're not doing any good here. Go to the doctor's room and go to bed," she said. I didn't need to be told twice. I was awakened the next morning by the nurse. "They're taking your wife to the delivery room, but you also have a telephone call." I dashed to the door of the delivery room to let Millie know I was here and then answered the telephone. "You have a patient ready to deliver," the voice on the other end of the line informed me. This was the delivery room nurse at St. Anthony Hospital on the south end of Terre Haute. I ran back to see how Millie was doing, and the doctor told me we were the proud parents of an 8-1/2-pound baby girl. With that, I dashed down to St. Anthony and delivered a fine healthy boy. We named our daughter Mary Katherine. It seemed I could never get my act together when it came to Millie's having a baby.

18

Highway Carnage

IN THE EARLY 1940s, construction of a new Highway 40 was started, beginning at the Mississippi River, the western boundary of the state. The new highway was designed eventually to become a four-lane highway. Sufficient right-of-way was purchased to provide for the addition of the eastbound lanes. The new highway skirted all of the towns across the state and was a vast improvement over the old highway, except that state officials failed to mark the dangerous spots.

I was called to the police station about 2:00 A.M. When I arrived, a group of people was standing around the back of a truck. Lying on the floor of the truck were two men. One was dead. The other one was still alive but was in poor condition. I had him placed on an ambulance cot and moved into the police station. His left arm was badly mangled at the elbow. He was in shock. I gave him morphine, started intravenous fluids, and splinted the arm. I rode to the hospital with the patient.

Closer examination of the patient at the hospital revealed that the elbow joint was completely destroyed and the upper and lower arm were attached only by some thin strips of tissue. Miraculously enough, the blood vessels were intact and functioning, providing for some circulation. After anesthetizing the patient, the surgeon began debriding the wound of pieces of bone and flesh and dirt. A decision had to be made quickly to amputate the forearm at the elbow or attempt to repair the elbow as best we could and hope the arm would remain viable without getting infected.

We decided we had nothing to lose in an attempt to save the arm. Meticulously, we pieced back the torn tissue and applied a plaster splint. When we finished, there was a fairly good pulse at the wrist. He continued to have a good pulse, and there was no sign of developing infection. He was later transferred to the veteran's hospital for long-term care and rehabilitation.

Checking later with the police, I got the details concerning the accident. Apparently the two men were from a town about fifty miles away and were out for an evening of fun. They had been drinking heavily and were headed east on Route 40. As they rounded a curve, the car swerved across the centerlines, sideswiping a westbound vehicle. The driver had his left arm on the window ledge, the elbow extending out. When the two vehicles sideswiped, his extended elbow was caught. The other man was thrown forward onto the gearshift rod. There was no knob on top of the rod, and it was driven completely through his body, killing him instantly.

I heard nothing more about the man with the elbow and wondered how he had fared. Some time later I was finishing up night office hours when I looked into the waiting room and saw two strangers, a man and a woman, sitting there. I asked them into my consulting room. "You don't remember me, do you?" asked the man. "I'm afraid I don't," I replied. "A few years ago you took care of me and saved my arm," he said. He took off his coat and rolled up his sleeve. The elbow was stiff, but the joint had been stabilized in partial flexion. He demonstrated how he was able to remove objects from his pockets and that his fingers and wrist worked perfectly. He had been retrained to do office work and was quite adept at using a typewriter and other office equipment.

He had a good job and was happy. He introduced his wife and told me she was the widow of the friend who had been killed in the accident. "Doctor, we just wanted to stop by and thank you for what you did. I know it would have been the sensible thing to amputate my arm, but you doctors decided that it was worthwhile to attempt to save it. Saving my arm has made my life worth living."

The accident rate and number of fatal accidents on Route 40 became alarmingly high. I was increasingly upset. "Surely something can be done to stop this slaughter," I thought. There were no yellow lines on the pavement nor any "No Passing" signs. I even met with the engineers of the district highway department but got no results.

One sunny afternoon a local ambulance pulled up to the back of my office. The driver informed me that he had a dead woman. Her husband was leaning against the side of the building, overcome by grief. I tried to console him and, after he had composed himself, I asked how the accident had happened.

He told me that he and his wife were driving from Ohio to St. Louis and just west of town, he started to pass two slower-moving vehicles. He was driving at a moderate rate of speed and, before starting to pass, he looked for a "No Passing" sign or yellow "No Passing" lines on the pavement. Seeing none, he moved to pass. Just then, a large truck popped over the crown of the hill just beyond. He had committed himself too far to get back so he made an abrupt turn to the left to avoid a head-on collision. His wife wasn't wearing a seat belt and was thrown violently against the door. The door flew open and she fell to the pavement directly in front of the truck and was killed instantly.

I was so upset over that needless death that I sat down that night and wrote a letter to the governor. I told him that people were being mangled and slaughtered on this highway because the highway department refused to mark the highway adequately. A few days later, I received a call from an official in Springfield. I was given the runaround, as I had expected. The official told me he would contact district highway headquarters and have their engineers call on me. I told him that I already had talked to them without getting any results and wouldn't be satisfied until the director of the state highway department or his authorized representative came to our town. He asked when I wanted the meeting, and I told him I would have to talk to the people in our community before I could give him an answer. "You mean you want a hearing?" he asked in amazement. "That's exactly what I want," was my answer. He hesitated and finally said, "Well, we've never done this before." "I don't care if you've never had a hearing before. That's exactly what I want now." Reluctantly, he agreed, and I told him I would let him know shortly when the meeting could be held.

I arranged for a meeting to discuss the highway problem in the private dining room at a local restaurant. Invited were some members of the state legislature, the captain of the state police for our district, and the media. Just a short time before the meeting was to begin, I had to go to the hospital for a delivery. The county highway engineer volunteered to conduct the meeting until I returned.

I was amazed when I entered the meeting room. It was packed. Every chair was filled and people were standing along the walls around the room. The official from Springfield and the engineer from the district highway department appeared to be uncomfortable sitting at the front of the room. Person after person voiced complaints about the lack of attention the highway department had given to safety. The meeting lasted over three hours; when it was over, we invited the engineers and Springfield delegation to take a test drive on Highway 40.

As he was approaching one of the dangerous spots, the driver purposely pulled into the left lane, simulating a passing maneuver. On several occasions an approaching vehicle suddenly appeared, and he swerved back into the right lane to avoid a collision. After he had done that a few times, the engineers were convinced. "You don't have to do that anymore. We can see perfectly well from the right lane," they said. After our test drive, the district highway engineer was instructed to call a crew immediately to measure all of the site distances. If it appeared there was even a remote possibility of a hazard, "No Passing" zones were to be posted. As an editorial that appeared in an area newspaper stated, "It has been proven that you can beat city hall."

There was a significant decrease in accidents and fatalities after "No Passing" zones had been marked, but it wasn't long until another problem arose. Interstate 70 had been designated to take over the major traffic that formerly had gone over Route 40. Standards had been changed completely from those that had existed when Route 40 had been planned to evolve into a four-lane highway. The interstate system had been designed to have limited access. Traffic could enter or exit only at interchanges that were miles apart. It was not practical to attempt to upgrade the existing Route 40 into an interstate highway so Interstate 70 was built over a new right-of-way.

Progress in the construction of Interstate 70 had been rather slow in Illinois but had proceeded at a rapid rate in Indiana. The entire highway was completed across Indiana from Ohio to the Illinois border where the traffic was funneled onto two-lane Route 40. The Illinois portion of Interstate 70 was completed from St. Louis to within fifty miles of the Indiana state line, where construction was stalled. From the west we also had traffic funneled from Interstate 70 to Route 40. Once again, in spite of all that had been done to mark "No Passing" zones, it became slaughter time on Route 40.

Most of the people traveling the highway were from other parts of the country. After driving for long periods of time on a four-lane highway, they often didn't realize they were now on a two-lane highway. When they came onto Route 40, they would attempt to pass, not anticipating any oncoming traffic. I wondered what the people could do to get the attention of the government.

I asked my attorney to prepare a petition to the governor to resume the construction of Interstate 70 to the Indiana state line. Next, I enlisted the help of my good friend Tom Comerford, the editor of a weekly newspaper in a neighboring town. He had written a number of excellent editorials condemning the deplorable safety conditions on Route 40. He printed the petitions. Our petition drive was publicized by mouth and through his newspaper. Only eligible voters in Illinois could sign. I was amazed at the response. People of all ages came to Tom's office and my office to ask to carry the petitions.

The newspapers featured numerous articles in support of our campaign. An Indiana television station invited Tom and me to appear on a half-hour discussion program. The station did a magnificent job of producing the program at no charge. Another station some ninety miles away in Illinois sent a news reporter and camera crew to Marshall for an interview, which we did at the site of an accident that had occurred just that morning.

We had gathered more than eight thousand names on the petitions. Also, we distributed opinion surveys at filling stations and restaurants along Route 40. Printed on the cards were such statements as "Route

40 is a good highway" and "Route 40 is a dangerous highway." At the bottom was space for remarks.

We had asked the governor for an appointment in October, shortly before an election. Although he refused to meet with us, he did agree to send an assistant. We attached the petition sheets end to end and had a ribbon between fifty and sixty feet long. The cards collected from the highway stops made a pile nearly two feet high. We selected a small group of about fifteen people from the area to make the trip to the state capital in Springfield.

The night before, a television crew came for a final interview before we went to the capital. We selected the headquarters of the local wrecker service as the site for the interview. That very day three women had been killed in an accident just east of town. The completely demolished compact car was still hanging from the boom of the wrecker when we arrived. We unrolled our ribbon of petitions and stretched it out in front of the mangled car.

My partner, the newspaper editor, had arranged for a photographer and reporter from the Associated Press News Service to be present at the meeting in Springfield. They were waiting for us when we arrived. We unrolled the petition ribbon and presented it to the governor's assistant in front of the camera. The "big guns" of the highway department and the administration were waiting for us and ready to shoot us down. We were told right at the beginning that there was no way that work could be started for at least three years to complete the interstate. None of us would accept that. There wasn't a bashful person in our group. We continued to fire back at them for nearly two hours. We gave them the gory details of the many accidents that had been occurring and told them that if there was any further delay in getting started they, along with the governor, would have to accept the responsibility.

The next day I was delighted to see the article and picture in the Chicago and St. Louis papers. The article filled a complete column. The reporter and photographer had done an excellent job. Our meeting was publicized across the Midwest. That was just the type of publicity a politician didn't like. The following day, late in the evening, I had just completed a delivery when I was paged. I answered the phone, and the governor's assistant was on the other end. "Doctor," he said, "I wanted to get the news to you quickly. I can't give you the details until the governor's news release tomorrow, but I'm sure you are going to be very happy."

The next day the announcement appeared in all the papers. The governor stated he was initiating a crash program to complete Interstate 70 and the first contracts would be let in two weeks. Instead of beginning the project in three years, the highway was completed and dedicated long before that time had elapsed. Again, the people all working together, along with the media, had triumphed. Yes, you can beat city hall! My only regret was that Tom didn't live to see the fruition of his effort. He had died of a brain tumor.

Soon after the governor had directed work be started on completion of I-70, the state highway department designated the fifty-mile stretch of Route 40 as the most dangerous highway in the state. I received a call from an official in Springfield informing me that a detailed investigation was to be made of each fatal accident occurring on that segment of Route 40. A team consisting of specially trained state troopers, highway engineers, psychologists, auto mechanics, photographers, and a doctor would investigate each accident. I was requested to serve as the doctor on the team. The title assigned to the group was the "Multidiscipline Fatal Accident Investigating Team." After all of the criticism I had leveled at the department, I felt I had no other choice but to accept the assignment.

At the organizational meeting held in Springfield, we each were told to develop our own protocol. No such team approach had been used before so there were no established procedures. My protocol provided for a thorough examination of the vehicle interior, with measurements to determine how much encroachment had occurred because of the force of the crash. The positions of the passengers after the crash and whether restraining devices were in place were also determined. Arrangements were made with the county coroner's office to approve complete autopsies, including a toxicological examination of the blood, stomach contents, and portions of the liver and brain. I was furnished a tape recorder to record my observations at the scene.

As soon as a fatal accident was reported to District Twelve state police headquarters in Effingham, each member of the team was notified. Our instructions were to proceed to the accident as quickly as possible. The dead and wreckage were to be left in place until we arrived, but the injured were removed from the site as quickly as possible.

My first call came at about midnight. The site of the accident was about thirty miles west of Marshall. As I raced down the highway, I tried to picture in my mind what I was going to find. Suddenly I had to stop because the line of traffic ahead was still nearly two miles from the wreck. I pulled out into the left lane, passing the solid line of vehicles on my right. Most of them were semitrailer trucks. I dodged the oncoming traffic until I arrived at the scene. It had been a head-on collision, and the two mangled vehicles, one a semitrailer truck, were in the middle of the highway. Lying on the pavement was the body of a woman. She had been thrown from the left front door. With floodlights set up, I examined the mangled body and directed the ambulance people to take it to the funeral home in a nearby town. After examining the vehicles, I went on to the funeral home, where I met the coroner and arranged for an autopsy.

The specimen of blood and stomach contents were to be sent to the state laboratory in Chicago. I arranged a relay of state troopers to carry the specimen to the lab. Driving back home I thought there must be a safer way to get to the wrecks without dodging traffic. I talked to the local sheriff the next day, and he loaned me a portable revolving red light. I mounted the light on the ledge of the back seat and plugged it into the lighter socket. I was amazed at the way cars got out of my way. There was no more dodging traffic.

In spite of all efforts to improve safety, there was no letup in accidents. The highway was totally inadequate to carry the traffic load. One collision was especially tragic. The westbound car, occupied by four adults and four children, collided head-on with an eastbound vehicle while trying to pass. The force of the crash was terrific. The front ends of both vehicles had been compressed within fifteen or twenty inches of the windshields. The steering wheel and column of the westbound car extended forward through the windshield. The back of the front seats in the westbound vehicle was within six inches of the instrument panel, and two adults and three children were jammed down on the floor between the front seat and the fire wall. One of the children survived until she reached the hospital despite having a compound fracture of the skull, her brain tissue protruding through the hole in the skull. One child had a large hole, measuring four by six inches, in the chest. The heart and lungs could be seen through the hole. It was determined that hole was probably made when the child was projected forward, striking a large tachometer mounted above the instrument panel. Only three people survived, and they remained in critical condition.

ONE SATURDAY NIGHT I was called to an accident only a mile west of Marshall. I could hardly believe what I saw—the tractor of a semitrailer truck sitting on top of what had been a passenger car. The car looked as if it had been run through a compactor. The top of the car was only about two feet above the surface of the pavement. A fire truck was on the scene, and floodlights were set up. On down the road about two hundred yards a large flatbed truck was upside down; along the road for another hundred yards were large chunks of what had been a heavy-duty farm tractor. There was not a sound coming from the car under the semi-tractor. Walking around, I could see a hand sticking out from the debris. When the semi was lifted from the car, we started looking for a body or bodies, but the metal on the top had been compressed, sealing off the interior of the car. I asked that the wreckage be lifted up and slung on the boom of the wrecker and taken to the salvage yard.

With the floodlights set up, we began prying away the top of the car as if we were tearing the top off a tin can. Finally, we could see inside. There was the body of the man who had been driving. It was split wide open, and scattered around the inside of the car were the mutilated bodies of three children. One child was jammed beneath the instrument panel.

It was a hot muggy night, and the smell of death was all around. We carefully removed the torn bodies from the wreckage. The following day, the owner of the salvage yard called to ask if I was through with the examination of the car. The stench was becoming unbearable so I told him to burn the car.

After gathering all the evidence, I was able to determine how that terrible accident had happened. The driver was a divorced father who was transporting his child and two friends to a lake in Indiana for the weekend. He had spent the evening in a tavern drinking heavily before he picked up the children. He was coming down a hill on Route 40 at high speed and veered across the centerline, striking the left front end of the flatbed truck. The man and his wife in the truck were returning from a tractor-pulling contest. The huge tractor was chained down to the bed of the truck. When the truck driver saw the car coming at him, he set the brakes. When the car struck the left front of the truck, the car acted as a fulcrum. It caused the truck to flip over forward. The impact and the violent force caused by the truck flipping over broke the chains and the tractor was catapulted through the air. The tractor was shattered by the impact of striking the pavement. That accounted for the large chunks of metal I saw scattered down the highway. After striking the truck, the car went into a slide down the highway. The driver of the semi saw what was happening and pulled off on the shoulder as far as he could and tried to stop, but the skidding car hit the semi. The semi-tractor came to rest on top of the car.

The day was clear and crisp, a beautiful fall day. A burned-out, flatbed semi-tractor sat on the shoulder of the road. Across the highway was the remains of a pickup camper truck. Witnesses described what had happened. The pickup camper was headed west, and the semi, loaded with lumber, was headed east. There was a long, gradual curve at that point. The camper had slowly veered across the centerline and struck the semi right at the point where the fuel tank was located. That caused a huge explosion and fire. The fire shot across the highway for nearly one hundred yards. The camper exploded. The driver of the semi and the elderly man and woman in the camper died instantly.

The remnants of the camper were scattered along the right-of-way. Since the bodies of the elderly owners were badly charred and had been taken to the morgue, I could not do a satisfactory autopsy. Searching through the debris, however, I found heart medication bottles belonging to the man. I confirmed that with his doctor in Pennsylvania. Blood analysis on the couple showed 80 percent saturation with carbon monoxide. Due to the cool weather, the couple was probably riding with the windows closed. Their truck was new, but it was possible there was a leak in the exhaust system that could gradually saturate the air in the cab with carbon monoxide. However, there was another possibility. The intense fire would also produce carbon monoxide. Would it be possible that the carbon monoxide in the pool of blood found in the man's thigh could have resulted from the intense fire?

I decided to try a crude experiment. I had my nurse collect a specimen of my blood. Then I put a portion in a glass cup. The exhaust pipe on my car curved down at the end. I set the cup of blood on a stool directly under the exhaust pipe and ran the engine for thirty minutes. All of the exhaust stream went directly into the blood. I sent the specimen to the laboratory, and only 8 percent carbon monoxide saturation of the blood was found. I was satisfied that the 80 percent saturation of the dead man's blood had to be there before the accident. My conclusion was that he had been overcome by carbon monoxide, causing him to veer across the highway into the side of the semi.

The last fatal accident we investigated occurred just a few days before the dedication and opening of Interstate 70 in late 1971. The study covered a period of approximately two years. During that time, we investigated approximately twenty fatal accidents along the fifty-mile segment of the two-lane highway. A number of them involved multiple fatalities. Approximately 50 percent were proven to be alcohol-related. Carbon monoxide was also something to be considered as a cause. We did not find one instance in which mechanical failure was the cause.

Sometime before I-70 was completed, the highway department took further steps to improve the safety of Route 40. New and improved guardrails were installed, and more "No Passing" signs were put in place. I had long urged the highway department to install larger "No Passing" signs on both sides of the highway. The driver of a car attempting to pass a truck, for example, might have his vision of a "No Passing" sign on the right side blocked but could easily see one on the left side. My suggestion was ignored until the new safety program was instituted. Then both sides of the road were posted with "No Passing" signs, each measuring four by six feet.

19

Citizen Politician

POLITICS HAD NEVER HELD much interest for me. Oh, I remembered a flurry of activity every four years when the presidential elections were held, when the teachers tried to tell us of the importance of our political system and that in a democracy all people had a right to participate in the elective process. After the election, though, we forgot about it to concentrate on more important things in our young lives—such as football, basketball, baseball, fishing, or how to get by without studying.

I do remember that my father, a staunch Democrat, changed parties after Woodrow Wilson was elected president in 1916. "He campaigned hard with the promise that if he were elected we wouldn't go to war," Dad grumbled, "so I voted for him. Six months later I was in the army. That's the last time I vote for a Democrat for president."

After I returned home from the service, I began to pay more attention to politics and found that the philosophy of the Republican party was most to my liking. In the 1960s I listened to the comments of my patients concerning the way things were going in the country, and some of their statements conflicted sharply with my beliefs. I hesitated to take issue because I didn't want to compromise the practice I had worked so hard to build. I wrestled with the problem until finally I decided that I was going to let people know my stand. After all, in a democracy, we have freedom of speech, and we have the right to disagree. I recognized the right of others to disagree with me, and I felt that, being sensible, they would not criticize me for saying what I had to say.

I began to speak out and discovered that I had been right in my thinking. I didn't have one patient leave me for another doctor because I had disagreed with them on political matters. I felt that shunning involvement in the political process only resulted in poorly qualified candidates being elected. The end result was having a substandard government with which we all had to live.

During the 1960s, the state medical society organized a political action committee. The membership of the society was given the opportunity of voluntarily becoming members of the organization by paying a small annual fee. That money was then used in support of candidates, regardless of party, who shared our philosophy.

It wasn't long before I was asked to serve on the governing board of the organization. I was becoming directly involved in the political arena. At a 1967 meeting, the chairman made an appeal for more doctors' becoming candidates for various offices. That appeal stimulated me immediately into thinking about becoming a candidate. I had been bitten hard by the bug of politics.

I decided to run as an alternate delegate to the Republican National Convention of 1968. Millie was surprised but agreeable. I began planning my strategy. Since I was an outsider, I knew I would need the support of active members of the party. As soon as I got home, I called my good friend John Lewis, who had been a Republican member of the state legislature for many years and was well liked by members of both parties. He immediately pledged his full support. Next I talked to the county chairman and later to the state chairman, who both were enthusiastic. Then I had to circulate petitions, which was accomplished with the cooperation of all the county chairmen in the district.

Shortly afterwards, the county chairmen met to discuss the candidates. The chairman from our county made a presentation on my behalf and asked for an endorsement. He called the next day to tell me I had received their unanimous endorsement. My petitions had to be filed at the state capital in Springfield. The county chairman went with me to file, and we were first in line. When the filing date ended, I was the only candidate to file. Two positions were to be filled, so I was automatically elected. Since no one else had filed, the vacancy had to be filled by appointment by the county chairmen. I suggested that a friend of mine, who had served in Congress and the state legislature, be appointed.

The convention was to be held in Miami in August. After the spring primaries, activity began to pick up. I had received the official document certifying my election. Then began a steady stream of correspondence from the national Republican headquarters, committees for the various candidates who would be in the race for nomination, special interest groups, and many others. I was wondering what I had gotten myself into, but I really was enjoying it.

In early summer, I received notice of a caucus of the delegation to be held at the Pheasant Run Resort near St. Charles. I had no idea of what to expect. I was really a boy from the country. All the others were total strangers, and I'm sure many of them were as uneasy as I was. It wasn't long before we became acquainted. Of course, all the leaders of the party were there. There was Senator Everett Dirksen, the grand old man, the last of the true statesmen; Senator Charles Percy, a young newcomer to party politics, who was in a hurry to gain more power within the party; and Richard Ogilvie, who in spite of the overwhelming dominance of the Democratic party in Chicago, had been elected sheriff of Cook County. Ogilvie now was the Republican candidate for governor.

I had met Senator Percy a few years before when he was a candidate for governor. He had had a successful career with Bell and Howell's, the photographic equipment company. In fact, he was one of the youngest men ever elected to the presidency of such a large corporation. During the primary campaign of 1964, Percy had come to Marshall with his wife and one of his daughters as the guests of Gene Spotts, who was the circuit clerk. I was invited to meet them in Gene's office at the courthouse. I was president of the school board at the time and was quite concerned about the lack of financial aid from the state. I asked Mr. Percy a number of pointed questions concerning his stand on education and what he would do to help in getting more aid for the schools. I liked his answers and agreed to support him. (Some time later the daughter who was with him that day was murdered by an intruder at the Percy home, and the murder was never solved.) Later, Percy asked me to serve as his finance chairman for our county and I agreed. Percy was defeated in the election that fall by the incumbent governor, Otto Kerner. The caucus at Pheasant Run was called to organize the delegation and elect the officers. We also discussed strategy for the upcoming convention.

Earlier that spring, Millie and I had gone with a delegation from the Illinois State Medical Society to Washington to lobby in Congress. We had a meeting with Senator Dirksen, who was the minority leader of the Senate. When we arrived at the Capitol, we were ushered into a large committee room. A door opened on the far side, and the rumpled figure of an elderly man, his wavy hair all ruffled, slowly made his way across the room and greeted us in a voice that was almost a whisper. All I could feel was pity for the poor man. Then he started to speak in a low voice. As he continued to speak, his voice increased in volume, until it was the deep, rich voice of a true orator. He continued for nearly an hour, still on his feet. The longer he talked, it seemed the stronger he became physically. The rest of us began to tire, and some of the women had to find seats. He gave us one of the greatest reviews of our government and how democracy works that I had ever heard. It was evident that he loved his country. I realized that I was listening to one of the true statesmen of our time. He knew exactly what was needed to make the democratic process work and was making a tremendous contribution toward that end.

After he had completed his remarks, he started walking slowly back to his office.

Since I was going to be a member of the delegation to the convention, our photographer requested a picture of the senator with me. That autographed picture hangs on the wall of my office.

Later that spring, at the annual meeting of the state medical society, I was asked to meet with Senator Dirksen. At the appointed hour, I arrived at the suite in the Hotel Sherman, where the officers of the society were awaiting his arrival. Soon the senator made his entrance, hobbling on a cane. "What in the world happened to you, Senator?" one of us asked. Answering in his deep voice, the senator said, "Well," he said, "Louella told me she wanted me to fix the light in the chandelier above the dining room table. I climbed onto the table and fell off, landing on the same damn hip I broke once before."

I remembered, a few years before, he went into Walter Reed Hospital for a checkup and fell out of bed during the night, fracturing a hip. "Would you like a drink, Senator?" "Oh, I guess I'll have bourbon and a little bit of branch water," was his reply. With his drink in hand, he took a seat on the couch, and I sat beside him. He asked me how my campaign was going, and I told him I guessed I already had won since I had no opposition. After he had finished his drink, three of us who were on the political action council asked him to step into the bedroom for a private meeting.

Since there were no chairs in the room, we sat on the beds. We gave him an envelope containing a check. He opened the envelope, looked at the check, and then thanked us. We told him he was free to use that money any way he wished. "No, that is not correct," he told us. Then he launched into a lecture on ethics. "You know one of my Democratic colleagues in the Senate right now is in trouble over the misuse of campaign funds." Then he mused, "You know he made two mistakes: first, he pleaded guilty and, second, he employed a corporation lawyer to defend him. You know I sat up until 2:00 A.M. writing out a defense for him, but he never used it." He continued, "I have been in politics for many years, as you know, and I have a ledger that I have kept since I first started. Every penny in political contributions I have received has been entered in that ledger along with the name of the contributor, and every penny that has been spent and what it was spent for has been entered. You know, one time I had a considerable sum left over after a campaign, so I thought I would donate it to the Salvation Army. First, however, I checked with the director of Internal Revenue. He told me that if I made the contribution I'd have to pay income tax on the money. I said to hell with that and just kept the money in the bank. But I had forgotten one thing. The money I had deposited earned interest, and I had to pay income tax on the interest."

The Republican party had a big dinner at the Hilton Hotel while we were in Chicago, so Millie and I attended. Ronald Reagan, who was governor of California at the time, was the speaker of the evening. The more than one thousand people in attendance were enthusiastic. I thought after hearing him that he had the qualities needed for a great president. After the dinner, we were invited to a private reception in Senator Dirksen's suite, where we met Governor and Mrs. Reagan.

After the caucus at Pheasant Run, we had our delegation organized and our officers elected. Senator Dirksen was the unanimous choice as chairman, and Richard Ogilvie was elected vice-chairman.

Not long after, I received a letter from Richard Nixon's office, requesting my attendance at a meeting for all delegates and alternate delegates in the Midwest. We got together in a large ballroom. Before the meeting started, I had an opportunity to get acquainted with some of the delegates from other states. Among those I met was Bud Wilkinson, the famous football coach from the University of Oklahoma. I remember one man I talked to was a farmer from Wisconsin, who told me that at 5:00 A.M. that morning he had finished milking his cows and hurried to get cleaned up and put on his good suit so that he wouldn't miss his plane to Chicago. I thought to myself, that truly is what our country is all about. People from all walks of life and diverse occupations are the ones who select the leaders to guide our nation. Mr. Nixon and his wife, Pat, greeted each of us individually with a handshake and a few words. A picture was taken. A few weeks later, I received the personally autographed photograph, "To George Mitchell, with warmest regards, Richard Nixon."

The time had come for us to leave for Miami. We had decided to go by train. We had received advance information concerning the schedule of events. Delegates paid all their own expenses. The Political Action Committee of the medical society had graciously voted me five hundred dollars to help with my expenses.

The Illinois delegates were assigned to a hotel almost ten miles from the convention center. The hotel was new and very comfortable. It was located on the beach just south of Fort Lauderdale. As we had planned, we arrived a day early. After we had checked in, we were visiting in the lobby with another couple, who were from Chicago, when a dapper gentleman wearing a bow tie came up to the desk to register. "You see that man," said my fellow delegate. "He could buy this hotel and not even miss the money." "Who is he?" I asked. "That, my friend, is W. Clement Stone. He is many times a millionaire and very influential in Republican politics in our state. He owns the Combined Insurance Company." Over the years, I was to see the extent of his influence.

I became well acquainted with Vic Smith, the state party chairman. He was a newspaper editor and lived in Robinson, only thirty miles from Marshall. Vic had been active in politics for many years and was highly respected.

We had a caucus the next day and received detailed instructions on everything that related in any way to the convention. Vic was kind enough to provide Millie with a guest ticket for every session. The following day we all piled into special buses and rode to the convention center. Each of us had an official delegate ticket, an identification card, and an official badge. As soon as we arrived, we were checked by the Secret Service and passed through another checkpoint before we went onto the floor of the convention.

The Illinois delegation was seated down front to the left side of the hall. The delegates and alternate delegates each had their own section. The elaborate opening ceremonies were quite impressive. I had never seen so many dignitaries in one place. After so many speeches, however, I began to get a little bored. It was late when we got back to the hotel, and we weren't able to get much to eat. The following morning, we started early, and I had time only to get a roll and coffee. We met in caucus all morning and heard from the various candidates—Nelson Rockefeller, Richard Nixon, and Harold Stassen. Richard Nixon was to meet with us privately later.

The state medical society had arranged a champagne brunch for the delegation. The announcement was made, and then it was discovered that the plans would conflict with the Nixon meeting. Clement Stone excused himself from the meeting. Soon he returned and told Senator Dirksen that he had just called John Mitchell, one of Nixon's advisors, and told him the Nixon meeting would have to be rescheduled. The brunch went on without a hitch and was a great success.

Security at the convention was tight. The local police, the FBI, and the Secret Service had saturated the convention hall and the surrounding area. Men armed with high-powered rifles could be seen prowling the catwalks high above the hall, and helicopters manned by police patrolled above the hall.

Television cameras were everywhere, and reporters constantly walked up and down the aisles interviewing delegates and dignitaries. I received a telegram from one of my doctor friends back home, ribbing me about being on television. I knew nothing about it, but apparently several times the camera zeroed in on me wearing the straw sailor on my head that identified the members of the Illinois delegation, cigar clamped firmly between my teeth, intently watching the proceedings on the podium. At least they didn't catch me sleeping.

After two or three days, being a delegate became real work—long days and short nights without much to eat. I began to think the only food available in Miami was the finger food that was served at receptions.

Our delegation agreed in caucus to cast most of our votes for Nixon.

A few of the delegates, however, were completely dedicated to Reagan and did not waiver. After all the speech making and pageantry, we finally came to the night when nominations were to be made.

The final results were in, and Nixon had won by an overwhelming majority. At that point, a motion was made, seconded, and passed to make it a unanimous ballot for the winner. When we arrived back at the hotel, it was 3:00 A.M. Millie and I sat on the side of the bed, exhausted. "Millie, do you know I'm starved? I haven't eaten all day, and there's no place to get anything to eat this time of night." Millie grinned and reached into her bag and pulled out half an orange and a candy bar. That was my dinner.

The last night was reserved for the nominating of the vice presidential candidate and the acceptance speeches. In the afternoon, we learned that Nixon had selected Spiro Agnew as his running mate. After the acceptance speeches, the convention was adjourned. Finally, we had a good night's sleep and the next morning a leisurely breakfast. We said our good-bys to our new friends and took the evening train home.

The incumbent, President Lyndon Johnson, had decided not to run for another term. The Democratic Convention in Chicago that year was a strange one. Bloody riots in the city and disruptions on the floor of the convention made it almost impossible to conduct the business of nominating a candidate. Hubert Humphrey was selected as the Democratic candidate.

The campaigns were grueling: each candidate crisscrossed the entire country, making speeches, attempting to sway voters. Constantly in the spotlight of the media, the candidates were scrutinized and dissected by the press.

It was an extremely close election; all through the night, polling judges worked to discover the outcome. On my way to the hospital the next morning, the winner was announced. Nixon had won by a narrow margin. The man who had been defeated in 1960 by young John Kennedy and who had announced with bitterness he would never run again eight years later had won—just barely.

He was inheriting a huge number of problems, not the least of which was the war in Vietnam, from the previous administration. There was a deep division in the country over the conduct of the war. Antiwar groups were active all over the country. Bloody riots, sit-ins, and bombings were occurring almost daily.

We had the opportunity to attend the inauguration on January 20 but decided against it. Then at the last minute we decided to attend the inaugural ball. We had the tickets but were too late to get hotel reservations. I called my cousin Dr. Earl Mitchell, who lived in Washington. He was going to be out of town that weekend but offered me his house. When I declined his invitation, he used his influence to get us into a hotel in Bethesda. When we arrived at the hotel, we found we had not just a room, but a suite.

Millie and I got gussied up, she in her formal and I in my tails, and Earl and his wife took us to dinner at the Chevy Chase Country Club. He told us President Nixon was a member. After dinner, he drove us to the Sheraton Park Hotel, the site of the ball. President and Mrs. Nixon made an appearance during the evening.

Early the next morning, we made the flight back, tired after our whirlwind trip, but thrilled that we had the opportunity to see and participate in the festivities of the inauguration.

Four years later, I was elected a delegate to the Republican National Convention. Governor Ogilvie was chairman of the delegation, and Senator Percy was the vice-chairman. The grand old man, Senator Dirksen, had passed on in September of 1969. President Nixon was in the race for a second term so the convention was a mere formality.

Hope McCormick, the wife of the president of International Harvester Corporation, was a member of our delegation, and she suggested we all wear jackets of the same color at the convention. We were all decked out in orange jackets, the state seal emblazoned just below the breast pocket. We spent a lot of our time attending receptions.

The big reception was the one hosted by our old friend Clement Stone. The entire terrace of the hotel was taken over and converted into a facsimile of a Hawaiian scene by landscape specialists, who even moved in sand and palm trees. The swimming pool was converted into a lagoon. By early evening, the transformation had been completed, and everything was ready for the big luau. All the top people in the Nixon administration were there. What an evening! I heard that Mr. Stone shelled out fifty thousand dollars for the party.

The convention was without controversy, but there were still some groups around the country trying to stir up trouble. We got word that a large group had set up camp in Miami. We didn't know what they were planning, but we kept on the alert. The last day of the convention arrived, and there had been no incidents. All that was left was the night session, when the President would accept the nomination, followed by the closing ceremonies. That afternoon, Millie and I took a cab to a shopping area near the convention center. We hadn't been there long when we were told the whole area was to be sealed off by the police. We ran out and fortunately got a cab. Other people piled in with us, and we raced away. Shortly, a convoy of old city busses began rolling in. The city of Miami had a large number of old busses stored at Fort Lauderdale. The busses were parked in single file encircling the convention center. That was the modern version of circling the wagons used by the pioneers as a defense against the Indians. We were a bit jittery as we rode to the convention that night. Along the way, we saw machine gun emplacements manned by National Guardsmen dressed in riot gear. The driver drove at high speed all the way without stopping, and we arrived safely. Another bus that was behind us wasn't as fortunate. They ran into a blockade of rioters. The driver tried to go around by driving over the parkway and sidewalk, but the rioters managed to jerk open the panel over the engine compartment at the rear of the bus and rip out the ignition wires. They pelted the bus with rocks, shattering the windows and scattering broken glass over the passengers. Fortunately, no one was injured, and shortly the police arrived and dispersed the rioters. The delegates were transferred to another bus and brought on to the convention.

Each group of delegates was given a specific location and time to board the busses to return to the hotel after the convention adjourned. Millie and the other wives of our group arrived at the loading point before I got there. When I left the hall, I could smell tear gas. When I got to Millie, she and the other women were standing there with tears streaming down their cheeks. The rioters had tried to break through the barricades formed by the old busses, and the police had used tear gas to drive them back.

The bus arrived almost two hours late. On the way back to the hotel, we again passed the machine guns and riot police. It was nearly 3:00 A.M., but another couple joined us for a quiet ride in a cab to a nice restaurant for a good meal far away from the rioting.

While at the convention, we had talked to Governor Ogilvie and his wife about his upcoming campaign for reelection and offered to help in any way we could. A few weeks later, we were asked to host a reception for Mrs. Ogilvie at our home.

Millie got to work planning the event. She had a lot of help from her friends, and soon the plans were completed, down to the last detail—a red carpet across the porch and down the steps to the driveway. A few days before the big event, a strange man came to the door. He asked if he could come in. At first, Millie was frightened, but he identified himself as a member of the Illinois Bureau of Investigation and had come to check out the house and grounds before Mrs. Ogilvie's visit.

It was a beautiful day. Mrs. Ogilvie arrived in her limousine, accompanied by her bodyguards, and walked across the red carpet into the house. There was a large group of women from the area, as well as local elected officials, on hand to greet her. Tables had been set up on the lawn, and refreshments were served. I came home from the office for a few minutes. I was surprised to see that my fellow delegate, Hope McCormick, had come all the way from Chicago for the event. Millie had done a superb job, and the reception was a huge success.

We went to Washington for the inauguration in January. This time we made plans well in advance and stayed with the Illinois delegation near the Watergate. We had reserved seats for the inauguration. Early that morning, with some friends, we took a cab to the Senate Office Building to attend the reception hosted by Senator Percy, then walked over to the Capitol to find our seats. We had excellent seats directly in front of the platform. We had reserved seats next to the White House to view the inaugural parade.

I knew it was impossible to get transportation so we walked. We had plenty of time and the weather wasn't bad, although it was a bit chilly. We were wearing insulated underwear and plenty of outer clothing, so sitting for two hours watching the parade wasn't uncomfortable. After the parade, we walked leisurely back to the hotel. That night we attended the inaugural ball.

After viewing the pomp of the inauguration, the parade, and the inaugural ball, I had a warm feeling of pride that I had played a small part in bringing it all to fruition as a delegate to the national convention back in August in Miami.

I have maintained close ties with many of those I was associated with during the convention and have continued to be fairly active in the political field.

IN THE EARLY 1950s, I was asked to attend a town meeting during which there was going to be a discussion of city planning. After the meeting, John Lewis and I stood on the corner and visited. He told me that some problems had arisen between some of the representatives and the medical profession. It seemed that the members of the legislature were becoming disgusted with the physicians because they never heard from them unless there was a complaint concerning some action affecting doctors. "Doc, I'll always back the doctors," said John, "but my colleagues are getting fed up. We need better cooperation and support from the doctors."

That complaint concerned me greatly and, as soon as I got home, I called Dr. Eugene Johnson, a good friend living in the nearby town of Casey. Gene agreed with me that the medical society needed a fire built under it. We got together a few nights later to plan our strategy. We had never attended a meeting of the House of Delegates, which was held each spring in Chicago, so we decided to go.

We knew we needed a resolution, but neither of us knew how to write one. We put our heads together and outlined what we wanted to say and gave it to our attorney. He came up with a beauty, with all the "whereases" and "wherefores" in the proper places. In effect, we stated that the relationship between the legislature and the state medical society stunk and something had to be done to correct the problem.

We appointed ourselves to represent the Clark County Medical Society. Johnson was delegate, and I was alternate delegate. Armed with our resolution, we packed our bags and went to Chicago.

The House of Delegates convened, and Johnson took the floor. He was recognized and proceeded to introduce the resolution. He was told the resolution was late. It should have been sent in to the society headquarters several weeks before in order to be considered. Neither of us had known that. The speaker finally ruled that by agreement of the delegates the rules could be suspended. The house voted to suspend so our resolution was accepted and referred to committee. When Johnson finished reading the resolution, a roar went up from the delegates. We couldn't imagine why our resolution had created such an uproar. After the house adjourned, several of the delegates commended us. They were elated that someone finally had built a fire.

One man remained after the others left. He asked if he could sit down and discuss the resolution with us. We walked down the hall and found an empty room. He introduced himself and told us he was hurt that we would bring up such a thing. He told us he was a member of the medical society staff in Springfield and worked for our best interests with all the members of the legislature. I asked him if he knew John Lewis. "I sure do," was his answer. "Well, he sure doesn't know you," I said and walked away.

Although our resolution died in committee, less than two months later the man who had talked with us was gone. The medical society began to become more active politically. We established a fully staffed branch office in Springfield and employed expert lobbyists to represent us. A political action committee was formed and contributions solicited from members to be used in support of candidates who were our friends.

Johnson and I continued to be active in the medical society and attended each session of the House of Delegates. It wasn't long before we became well acquainted with many of our colleagues around the state. Johnson was a good speaker and loved to debate. He was highly respected by his colleagues and served several terms as secretary-treasurer; he was a member of the board of trustees for many years and eventually was elected president of the society. I work better one-on-one rather than speaking or debating in the House of Delegates. I have made many friends in the society and in the legislature, and I value those friendships.

We have developed a "key man" program in the society. A key man knows his legislator. Sometimes the legislator is a patient of the key man. The key man keeps abreast of all legislation of concern to the medical profession and keeps the legislator appraised of the profession's position and enlists support for that position. This has been quite effective combined with the expertise and efforts of our professional lobbying staff.

Johnson and I have been the subjects of a lot of good-natured ribbing by our colleagues around the state, particularly our Chicago brothers. Clark County has a population of sixteen thousand, and at most in recent years, we have had five members in the medical society. Although we are entitled to one seat in the House of Delegates, a few years ago we had three. At that time, Johnson, as secretary-treasurer, and I, as vice-president of the state society, each were entitled to a seat, in addition to the one regular seat.

It's been a long time since we made that first trip to Chicago, but we have come a long way. I always tell our colleagues that Johnson is the man who does the work and I'm his "bag man." I carry his bag. It's been fun working together, and we feel well rewarded because the state society now has the top lobbyist in the Capitol and has the respect of everyone—governor and entire legislative body.

A few years ago, Johnson decided the society needed to own its own headquarters building in Springfield, so we introduced a resolution in the House of Delegates authorizing the purchase of a building. The resolution passed easily. When a reception was held to celebrate the opening of our new headquarters, Johnson and I were asked how we liked our very own building.

Over the years, we have had excellent people in Springfield representing us in the legislature. One of them was James Brady, who later went on to become press secretary to President Reagan and was nearly killed during the assassination attempt on the president's life. Bernie Robinson succeeded Brady, and Bernie has gone on to become corporate director for Philip Morris. He lives in Switzerland now and is responsible for the operations of the Philip Morris Corporation in over eighty countries. Having men of such caliber working for us is proof that we have made some great steps in promoting the interests of medicine, which, incidentally, are not just the selfish interests of the doctors but the interests of the public—laws to protect the people and to promote better health care.

Although I'm not active in the House of Delegates (I have passed that on to a younger man), I still sit on the Committee for Governmental Affairs, which deals with medical legislation, and retain a seat on the IMPAC Committee to keep my hand in the political field. It has been a long time since I first became interested in the political process, but I haven't been disillusioned. I feel the same now as I did then. Unless we become involved, we have no right to complain if government doesn't perform as we think it should. In a democracy, everyone has a right and, yes, a duty to participate.

20

A New Concept in Rural Health Care

WHEN I CAME to Marshall to begin my practice, I became the sixteenth doctor in a county with a total population of sixteen thousand. There were two doctors in West Union, with a population of between five and eight hundred, and at least one doctor in Westfield, Casey, Martinsville, and Marshall. As the years went by, the older doctors died or retired, and others left to return to school for specialization or moved on to other locations. By 1968 the number of doctors in the county had dwindled to five—two in Casey, one in Martinsville, and two in Marshall. The total population had remained stable.

The five remaining doctors discussed the possibility of forming a corporation. An attorney who was an expert in the field of corporate law was contacted, and a meeting was held to explore the idea. It was decided to call another meeting the following night. Dr. Illyes, the other doctor in Marshall, told us he would not be able to attend the next meeting but was agreeable to any decision made. I had been home less than two hours when I received a call from his sister-in-law informing us that he had suffered a heart attack and died.

We now had only four doctors in the county. It was estimated that Marshall and the immediate area had a population of six to seven thousand people, and I was the only doctor available to service the area. The people were anxious. They had never thought they would find themselves in such a predicament. They suddenly realized that doctors do die. Some of the leaders called a town meeting at a local restaurant, and I was asked to attend. I sat and listened to the discussion. Everyone had ideas on solving the problem, but when all their ideas were taken together, they simply were saying, "We must go out and get another doctor—quickly."

Finally, they asked for my ideas in solving the problem. First, I told them it made me feel good to see that they were concerned and that they wanted to move quickly to solve the problem, but the day was long past when they could entice a young doctor to come to a rural area to set up a solo practice even if they offered a home and office free of charge. The new breed of doctors wanted to be in a center with a group of doctors and have access to a well-equipped hospital.

Furthermore, doctors wanted free time and, therefore, needed to be closely associated with other doctors so that coverage was always available when they wanted to be away from their practice. The days when a doctor devoted seven days and nights a week to the care of patients, as all of us in solo practice had been doing so long, were past. Also, a county with a population of only sixteen thousand could not support a well-equipped and staffed hospital.

Our people already had access to good hospitals. Terre Haute to the east had two large hospitals. Paris to the north had an excellent community hospital, as did Robinson to the south. There was a hospital in Olney to the southwest, Effingham to the west, and Charleston to the northwest. The county medical society fortunately had been studying the problem for some time, and two of the members, the Johnson brothers of Casey, had come up with a unique proposal. Their plan was to build two medical centers—one in Marshall and one in Casey, sixteen miles to the west. Although they would not substitute for hospitals, medical centers would constitute more than solo doctors' offices. They would each be equipped with a complete laboratory, hospital-type X-ray facilities, an emergency room, a physical therapy department, and several beds available for short-term observation of patients. It would be up to the people to raise the funds needed to put the plan into operation.

I then outlined the medical center concept. I pointed out that with such facilities doctors would be attracted more easily. With a fully-equipped medical center, there would be no need for a young doctor to invest in expensive equipment. With all doctors located in the same facility, they could work as a team and provide coverage for each other.

The populace liked the idea. More meetings were scheduled, not only in Marshall but throughout the rest of the county. The medical society decided that before things went any further we should consult with colleagues to determine if our plan was sound. Dr. Eugene Johnson went to Chicago to talk with physicians at the headquarters of the Illinois State Medical Society. It was with great difficulty that he finally got it through their heads he wasn't talking about building a hospital. When they finally realized what he was trying to describe, they were enthusiastic. Nothing like this had ever been done before.

He and the people from the medical society went over to the headquarters of the American Medical Association and described our plan to them. They, too, were enthusiastic. The state medical society provided the funds for a feasibility study. During the time the study was being done, more meetings of citizens were held, and an informal organization was formed.

Ours is not a wealthy county. Our population is made up of hardworking people, some engaged in business, some in light industry, and a large number in farming. Regardless of their political persuasion, most could be considered conservative and fiercely independent. They don't take kindly to government intervention into their personal business. Thus, it was no surprise that they decided immediately that no government or tax money would be sought to finance the project, nor did they want any invested money. The financing was to be by donations from the people. Ours was to be purely a "people project." Finally came the day when the feasibility study was completed and presented to the citizenry. The consultant simply reported that the project was viable and that all of the preliminary planning was sound. His final recommendation was, "Get going."

There had always been a rivalry between the east and west sides of the county, and I wondered if that was going to hamper development of the medical centers, but I was pleasantly surprised. This was one of the rare occasions when people from the entire county came together as one and moved on to bring the medical centers into being. It was decided to build each of the centers adjacent to and connected by a corridor to the existing nonprofit nursing homes in Casey and Marshall. Each of the nursing homes had in excess of a hundred beds. The idea was to group medical facilities together and also to provide easy access to diagnostic services for patients in the nursing homes.

Fund drives were organized. Everyone seemed to want to help. Children's groups sold candy. Pledge cards were made available, and people were contacted. Industries in the area were given an opportunity to contribute. A wealthy gentleman who resided in Casey had bequeathed the money to build the nursing home, and there was a considerable amount remaining, so the extra funds were earmarked for the Casey Medical Center. An elderly woman in Marshall made a sizable bequest that was designated for either the expansion of the nursing home or a new medical facility. She stipulated that if the money were used for a medical facility it would be named for her husband.

As an example of the way people supported the project, I called on an elderly friend of mine one afternoon to explain what we were doing. I had a pledge card in my pocket and, after I completed my presentation, asked if she would like to make a pledge. She took the pledge card and excused herself. In a few minutes, she returned and handed me the blank pledge card and a check for ten thousand dollars. She stipulated that the public was not to know she had given the money, so on the plaque that hangs in the medical center today, her donation is recorded not by her name, but by the word "Anonymous."

The same architect was employed to design both medical centers, and construction was started at nearly the same time. While all of that was going on, we still had patients to care for and only four of us to handle the job. The other three doctors decided that I needed help on this side of the county so a countywide call system was set up. At least it was now possible for all of us to have an occasional night off. One doctor was designated on call for the entire county each night. The public was informed through notices in all the papers that it was only necessary to call one of the two nursing homes and a doctor would be provided. The only drawback to the plan was that the doctor on call sometimes had to drive all over the county seeing patients.

Jim Buechler came in one day to see me. I had been his family doctor since he was a small boy. He had just finished his junior year at Illinois Tech, where he was majoring in physics. He was an extremely intelligent young man and had received a full scholarship to college. He had come in to discuss going into medicine.

It was his intention to finish his senior year at Illinois Tech and then enter medical school. I was convinced he was dead serious. I told him it wasn't easy to get into medical school. Competition for a place in any freshman class is fierce. I thought his best chance of gaining admission was to apply through the Illinois Farm Bureau. There was a serious shortage of doctors interested in practicing in the rural areas of Illinois. The Illinois State Medical Society had come up with a unique plan to fill the need for doctors in rural areas. The medical society had enlisted the aid of the farm bureau, and the two organizations formed a partnership and then sold their plan to the legislature. Through legislation, a certain number of places in the first year of the University of Illinois School of Medicine were reserved for students selected by a committee of the state medical society. The farm bureau provided low interest loans, and the students agreed to serve a specified number of years in an Illinois rural community after finishing their training.

Jim liked the idea. I called my old friend Dr. Harlan English, the president of the medical society and the father of the medical society-farm bureau plan. He told me to have Jim meet with the registrar of the medical school and that he would call the registrar to let him know that Jim would be contacting him. It was all set before Jim left my office. He had no trouble getting accepted and a year later started his medical career. He did well in school and, during his infrequent visits home, usually gave me a progress report. It seemed the time flew by and before I knew it, he had graduated. Of course, I was hoping he would go into family practice and would return to Marshall to join in my practice, but that was not an assured thing. I talked to him about it but did not use any pressure. I felt the decision was up to him entirely. After graduating, he took a three-year residency in family practice.

Jim visited me after finishing his residency. I was then the only doctor in town. I was working seven days and nights, although the people were trying to cooperate by putting off calling at night because they wanted me to get my rest. People actually were asking me how I was feeling. At times, they were more concerned about my health than their own.

I asked Jim if he would be interested in coming in with me. Then he dropped a bombshell. He told me that he would be happy to join me but that he had joined the Marine reserves while in medical school and was committed to three years' active duty. He was to report to Camp Pendleton, California, in a month. "If I can get you out, would you come back here?" I asked. "Of course," he said, "but there is no way anyone can get out." "Let me give it a try," I replied. "Nothing is impossible." I started my campaign immediately. Now was the time to make use of my political contacts. I contacted my congressman, Senator Everett Dirksen, and President Nixon. I also wrote to the director of Selective Service and the Secretary of the Navy.

In the meantime, I talked to Jim nearly every week; just as I had expected, there were so many doctors that Jim never saw more than three or four patients a week. He was bored, and his morale was dropping fast. I kept feeding this information back to my political contacts. Another part of my plan was to gather petitions from the people. This was easy. I got a tremendous response from the public. I remember one petition that was on yellow paper. All the names were written with a pencil. This was the petition from the Coon Hunters' Club. I kept the pressure on and was finally rewarded by a call from Jim on New Year's Eve. He was jubilant. "I received my discharge and will be home next week." That was the best New Year's gift I ever had. A few days later, Jim called to tell me he was home. "When do you want to start work?" I asked. "How about tomorrow?" he answered.

This was to be an entirely new experience for me. For all those years that I had been in practice by myself I ran things the way I wanted. Now I was going to have another doctor working with me. I guess it was like being single for many years and finally getting married. I turned a storeroom into an office and hired an extra receptionist. At first, Clara, my nurse, worked with both of us. After Jim's practice grew, he then had his own nurse. We agreed at first that he would be paid a salary equal to his salary in the Marines. As the practice grew, we separated the practice so that the fees from the patients he saw went to him and the fees from my patients went to me. That worked very well. After all the years when I had no one to cover for me, I now had a doctor who could take calls, and I could have some free time. The first night Jim took call, I was like a bird freed from its cage. I felt like a heavy load had been lifted.

Jim was an excellent doctor and got along with his patients extremely well. I felt comfortable with him and knew that he would give my patients the best of care. Jim was aware of the efforts being made to improve the delivery of health care in our county and was looking forward to the day when a modern, well-equipped facility would become a reality.

Shortly after Jim joined me in practice, I received a call from the office of the American Medical Association in Chicago, asking if they could send a writer and photographer to spend a few days with us to write a story about physicians in rural America.

Jim was agreeable so we gave them our consent. We were both puzzled. Why were they selecting us from the many thousands of doctors across America? We never did get the answer to that question. Here are excerpts from the story that appeared in the October 19, 1970, issue of *American Medical News*, which was received by doctors throughout the United States.

> It was his day off, and he had been up most of the night at the hospital, but James R. Buechler, M.D., was on his way to the office to see patients.
>
> "I have a house call to make on the way to town," he said, turning down a gravel country road. "Yes, we make house calls. We do it if it is really hard for someone to come to the office."
>
> Dr. Buechler parked in front of a large frame house and was soon inside examining an 84-year-old farmer, who had a kidney infection. He wrote out a prescription and suggested that a urine specimen be brought to the office later.
>
> For the house call, the physician charged the usual $6.
>
> Fees are just one of the differences between a rural medical practice and a practice in a metropolitan area.
>
> Dr. Buechler, 29, had been practicing since last February when he returned to his hometown of Marshall, Illinois, after serving as a physician in the Navy. He is associated with George T. Mitchell, M.D., a 56-year-old general practitioner who had been in Marshall nearly 25 years. The two share facilities and expenses but have separate practices. Together, they serve nearly 7,000 people.
>
> Here in East-Central Illinois, 190 miles south of Chicago, rolling fields of corn, soybeans, and wheat stretch for miles, with only an occasional

wooded area or cluster of farm buildings breaking the pattern.

Life for the 3,000 inhabitants of Marshall is unhurried and relaxed. There is little crime other than what the mayor calls "mischief." The town's frame homes set on quiet tree-lined streets are seldom locked. Most of the porch lights burn all night under a unique arrangement where the city-owned power company supplies free electrical service for one outside light.

Chiefly a farming community, Marshall has two industries, a chemical plant which manufactures adhesives and paper coatings, and an electronics component plant. The two firms employ about 600 persons.

The business district consists of a couple of blocks of two-story buildings, two banks, a savings and loan, a few "cafes," and the courthouse square.

Religion is important in this predominantly Protestant area, and there are no less than 13 churches in the community. Racial strife is unheard of.

There is no drug problem among Marshall's teen-agers.

For the most part, life in Marshall and surrounding Clark County is simple and stubbornly independent. The biggest concern this year has been the corn blight, and the effects will not be known until all of the feed corn now drying on yellowing stalks is harvested.

Besides Dr. Mitchell and Dr. Buechler, Clark County has three other physicians and two dentists serving a total population of 16,000. Clark County has no hospital, but excellent facilities are available in Terre Haute, Indiana, 17 miles to the east and Paris, Illinois, 16 miles to the north.

Marshall's residents also take pride in their modern 110-bed nursing home, built with donated funds and run by a board of directors made up entirely of local people.

Mayor Hubert O. Ferris likes to point to the town's many assets: a swimming pool built with funds raised by the Lions Club; a large state park with a lake and camping facilities; its friendly people, and of course, its "suburbs"—really subdivisions that have not yet been annexed.

The community is currently in the midst of a fund drive to raise $400,000 to build a much needed medical center.

Dr. Mitchell is part of a medical family. Besides his father, who started practicing medicine in Marshall in 1907, Dr. Mitchell has an uncle who was also a physician, and another uncle who was a dentist in the town. A cousin practices medicine in Washington, D.C., and three cousins are dentists. His wife and one daughter are nurses, and another daughter is a speech and hearing therapist.

"My father was a horse-and-buggy doctor," Dr. Mitchell said. "But he got an automobile as soon as he could afford one." The original stable where his father kept a team of horses still stands behind the physician's ivy-covered brick office built by the senior Dr. Mitchell and his brother in 1910.

Actually, Dr. Mitchell never had any intention of becoming a physician, much less a general practitioner in Marshall. He earned a degree in mechanical engineering at Purdue in 1935.

"When I came out of college, we were still under the effect of the depression, and I could see that jobs were hard to get for engineers, or anybody else," he recalled. "I began to think more about going into medicine."

Dr. Buechler was born in Chicago, but his family moved to the Marshall area while he was in elementary school. His parents operated a restaurant in the community.

Somewhat like Dr. Mitchell, he, too, had not planned to be a physician. He spent 2 1/2 years studying physics at Illinois Institute of Technology in Chicago before deciding he didn't like it. After talking to friends, and to Dr. Mitchell, Dr. Buechler embarked on a career in medicine.

He attended the University of Illinois College of Medicine in Chicago, interned at St. Joseph's Hospital in South Bend, Indiana, and followed that with a year in a general practice residency at the same institution.

Dr. Buechler entered the Navy and was attached to a Marine division at Camp Pendleton, California. Through the efforts of the community, including a 3,500 signature petition to the Secretary of the Navy, he was released from active duty early to return to Marshall to practice.

"The practice of medicine in a rural area is considerably different from that of the urban areas," Dr. Mitchell said. "I think one of the big differences is that you are closer to the people here. You're not just a doctor, you're a friend."

The way of life is "much more relaxed" in rural communities than in the city, Dr. Mitchell pointed out.

"You're not confined to an area where there's nothing but buildings, people and crowds, heavy traffic, noise, and all the other types of pollution. You have more freedom to move about, you have trees and flowers, fields of corn and wheat."

"It's a nice place to live," said Dr. Buechler, as he gazed out the window at his 10-acre "farm" two miles outside of Marshall. The barn behind the home is empty now, but the Buechlers hope to get a couple of horses next spring.

"There is none of the hustle, bustle of the big city here," the physician remarked. "It's a slower pace. You can go down on Friday night in the summer and listen to the band concert. It's just a nice life." Both physicians concede they work hard at times, but they usually manage to get a day off during the week, besides Sunday, and do not have regular night office hours. They list their home telephone numbers in the local directory and on prescription forms, and they are readily accessible to their patients.

And they do make house calls, or will go down to their office to see patients at any time, if it's necessary. They also make it a point to see patients at home who have a difficult time coming to the office—mostly bedridden or elderly persons, or "if someone really gets sick at night," Dr. Buechler said. Surprisingly, it's rare for them to be called in the middle of the night. "The people here are considerate," Dr. Buechler said.

"They know they can depend on me, but they don't call you up as much as you might expect."

People living in large metropolitan areas would consider their fees something from another era. The physicians charge $4 for an office visit, and $6 for a house call. When they are called out at night, they may charge $8 for a house call. They also have a mileage charge for trips out into the country—50 cents a mile, one way.

While their fees are modest, both physicians are convinced there is a good living to be made in small towns. Besides, it doesn't cost as much to live in small rural communities. "Money was not a prime consideration," Dr. Buechler said, in discussing his reasons for returning to Marshall. "I'd say I've had a reasonably comfortable time of it from a financial standpoint," said Dr. Mitchell. "Anybody who would want to come out, and work and live in the rural area, I don't think he would have to worry financially."

"I am not rich by any means, and anyway, I don't think you can measure wealth entirely in the amount of money you have in the bank, or the number of stocks and bonds you own, or the amount of land you control. I think you have to consider other things . . . the advantages that you have, the friendships that you make, the experiences you have in a small community.

"The things you may have done to help people, or to make the community better. . . . I think these things have to be taken into consideration in counting up your wealth. In that respect, I feel I am pretty well-to-do."

Although he no longer delivers babies, Dr. Mitchell feels obstetrics has been one of the most rewarding parts of his practice. (He figures he has delivered about 1,400 babies during his career.) "Babies are still born in the county the same as in the city, or anyplace else," he laughed.

When he started out in Marshall, all of the deliveries were at home. But this "was too much horse and buggy," and later all deliveries were made in hospitals in Terre Haute and Paris.

Dr. Mitchell feels there is little a rural physician misses in the way of professional challenge or advancement. He estimates that he and Dr. Buechler can handle 95% of the cases they see; the others are referred to specialists.

"In a country practice, we don't get as much of the trivia as I saw in the cities," Dr. Buechler asserted.

Dr. Buechler said he puts in about a 62-hour week, but doesn't feel he's overworked. His practice is still growing, but he averages about 30 patients a day in the office.

Both physicians feel they have a real advantage over some rural areas in being within easy driving distance of Terre Haute and Paris. It gives them access to good hospitals, and makes specialists available for consultation or referral.

"We see everything," Dr. Buechler said. "We have some unusual things, too, many things I haven't seen before." One man came in for treatment of a leg wound which Dr. Buechler diagnosed as a brown recluse spider bite.

"We see a lot of emotional problems," he continued. "Venereal disease is a problem here like it is everywhere else."

Drugs have been kept out of Marshall . . . at least so far.

One of the reasons drugs have not been a problem in Marshall, according to Dr. Buechler, is that "in general kids here are a little more obedient to their parents, and they respect their wishes a little more."

Because Marshall is on Route 40—considered one of the most dangerous highways in the nation, and because the area is predominantly farming—the two physicians treat a lot of accident victims.

The highway accidents usually are "very serious," and there is little the physician can do because of the lack of hospital facilities.

The area is blessed with an efficient ambulance service, however. Both funeral homes in Marshall provide staffed ambulances 24 hours a day. In fact, every community of any size in Clark County has a well-equipped ambulance. Lacerations and broken bones comprise the majority of farm injuries, but few of the accidents are fatal, as they were 20 years ago, because more safety devices are built into farm equipment today.

"We do see a lot of serious injuries where people lose fingers or toes, or have cut tendons, or broken bones," Dr. Buechler reported.

Neither physician feels he or his family is deprived socially or culturally because they live in a small town.

"During my time in the big city, I had a small group of close friends like everybody else," Dr. Buechler remarked. "I didn't know people all over town. It is similar here."

Culturally, they feel there is plenty of opportunity to attend events in Terre Haute, especially since Indiana State University is located there. They also do not feel it's impractical to drive to Indianapolis or Chicago for special events.

Dr. Buechler, who has two young children, is convinced that a small town is the best place to raise a family.

"The schools here in our community are just tremendous," he said. "We've got good facilities (four new schools have been built in the last 20 years), and good teachers. They don't offer everything that maybe the schools in the great cities offer, but they are very progressive."

But Dr. Buechler's pretty wife, Jamie, is not completely sold on small-town living. She grew up in Aurora, Illinois, a city of about 70,000 people west of Chicago, and is still adjusting to rural life.

"It's taken a lot of getting used to," Mrs. Buechler said. "It has its advantages, but if you're not used to it, it's hard."

Mrs. Buechler, who also is a nurse, believes she would probably enjoy the community more if she had the companionship of another young physician's wife. Another physician, too, would give Dr. Buechler more time off so they could do more of the things they like.

The two physicians, as well as the people of Clark County, are also concerned about the future.

As Dr. Mitchell observed, "I think rural medicine has been neglected for a long time because doctors coming out of medical school don't realize that maybe there are people—good people—who need medical care in the rural areas as well as in the city.

"And unless we get doctors out here in the country, I don't know what's going to happen."

The Cork Medical Center was opened in 1972, and we moved there from our downtown office, which was eventually sold to the Christian Church.

The two medical centers, the Cork Medical Center in Marshall and the Casey Medical Center in Casey, were hailed as a "new concept in rural health care." Articles appeared in national health publications as well as in a number of newspapers.

One such article, which I was asked to submit to *The Family Practice News*, appeared in the August 15, 1973, issue. Here is an excerpt from "Cooperation Insures Quality Medical Care in Rural Illinois Area":

> Quality medical care can be practiced properly in the rural areas, and there is no reason that the people in these areas should not be given this type of care. To say it cannot be done and walk away is being unfair to them.
>
> This problem will never be solved satisfactorily by the bureaucratic process; instead, to be successful, it must be a grass roots effort—a total community involvement. The people themselves must be made aware of the problem, and the local medical society must provide the necessary leadership and guidance.
>
> Working together in partnership, the community will be assured of continuing quality medical care, and new doctors will be attracted.

Our community, as well as the majority of the communities throughout the country, except for the large metropolitan areas, had always depended upon the local funeral directors to handle the ambulance service. With the tremendous advances that were being made in handling medical emergencies, however, that model of service was rapidly becoming outmoded. For the most part, the morticians were eager to get out from under the responsibility.

In the first place, it was sometimes time-consuming and, in many cases, an added expense because many people believed that it should be a free service provided by morticians in return for a future funeral. Secondly, with the increase in liability suits, a funeral director was more vulnerable to litigation than he had been in the past.

The emergency medical technician (EMT) program had been initiated in Illinois, and more and more volunteers were receiving an intensive course in the care of medical emergencies. There were EMTs manning the modern well-equipped ambulances, operated by both private and public agencies. Our local funeral directors were caught in a dilemma. They secretly wished to be out of the ambulance business, but many of their potential clients were making statements such as, "If he can't carry me, he won't bury me." It had become a matter of educating the public to the necessity of bringing the ambulance service up-to-date, and that was a slow process.

Dr. Buechler and I were both anxious to get the service upgraded, so we started by getting volunteers enrolled in the EMT program. The next problem was getting an ambulance service started. Money was the main obstacle. Should the ambulance be operated by a private service, or should the service be provided by a government entity?

In a rural area with a small population base such as ours, we didn't think a private service would survive. It seemed logical that such a service could be provided by the fire district, but we had the problem of convincing the governing board that it should assume that responsibility. In proposing the plan, we got a lukewarm— really, a cold—reception from the board. Jim and I had looked at the law concerning ambulance service provided by a fire district. It was an excellent law. Service would be provided both within and without the boundaries of the district. That meant that if an emergency occurred on the other side of the boundary and another ambulance wasn't available, the fire district ambulance could make the run.

Financing for the ambulance would come from a levy up to twenty-five cents per hundred dollars' assessed valuation. That was subject to the passage of a referendum by the voters within the fire district. The Marshall fire district had an adequate tax base to support an ambulance service. Jim and I prepared an outline of procedures for operating such an ambulance service and discussed it with the board, but the proposition was not accepted, so we stuck our plan back in the files.

I had the opportunity to discuss the plan with the woman who had been the anonymous donor of a ten-thousand-dollar gift toward the construction of the medical center. She responded enthusiastically. The next day I received a thousand-dollar check in the mail from her, an anonymous gift to be used for an ambulance service. The check was deposited for future use for the project.

The local funeral directors finally got together and bit the bullet. A public notice appeared in the local papers in June announcing that they would discontinue furnishing ambulance service as of midnight

December 31 of that year. That created quite a stir among the public, but no one seemed to believe it would happen. A series of public meetings was held, but no decisions were made. The rest of the county was not under the same pressure as was Marshall.

I purposely did not attend any of the meetings because I thought I would be a divisive influence. I felt that people at times looked upon me as being too assertive when it came to safety or health problems. The mayor of Marshall, a close friend, attended all the meetings and kept me posted. By fall, he said that they still couldn't come to any decision. I told him about our plan for a Marshall fire district ambulance service, and he liked it. I offered him the plan we had on file to take to the next meeting but told him by all means not to reveal the source of the plan. "It's your plan, Frank, and present it as such," I told him.

At the next meeting, he presented "his" plan and received an enthusiastic endorsement. Pressure was applied to the fire board, and they reluctantly agreed to hold a referendum for the purpose of authorizing the creation of a fire district ambulance service, supported by a separate tax levy. By that time, it was late fall.

The fire board complained that they didn't want to spend the money for holding an election, so the mayor told them the city would foot the bill. The election was held on Saturday, December 13. There had been little, if any, publicity concerning the election, and I had heard few people talking about it. On election day, I had a meeting to attend in Springfield. On the way back from Springfield, I told Millie I was sure the referendum had failed. To my surprise, when I arrived home, I learned that the authorization was passed by a huge majority. Now we had to get into business in less than three weeks.

The following week, the mayor called a town meeting, and I was asked to attend. The mayor, the city council, and a large number of private citizens were present. A new, fully equipped ambulance was parked in front of City Hall.

Before the meeting, the mayor called me aside and said he already had had a meeting with the council in the corridor leading to the restroom, and they had voted to purchase an ambulance just like the one on display and give it to the fire district for one dollar.

The council assembled in the council chambers, and the meeting was called to order. The council voted in public to do what they had already decided in the corridor. The people were told that we had a large group of certified EMTs ready to operate the ambulance. The question arose as to who was going to supervise the operation of the service.

Young Jim Turner was in the room. Jim had completed part of his premedical education but was going to lay out awhile until he could afford to continue his education. He was a certified EMT and had considerable ambulance experience. He enthusiastically accepted the position as ambulance supervisor.

The new ambulance wouldn't be available for several weeks, but the company provided a substitute ambulance at no charge. The next day, Turner went to Indianapolis and brought it back to the medical center, loading it with all the needed supplies.

There was still one big problem. Where was the money coming from for fuel, upkeep, and supplies for the ambulance? No tax money would be coming in for another year and a half at least. The fire board agreed to anticipate against next year's taxes, but that necessitated the publishing of a public notice plus a waiting period for the public to petition against it.

I then remembered the generous donor's gift. I told Turner that one thousand dollars would be available to finance the service until tax funds were available. He had everyone completely organized in less than two weeks, and shortly after midnight, December 31, they made their first run. The service has run smoothly since its inception under the supervision of several different directors over the years.

Training of EMTs has been upgraded, and new EMTs have been added to the rolls. A new building was constructed to house the ambulances and to be used as headquarters. Another component has been added to work in cooperation with the ambulance service: an emergency rescue service with trained and equipped scuba divers. They are equipped and trained in the use of state-of-the-art equipment to extricate victims from wrecked automobiles and buildings. All vehicles are linked to the medical center and area hospitals by radio. I'm sure a number of people are alive today only because of the ambulance service.

Shortly after our service was set up, the county board organized a county ambulance service for all the area outside the Marshall fire district. Trained, well-equipped EMTs operate the service out of the other towns and villages in the county. Even though the county and fire district are separate entities, there is complete cooperation, and they provide backup for one another.

At the present time, the Marshall Ambulance Service is again going to upgrade the service by working with Union Hospital in Terre Haute. An agreement has been made with the hospital to provide ongoing training that will advance our EMTs to the EMTI (Emergency Medical Technician Intermediate) level, which means our ambulance personnel will be trained to start IVs and do other more detailed procedures in caring for the patient. Those treatment procedures will be under the supervision of hospital personnel, who will be in communication by radio.

LOOKING BACK OVER the last fifteen years, I recognize that we have made great strides in bringing up-to-date quality medical care to the people of our community. During the period from 1972, when the Cork Medical Center opened, to 1989, we have had a number of physicians associated at various times with the medical center. Of course, Dr. Buechler was with me until he left to become director of Medical Education at Union Hospital in Terre Haute, where he organized the Family Practice Residency Program. Prior to his departure, Dr. Paul Banning joined the group. Others included Drs. Vasu and Dinker Patel, Dr. Steven White, and Dr. Cecil Watson.

Dr. Steven Macke joined me in 1979. He was born and raised in the community and had just completed his three-year family practice residency when he started his practice. There was a great amount of competition from other towns around for his services, but he finally decided on Marshall, for which I have been grateful. He is a fine, well-educated, hard worker, dedicated to the care of his patients. He has a fine family and has fit right into the life of our community.

Dr. James Turner, the young man who first ran our ambulance service, has completed his three-year residency in family practice and has joined Steven and me here in the Medical Center. Jim is also a hometown boy. So far the medical center concept is working. As doctors get older, younger doctors come in to assure the people of having quality medical care readily available.

THE RAPID DEPLETION in the number of doctors we faced in Clark County in the late 1960s has become a problem for all of rural Illinois. As the older doctors have died or retired, fewer younger doctors are willing to locate in the rural areas. Several reasons can be given for the shortage of primary care physicians.

Fifty years ago, when I became a doctor, malpractice suits were a rarity. In recent years there seems to have been a radical change in public attitude. We have seen a meteoric rise in the number of suits filed and the size of the sums awarded to the plaintiffs. In my own case, my present premium is over 150 times as much as I paid when I began practice and I'm considered a low risk. Illinois has no cap on awards for noneconomic damages, which results in extremely high premiums for doctors, particularly those with obstetrical patients.

Before Medicare and Medicaid, all doctors provided care for the elderly, regardless of their ability to pay. Each county had funds provided through local taxes that were used to provide medical care for those who couldn't pay. Physicians reduced fees in those instances, but sometimes the county funds were exhausted, in which case services generally were provided without charge. Every doctor expected to do a certain amount of charity work. Then along came Medicare and physicians were told that they would be expected to charge usual and customary fees. It wasn't long before the government discovered it had bitten off more than it could chew and the costs of these programs began to escalate. The government's solution to the problem was to cut back on the fees paid to doctors and the allowances made to hospitals. Rural Illinois has a high percentage of elderly people and, in some areas, a large number of Medicaid recipients. The fees paid for such services are considerably less than fees received from private-pay patients and sometimes don't cover doctors' expenses.

In the past, most people in the rural areas had ready access to a community hospital. Most of the hospitals were small but provided adequate care for acutely ill patients. Today, rural hospitals are disappearing rapidly, with the improvements in roads and the availability of good transportation. Rural residents now have access to larger, better-equipped hospitals and travel a greater distance because they believe they will receive better care. It is true that tremendous advances have been made in the last twenty-five to thirty years in the development of sophisticated diagnostic equipment and in the treatment of patients, but the cost of the equipment is prohibitive for a small hospital. To be cost-effective, a hospital must have a large patient capacity, and the beds must be occupied. The small hospital has seen a dramatic drop in the number of patients served. Often, a large percentage of the patients are those covered by Medicare and Medicaid, and reimbursement to the hospital does not equal the actual cost of operations. There is still a need for the small rural hospital, particularly for acute care and obstetrical deliveries; however, if the hospital is to remain viable, there must be a change in regulations and adequate funding for non-private-pay patients. For a doctor planning on going into practice in a rural area, access to a hospital is a "must."

The days are past when country doctors were "married" to their practices and worked seven days and nights a week serving patients without regard for personal time off. Solo practitioners isolated from colleagues, with no one to cover for them, are no more.

Family life is also important. Spouses and children must be considered when a doctor wants to locate in a rural area. In my opinion, it is important for the community to work hard to welcome physicians and their families. Rural communities have a lot to offer, including a more relaxed life-style and a warm friendliness that sometimes is hard to find in the city.

The deterioration in the availability of health care in rural areas has become a crisis. Currently, there are fifteen counties in downstate Illinois without a hospital, with a total population of forty thousand women in the child-bearing age group. Those women must travel long distances to be delivered and often have had inadequate prenatal care that puts them at risk.

During recent years, the rural population has awakened and recognized the problem. The Illinois Farm Bureau formed a Rural Health Task Force, composed of lay people and health professionals. Another group, the Lieutenant Governor's Task Force, was formed and conducted a study. About the same time, the Illinois Rural Health Association was organized. Early in 1990, the Illinois State Medical Society formed the Rural Health Initiatives Subcommittee, which I chaired. The subcommittee has been upgraded and expanded into the Committee on Health Care Access and its scope expanded. Closely allied with the farm bureau task force, the committee works together pooling resources, expertise, and influence to move forward. We have one common goal—the revitalization of the health care system in Illinois and the provision of quality medical care.

In attending the meetings of these groups, I have found that there seems to be considerable interest in developing a model similar to that which we have in Clark County: a primary care center adjacent to an extended care facility, with a good transportation system (ambulance) linked to a large hospital or hospitals. Also, the suggestion has been made that small hospitals could be converted to primary care centers and extended care facilities. Consideration is being given to developing birthing centers, perhaps in some of the hospitals that have stopped providing OB services for economic reasons. Present regulations require the same staffing, equipment, and space that is required in a large hospital. With a change in regulations, the centers could provide "level one" uncomplicated deliveries without endangering the life of the mother or baby. There would be a direct link to a larger hospital with the personnel and equipment necessary for "level two" and "level three" deliveries. Transportation would be provided by ambulance or helicopter.

Under consideration also is using nurse midwives and nurse practitioners to augment services to patients. Of course, health professionals would be under the supervision of a physician. Staff members at Southern Illinois University School of Medicine are working closely with us to upgrade and increase the availability of continuing medical education for physicians. It is also the intent of the medical school administration to provide preceptorships for medical students, in which they can work alongside physicians in rural areas. Possibly there will be a rotation in a rural setting required as part of residency programs. They may like what they see and come back to set up practice when they have finished their training.

It is not going to happen overnight, but I am full of optimism. I think we have a good start in resolving the health care problem in rural Illinois and before too long our rural residents once again will have quality health care readily available.

21

Some Final Reflections

I HAVE ATTEMPTED to paint a picture of my life with words. Some of the picture is pretty and some of it is not, but I guess that is the way life is. There is happiness and sadness, success and failure, and the thought that a lot of things should have been done differently; but any other way wouldn't be life.

Seventy years ago when I was a small boy, life in rural Illinois was simple but rugged. Most of the food eaten by people in the rural areas was grown on the farm and processed in the farm kitchen. Row upon row of canned food was stored on the shelves. Hogs were butchered and processed into hams and bacon, then cured in the smokehouse. Milk came fresh from the cow, and butter was made from cream. A by-product of the making of butter was cottage cheese, commonly called *schmierkase*. The water supply came from a well behind the house. It was pumped into a bucket and carried into the kitchen. The Saturday night bath ritual was carried out in the kitchen. The water was carried in and heated on top of the wood cookstove.

The toilet was located in the outhouse or privy. It was customary for the door of the privy to be decorated with a cutout of a new moon. The toilet seat was a round hole cut in a wooden plank—a large hole for grown-ups and a small hole for the children. Toilet paper consisted of strips of old newspaper or pages from last year's Sears Roebuck or Montgomery Ward catalogs. (The harness section was used only as a last resort because it was slick.) A bucket containing either ashes from the cookstove or lime was always nearby, along with a shovel; a small shovel-full of the contents of the bucket was sprinkled down through the hole in the seat after each visit. Heat was supplied by stoves or fireplaces. When the weather was cold, there were many areas in a house that heat could not reach. Also, there was no insulation in the walls or roof. The common practice was to hover close to the stove or fireplace until bedtime and then to make a mad dash to the bedroom, carrying some hot bricks covered with flannel or maybe a hot water bottle to warm the bed. Some people used a bed warmer, which was a long-handled covered pan filled with charcoal. The pan was pushed under the covers before going to bed; by bedtime, the bed was nice and warm. The bed warmer was then removed. The brick or hot water bottle was left in bed and soon became cold during the night, giving occupants a thrill when they accidentally hit it with bare feet.

Kerosene lamps were the source of illumination inside the house, and a kerosene lantern was carried when making a trip outside during the night.

Horses furnished the motive power for farming. They pulled plows, discs, and the harrow when preparing the soil for planting. They pulled corn planters and seed drills when farmers planted, and they pulled binders when it was time to harvest wheat and oats. Horses pulled mowers when hay was cut and then rakes to put the hay into windrows. They pulled wagons to haul the crops in, and they pulled buggies when families rode to town.

Very few people had any refrigeration. It was difficult to get ice out from town before it melted. Some people did have icehouses, their walls and roof heavily insulated with sawdust. During the cold winter months, huge slabs of ice were cut from a pond and stored for later use. Most people relied on other means of refrigeration. Perishables were placed in buckets and suspended down to the cold depths of the well just above the water level. Fortunate people had a natural flowing spring that emitted a stream of cold water. A small building was constructed and containers of food were set on rocks, a process that allowed the cold water to circulate around the containers.

Clothing not made at home and other essentials were purchased in local stores or quite often ordered from catalogs. There were few good roads, and it was difficult to travel more than a few miles from home. Social life revolved around the neighborhood, the church, and the country school. Most news came from the weekly papers, but a goodly amount of news was circulated by the telephone party line.

The people did not call on "Old Doc," the family practitioner, unless there was a serious accident or a life-threatening illness. They instead relied on home remedies to take care of their health needs. Each family was sure to have a good supply of patent medicines, ointments, and liniments (sometimes horse liniment was used on the owner's own sore muscles). I remember my grandfather's favorite treatment for a minor cut or scrape was a cud of chewing tobacco, and I had the treatment from him on more than one occasion.

The family farm life I have described was less complicated than the farm life of today. Fortunately, there has been little change in the neighborliness that was prevalent in the past. Farm families still have a concern for their neighbors and are quick to respond to help a neighbor in distress. The farm organizations remain strong, and their members work hard for the benefit of all.

Today, farming has become a major industry. The small farm is disappearing. One family now can farm hundreds of acres. Large, powerful tractors have replaced the horse. Huge combines harvest grain. No more shucking of corn by hand, no more cutting wheat with a binder and thrashing it by a separator. Modern machinery is very expensive. It is not unusual for a combine to cost upwards of $200,000 and a tractor $50,000. What took many steps to accomplish in the past is now done in a single operation. Today's farmers buy most of their food at grocery stores or supermarkets. They have the same modern conveniences as their city cousins—electricity, central heating, air-conditioning, water supply, and modern plumbing. No more kerosene lamps, outhouses, and buckets of food hung in the well.

Today's farmers must be smart business people. Computers are used extensively. Television and radio furnish up-to-the-minute market information as well as other information vital for a good farming operation. Sophisticated fertilizers and herbicides have replaced the manure, the cultivator, and the hoe. Large trucks speed farm products to markets over a modern network of good roads.

The farm family is no longer isolated. With modern automobiles and good highways, they are not limited to short-distance travel. It does not take long to make a trip to a major city or to Florida or California for a vacation. Air travel has brought many changes. It is not unusual to see a landing strip near a farmhouse, with an airplane parked in a shed out by the barn. Many of my farmer friends who once spent a lot of time behind a horse now vacation in England or Germany, or even Russia or the Far East.

Instead of making house calls through all kinds of weather, physicians now see patients at medical centers, except in rare emergencies. Utilization of medical care has increased tremendously. Having access to all sorts of health information, people are more concerned about their medical well-being than in the past. They also expect to have access to the most up-to-date diagnostic procedures and treatment. There is nothing wrong with that, and I am happy that we have made so much progress. However, how much have we benefited from the progress that has been made? People are living faster lives, beset by tensions and frustrations not apparent in past years. In most cases, they have much better incomes and enjoy much they never had the opportunity to enjoy before. Unfortunately, in order to maintain those standards, they must work harder, invest more, and worry about paying their bills. Maybe now is a good time to slow down and take time to reflect.

I have been privileged to live during some of the most exciting times in recorded history and have experienced the days of the horse and buggy transformed into the age of space travel. I have watched the orbiting of astronauts around the earth and seen satellites in space and probes by space vehicles to Mars and Jupiter. Humans living and working for long periods of time in space have become a relatively common occurrence. Tremendous advances have been made in all fields—from the crank telephone to instant communication by satellites, from the adding machine to the computer, from elixirs and powders to antibiotics and other highly sophisticated pharmaceuticals. We have seen the virtual elimination of tuberculosis, smallpox, diphtheria, whooping cough, measles, mumps, polio, and many other diseases that have plagued the earth. Surgeons perform bypass heart surgery as well as heart, liver, and lung transplants. Sophisticated procedures and equipment have been developed to aid in diagnosis. The list could go on and on. These achievements have all contributed to improving life on the planet.

On the other hand, I have lived through some of the most terrible conflicts in the history of the world—World War I and World War II, the Korean conflict, and the Vietnam war. The major powers have remained armed to the teeth, including the nuclear weapons developed after the splitting of the atom.

With all the great advances made by human beings during this century, there is still a major problem that hasn't been resolved. That is how to get along with one another and live in peace, trusting one another with mutual respect and friendship. After I'm gone from this earth, I wonder what will happen. Will advances continue to benefit humankind? Or will there be a war that will actually be a war to end all wars—total destruction of life on this planet?

I have enjoyed my life and feel privileged to have been able to do what I have done. The life of a country doctor, which I'm proud to be called, has been most rewarding. I have been privileged to share in the joys of my patients, but at times have also grieved with them. Life in a small town has been especially good. I have enjoyed being involved in the community, doing things unrelated to the practice of medicine.

My chief regret is that I didn't spend the time with my family that I should have. For many years, I spent most of my time caring for patients, taking only two weeks a year away on vacation. As a result, my family was neglected. My reason for this (not really a valid one) was that providing for my family was the most important thing I had to do. If I weren't available twenty-four hours a day to my patients, I would not have had a practice. I realize now I was wrong—very wrong. I seldom got home to enjoy a meal with my family, but when I finally arrived home, Millie would be patiently waiting up for me.

She never once complained. Our daughters tell me they didn't know me during their childhood. A recital, school play, or dance, any other event so important to a child, I missed, most often because some emergency would arise. But Millie was always there. She has been at my side since our wedding day, sharing with me the joys and sorrows of life. She came to live in a strange town among strange people, giving up the dream of my becoming a specialist and our living in Indianapolis. In her quiet way, Millie made many friends and came to be loved by all. She never refused to take part in any community or church project but preferred to remain in the background.

Now, when we should be able to spend time together doing things we want to do, Millie isn't able. Her health began to deteriorate a few years ago, and she was diagnosed as having Alzheimer's disease. I have hoped that some cure, or at least something that would restore some of her mental functions, would be found, but to no avail. She has reached the stage where she requires total care. Her condition breaks my heart. My sweetheart throughout all these years, who deserves to have everything, who has always thought of others, is now condemned to live out her life in this state.

It has been over fifty years since I graduated from medical school, and I'm still practicing medicine in Marshall. A few years ago the good people of Marshall and the surrounding area honored Millie and me by having an all-day celebration—"Dr. George and Millie Mitchell Day." There was a noontime barbecue and a banquet that night. We were overwhelmed by the whole affair. There were speeches, entertainment, and presentation of gifts and mementos. A tree was planted, and the mayor and city council gave the name "Mitchell" to a street. After this event I should have retired, but I didn't.

I don't work the long hours I used to, however. I see patients four afternoons a week but do no night work or take calls. On a recent afternoon I saw several patients with arthritis, treated a child with tonsillitis, counseled a young woman having marital problems, examined two or three patients with hypertension, treated a case of gout, reduced a dislocated shoulder, did surgery on a neck to remove a tumor, diagnosed and prescribed for a case of scabies, and treated a burn. This is a typical day in the life of a country doctor. My patients have grown old with me, and many still rely on me when they have a problem. Recently, an elderly woman, a longtime patient, came in for her yearly checkup, and everything checked out all right. I inquired about her daughter, who was one of my classmates in high school. "Oh, she's in much worse shape than I am. She has bad arthritis." As she was leaving, I complimented her on her long life. "Well, I'll tell you this—getting old is not all it is cracked up to be," she said as she walked down the hall. She will be 102 her next birthday.

It is hard to let go—and I have no plans to retire. My nurse Clara has retired after more than forty years of service. I feel it is important to keep active and plan on working as long as my health will permit.

I also enjoy my outside activities—the bank, the farm, serving as a member of the Board of Trustees of Lake Land Community College, trustee and member of the Building Committee at the Methodist Church, and the occasional trip to Chicago to attend a meeting of the State Medical Advisory Committee to the Department of Public Aid or a meeting of the medical society's political action committee.

One of these days I know I'll have to hang it up or maybe I'll die with my boots on. Only the Lord knows, but whatever happens, I have had a most interesting and rewarding trip through this life.

Index

Index

George T. Mitchell, M.D., was born and has lived most of his life in Marshall, a small town in rural southeastern Illinois where his father came to practice medicine in 1907. After receiving a B.S. degree in mechanical engineering from Purdue University, Dr. Mitchell went on to receive an M.D. degree from the George Washington University School of Medicine. After completing an internship at Methodist Hospital, Indianapolis, Indiana, he volunteered for service in the medical corps of the Army Air Corps in early 1941. Following nearly five years of military service, Dr. Mitchell returned to his hometown in 1946 to start a practice as a country doctor in his father's old office, where he has continued to serve the rural community of Marshall.